CRISIS INTERVENTION WITH CHILDREN AND FAMILIES

THE SERIES IN CLINICAL AND COMMUNITY PSYCHOLOGY

CONSULTING EDITORS

Charles D. Spielberger and Irwin G. Sarason

CRISIS INTERVENTION
WITH CHILDREN
AND FAMILIES

Edited by
Stephen M. Auerbach
Arnold L. Stolberg
Virginia Commonwealth University

HEMISPHERE PUBLISHING CORPORATION, Washington
A subsidiary of Harper & Row, Publishers, Inc.
Cambridge   New York   Philadelphia   San Francisco
London   Mexico City   São Paulo   Singapore   Sydney

CRISIS INTERVENTION WITH CHILDREN AND FAMILIES

2 3 4 5 6 7 8 9 0 B R B R 8 9 8 7

This book was set in Press Roman by Hemisphere Publishing Corporation. The editors were Christine Flint Lowry and Amy Whitmer; the production supervisor was Miriam Gonzalez; and the typesetter was Rita Shapiro. Braun-Brumfield, Inc. was printer and binder.

Library of Congress Cataloging in Publication Data
Main entry under title:

Crisis intervention with children and families.

(The Series in clinical and community psychology)
Includes bibliographies and indexes.
1. Child mental health services. 2. Life change events—Psychological aspects. 3. Mental illness—Prevention. 4. Crisis intervention (Psychiatry) I. Auerbach, Stephen M., date. II. Stolberg, Arnold L., date. III. Series. [DNLM: 1. Child Psychology. 2. Crisis Intervention—in infancy & childhood. WS 350.2 C932]
RJ499.C684   1987   618.92'89   85-30536
ISBN 0-89116-395-6
ISSN 0146-0846

To Our Wives

Jan Auerbach
Martha Schulman

and

To Our Children

Robby Edwards
Jennifer Auerbach
Amanda Auerbach
Joshua Stolberg

Contents

Contributors

STEPHEN M. AUERBACH, Department of Psychology, Virginia Commonwealth University, Richmond, Virginia

SANFORD L. BRAVER, Department of Psychology, Arizona State University, Tempe, Arizona

JOSEPH P. BUSH, Department of Psychology, Virginia Commonwealth University, Richmond, Virginia

EMORY L. COWEN, Department of Psychology, University of Rochester, River Campus Station, Rochester, New York

ROBERT D. FELNER, Department of Psychology, Auburn University, Auburn, Alabama

BRUCE S. FOGAS, Department of Psychology, Arizona State University, Tempe, Arizona

KATHERINE M. GARRISON, Richmond Center for Independent Living, Richmond, Virginia

NORMAN GOLDWASSER, Department of Psychology, Virginia Commonwealth University, Richmond, Virginia

A. DIRK HIGHTOWER, Department of Psychology, University of Rochester, River Campus Station, Rochester, New York

NANCY J. KERR, Department of Educational Psychology, Arizona State University, Tempe, Arizona

DIANE J. KILUK, Richmond, Virginia

MARY JO KUPST, Department of Child Psychiatry, Children's Memorial Hospital, Chicago, Illinois

BARBARA G. MELAMED, J. H. Miller Health Ctr., University of Florida, Gainesville, Florida

RICHARD T. ROWLISON, Department of Psychology, Auburn University, Auburn, Alabama

IRWIN N. SANDLER, Department of Psychology, Arizona State University, Tempe, Arizona

ANTHONY SPIRITO, Department of Psychiatry, Rhode Island Hospital, Providence, Rhode Island

ARNOLD L. STOLBERG, Department of Psychology, Virginia Commonwealth University, Richmond, Virginia

CAROLYN F. SWIFT, Stone Center for Developmental Services and Studies, Wellesley College, Wellesley, Massachusetts

LISA TERRE, Department of Psychology, Auburn University, Auburn, Alabama

SHARLENE WOLCHIK, Department of Psychology, Arizona State University, Tempe, Arizona

Foreword

It is both ironic as well as appropriate that these remarks are being composed during the final week of November, since November 28, 1942 commemorates the anniversary of the Cocoanut Grove fire in Boston in which 492 persons lost their lives. That horrible tragedy served as the stimulus for Erich Lindemann's naturalistic experiment with the survivors who lost loved ones in the fire. Lindemann's observations from his clinical interviews and his subsequent orderly analysis and presentation of the information obtained served as the vehicle for the development of crisis theory and its practical applications, crisis intervention.

More than four decades later we have a rather unusual volume that advances not only the theory of crisis intervention, but also presents data-based preventive interventions that invite adoption and adaptation in communities across the nation.

Crisis theory and crisis intervention have been subjects of controversy among primary prevention advocates. Some persons have suggested that since those experiencing a crisis are symptomatic, interventions either fall into a "grey" area somewhere between primary and secondary prevention, that is, early preventive intervention, or that these interventions are clearly secondary prevention since they involve early diagnosis and treatment for the purpose of forestalling the progression of an already present disorder or dysfunction. What appears to have been lost in such thinking is that a crisis is a period of temporary disequilibrium and that the behaviors experienced and demonstrated are within the normal range, given the circumstances, and that diagnostic labels are inappropriate. Clearly, this writer sides with Lindemann and Caplan, who have advocated that crisis intervention is a form of primary prevention.

However, more importantly, what is frequently obscured in the debate over crisis intervention as primary or secondary prevention (or somewhere in between) are the theoretical constructs of crisis theory, which provide a mechanism for developing anticipatory guidance programs, definitely primary preventive in nature and scope. Such programs are based on the observations that some crises are pre-

This Foreword was written by Dr. Goldston in a private capacity. No official support or endorsement by the National Institute of Mental Health is intended or should be inferred.

dictable, normative, and developmental, and that the skills and strengths needed to cope and adapt effectively can be provided to specific populations at risk long before the crisis occurs—such efforts are primary prevention par excellence.

Each chapter in this volume emphasizes basic principles of primary prevention while extending knowledge of opportunities to conduct effective preventive interventions. Some years ago, this writer emphasized that "all primary prevention activities must be characterized by *specific* actions directed at *specific* populations for *specific* purposes" (Goldston, 1977). The studies reported herein emphasize the imperative of determining which intervention is to be used and directed at which persons at what point in time. The message is clear but bears repeating from the vantage point of preventive service providers—all persons who experience a critical life event are not at risk for disorder or dysfunction. Rather, specific subpopulations that research has identified as being at high risk should be the targets of preventive interventions. These chapters highlight the tasks awaiting researchers in enumerating specific subpopulations, and subsequently developing and testing out interventions. Practitioners will benefit from this information by becoming increasingly aware of the importance of designing interventions for discrete subpopulations and carrying out efforts to recruit these persons into service delivery efforts.

Most of the crisis intervention literature has been directed to adult populations. This book addresses a gap in knowledge by focusing on children and their families. The authors remind the reader that not only do persons in crisis require a "map of the territory" in order to facilitate coping and adaptation and the acquisition of appropriate skills, attitudes, and behaviors, but that where children are involved, knowledge of the developmental needs of youngsters is essential. Once again, preventionists are reminded of the virtually untapped lodes of riches in developmental and educational psychology which can be used to develop and implement primary prevention programs (Cowen, 1981).

Viewed from a national perspective, many of the problem areas to which individual chapters are devoted have been of concern in the developing prevention program at the National Institute of Mental Health. During its initial year of operations in 1980, the Office of Prevention prepared an announcement inviting grant applications focused on the impact of marital disruption on children. In subsequent years, NIMH prevention grant announcements about children, youth, and their families have dealt with such subjects as the effects on children of severely disturbed parents, high-risk factors in depression, and infants at risk. Contract studies have dealt with mental health practices in pediatric settings, and the health consequences of the stress of bereavement. Research planning workshops involving a concern with children and youth have been convened on the following topics: preventive interventions to reduce the harmful consequences of severe and persistent loneliness; preventive intervention programs for family units with a mentally ill relative; conquest of two agents that endanger the brain, measles and rubella; prevention and mental health promotion, the interpersonal cognitive problem-solving model; preventive aspects of suicide and affective disorders among adolescents and young adults; research on preventive child psychiatry and childhood chronic illness; assessing and promoting healthy family functioning; primary prevention of aggressive and violent behavior; and roles of the core mental health professions in preventing and reducing the incidence of black homicide.

Moreover, the NIMH Center for Prevention Research, which plans and administers the prevention research grants program, issued a research program notice in 1982 stating:

Increasingly, research is making evident the contribution of episodic (e.g., a brief traumatic event) or enduring (e.g., an emotionally ill parent or family instability) stressful life events to the onset and maintenance of disorders and dysfunction. The Center for Prevention Research is interested in research specifically linking stressful life events to individual vulnerability and resistance to specific disorders or dysfunctions with the intent of applying these research findings directly to the development of preventive interventions. Also encouraged is research assessing the impact of preventive interventions on at-risk individuals which enables them to cope effectively with the emotional consequences of stressful life events or ameliorate their pathogenic influence.

In short, the area of prevention, as reflected in Federal research priorities, is emphasizing preventive *interventions*. Similarly, this book also focuses on interventions, and thereby makes a welcome and significant contribution to the prevention literature by contents recording data-based approaches that work with children and their families faced with life crises.

Stephen E. Goldston
Office of Prevention
National Institute of Mental Health
Alcohol, Drug Abuse,
and Mental Health Administration

REFERENCES

Cowen, E. L. (1981). Choices and alternatives for primary prevention in mental health. In M. J. Goldstein (Ed.), *Preventive intervention in schizophrenia: Are we ready?* (DHHS Publication No. (ADM 81-1111). Washington, D.C.: U. S. Government Printing Office.
Goldston, S. E. (1977). An overview of primary prevention programming. In D. C. Klein & S. E. Goldston (Eds.), *Primary prevention: An idea whose time has come.* (DHEW Publication No. (ADM) 77-447). Washington, D.C.: U. S. Government Printing Office.

Preface

Crisis intervention focuses on otherwise "normally" functioning persons exposed to stressors that are eliciting high level emotional distress and straining coping capability. Conventional psychotherapy, in contrast, is more oriented toward dealing with maladaptive behavior and emotional problems associated with long-standing disturbance where the environmental presses are more diffuse and play a less central role. Given this "situational" orientation, developing a taxonomy of crisis intervention techniques that specifies which procedures to use for particular stressors should be a comparatively manageable task. If one assumes that the patterns of maladjustment predisposed by major stressful events can be identified, then points of intervention, types of procedures to use, and outcome goals should be apparent. As Cowen and Hightower (Chapter 4) note, some of these crucial stressor-maladjustment reaction patterns have in fact been identified (e.g., the relationship between parental separation/divorce and school adjustment problems) and have led to successful implementation of intervention programs. Indeed, one of the goals of this volume is to present examples of programs in which operationalized intervention procedures are applied to children and/or families experiencing common stressors with an eye toward shedding light both on the nature of the stressor-maladjustment relationships and the effectiveness of the techniques designed to short-circuit them.

Nonetheless, the task of developing such a taxonomy of crisis intervention techniques is complex and difficult, and for numerous reasons. First, the apparent simplicity of being able to orient intervention procedures around unambiguous, well-defined stimulus events of known impact is illusory. As noted by Auerbach (Chapter 1), based on current research findings, many crisis-level stressors do not eventuate in predictable patterns of response either from a qualitative or quantitative standpoint (for many critical stressors the necessary systematic longitudinal research either has not been undertaken or is currently being conducted). Individuals differ in their response to even the most disruptive stressors as a function of differences in dispositional traits, reinforcement histories, and so on, as well as situational moderators such as social support. As Cowen and Hightower (Chapter

4) put it: Confronted with "the most profound adversities imaginable . . . stressors of marked gravity . . . some children not only surmount (them), but are competent and well adjusted . . . . What factors make them invincible despite overpowering odds against them?" Isolating such differentiating factors is one of the crucial challenges for those who hope to develop a "science" of crisis intervention.

A second related aspect involves recognition of the fact that crisis-level stressors are not homogeneous unitary entities, but rather subsume multiple substressors that are likely of differential impact in producing emotional disorder. For example, Melamed and Bush (Chapter 6) identify a "taxonomy of stressors" facing a family entering the health care system. Hospitalization for surgery involves "not only anesthesia induction when the patient is about to be operated on, but also post-operative recovery, hospital admission, separation from significant others, a variety of presurgical procedures such as injections and sometimes highly invasive examinations, and the initial learning that surgery needs to be done" (p. 140). Kerr (Chapter 10) points out the particular complexities involved in coping with physical disability, which is not a "temporally confined event that occurs and then disappears." Adjusting to physical disability involves coping with a continuous series of stressors that are "rare or unknown to other children." As Sandler, Wolchik, Braver, and Fogas (Chapter 3) point out, one of the preconditions for the development of effective intervention is a "thorough understanding of the specific events occurring in a particular risk situation," and in their chapter they provide us with a methodology for "describing the multiple stressors of risk situations" using children of divorce as an example.

Another clearly important determinant of the appropriate crisis intervention technique to use in a particular situation is the temporal relationship of the individual to the crisis-inducing stressor (Auerbach, Chapter 1). Many of the chapters in this volume exemplify how not only the nature of the intervention technique, but also the type of individual conducting the intervention, and the intervention goals (i.e., appropriate outcome criteria) vary as a function of this factor. With some stressors persons often experience a sequence of temporal stages, and interventions may be instituted at any or all of these stages. For example, Stolberg, Kiluk, and Garrison (Chapter 5) identify four stages of the divorce adjustment process (predecision, final separation, adjustment to separation, and recovery/redefinition), typically covering a period of several years, and note the differing intervention needs of children and divorcing parents at each of these periods. Kupst (Chapter 8) identifies five time-linked stages that comprise the crisis of pediatric leukemia (for the ill child, siblings, and family members) and describes how the nature of the intervention (e.g., relative emphasis on emotion-focused support versus problem-focused information and planning for specific tasks), the roles of the various intervenors (counselors, physicians, and external support persons) and the goals of intervention vary as a function of the stage of the crisis.

In the area of child sexual abuse, Swift (Chapter 7) spells out specific interventions and intervention targets that are appropriate at each of the four temporal stages identifed by Auerbach. For example, Type 1 distal prestress educational programs designed to prevent sexual victimization of children are appropriate for all children, parents, and teachers, but are particularly relevant for siblings of incest victims who are at high risk for sexual abuse. Type 2 proximal prestress programs may involve forced separation of the victim (and siblings) from the abuser, or teaching children escape or defensive behaviors. In contrast, Type 3 proximal poststress interventions may involve case monitoring activities by professionals, and Type 4 distal poststress interventions include more traditional counseling or therapy approaches. Melamed and Bush (Chapter 6) note that in the case of a relatively focalized stressor such as impending surgery, even within a temporal stage the timing of intervention may be very important. "Preparation either too far in advance or too immediately prior to the stressful event results in arousal which is less likely to be used in adaptive coping efforts" (p. 139).

Clearly, the most desirable interventions are those conducted as early as possible, preferably prior to exposure to the stressor. However, in many cases the stressor is difficult or impossible to anticipate or prepare for (e.g., physical disability, concentration camp internment). With other relatively low frequency stressors (e.g., natural disaster) it is difficult to motivate people to engage in early (Type 1) preventive interventions, and this is complicated by the fact that we often ignore (deny?) or misinterpret warning cues and concentrate on stresses immediately impinging on us (see Swift's chapter for an example of this phenomenon in child sexual abuse). But as Kerr (Chapter 10) points out, though it may not be feasible to expect people to prepare for a large number of aversive situations that may never occur, parents may teach children "survival skills" as they encounter developmentally sequenced "mini-crises." In addition, they may expose them to attitudes and teach them cognitive sets (e.g., to search for new ways of reaching a goal when a conventional path is blocked), which, one would hope, will generalize and serve them adaptively when confronted with future stresses. Outside of such general preparation, the total intervention focus with some low-frequency cataclysmic stressors (e.g., surviving Holocaust victims) is of necessity on the poststress periods.

Many of the common themes of the fairly diverse group of chapters in this volume indicate those aspects of crisis intervention which reflect its historical association with community psychology and which differentiate both of these from more traditional approaches. There is strong emphasis on the role of the family and other indigenous support systems as stress moderators. The interventions described with few exceptions involve parents and other family members as well as the children who are usually the direct targets of the crisis-inducing stressor. The role of professionals as direct service providers is deemphasized with many of the interventions described capable of being administered by paraprofessionals or persons who are not mental health professionals (e.g., teachers) in community environments (e.g., schools, hospitals, community centers, police departments) rather than traditional office settings. Consistent with the model outlined in Chapter 1, prevention of psychopathology per se is deemphasized. The focus is on identifying and effecting change in those indicants of adjustment, competence, or maladjustment that are relevant outcomes depending on the nature of the stressor, the individual(s) that is the target(s) of the intervention, and the temporal relationship of the individual(s) to the stressor.

We have solicited, where possible, chapters that describe specific intervention procedures and present empirical data on the effectiveness of those procedures. This book will be of interest to behavioral scientists working in the areas of stress, coping, and crisis intervention, and would be appropriate as a textbook for graduate level courses in those areas. In addition, clinical and school psychologists, pediatricians, pediatric nurses, and other service providers working with children and families will find useful suggestions for dealing with stresses associated with particular situations or problem areas.

This volume grew out of a conference entitled *Children's Life Crisis Events and Preventive Intervention Strategies* presented in April 1983 at Virginia Commonwealth University and sponsored by the Department of Psychology's Clinical Training Program. The conference was partially supported by an NIMH research grant to Arnold Stolberg (Primary Prevention of Psychopathology in Children of Divorce, 5 R01 MH34462) and by the Clinical Psychology Program's NIMH Training Grant (5 T01 MH15645; Stephen M. Auerbach, principal investigator). The chapters in this volume by Auerbach, Sandler et al., Melamed and Bush, and Stolberg et al. are based on presentations made at that conference. The remaining chapters were independently solicited.

We would like to thank David Hartman and Mary Hester for help in organizing the conference that served as the impetus for this volume, and Diana Rawls for typing and clerical assistance. We would also like to express our gratitude to Charles D. Spielberger for his support and encouragement throughout all phases of bringing this work to fruition.

Stephen M. Auerbach
Arnold L. Stolberg

I

INTRODUCTION

Among the areas of major concern to mental health professionals, crisis intervention is unique in that it focuses on treating psychological problems resulting from exposure to highly stressful events in otherwise "normally" functioning individuals. As noted in Chapter 1 by Auerbach, crisis as a theoretical construct is still in the formative stages. As empirical data accumulate, widely held clinically based assumptions regarding the effects of crisis, and the determinants of whether a given event is perceived as a crisis-level stressor, and the effectiveness with which it is coped, will need to be modified. The field of crisis intervention, similarly, is in a state of flux with no widely accepted model to guide clinical and research efforts. The temporal model developed in Chapter 1 is an attempt to provide an organizational framework for conceptualizing and implementing crisis intervention procedures. In developing this framework, the diversity of treatment approaches relevant to crisis intervention is exemplified, while at the same time it is demonstrated that certain classes of intervention procedures are particularly appropriate depending on the temporal relationship of the individual to the crisis-inducing stressor.

In the second chapter of the introductory section Felner, Rowlison, and Terre review the theoretical roots of modern crisis theory and attempt to clarify the conceptual confusion that has arisen from the interchangeable and nondiscriminating use of the multiple terms associated with stress, crisis, and life events. In addition, they address the question of which aspects of life events have the most impact in defining them as stressful, and outline attempts to account for the relationship between the occurrence of stressful life events and the onset of emotional disorder. In Chapter 3, Sandler, Wolchik, Braver, and Fogas, using the example of children of divorce, describe a methodology for evaluating the impact of different stressors associated with a given crisis situation. Their findings illustrate the need to conceptualize crisis situations as being composed of multiple events, each component of which has differing impact and likely poses different adjustment demands for given individuals.

1

Assumptions of Crisis Theory and a Temporal Model of Crisis Intervention

Stephen M. Auerbach
Virginia Commonwealth University

The predominant attitude toward the assessment of a state of crisis is similar to that expressed by a retired Supreme Court justice when asked to give his criteria for defining pornography: "I know it when I see it." Despite widespread usage, crisis remains an elusive hypothetical construct without a well-defined nomological net, "a convenient catch-all concept within which to organize certain brief, identifiable, and transitory experiences" (Schulberg & Sheldon, 1968). Nonetheless, "crisis theory" is often referred to as if there existed an established conceptual model that has been validated to the satisfaction of the most stringent requirements, and crisis intervention is similarly referred to as if it denoted a well-accepted set of techniques based on the "established tenets of crisis theory." The major theses of this chapter are that (*a*) a number of assumptions that have accrued to the crisis construct have been accepted uncritically without reference to relevant empirical findings and (*b*) crisis intervention, rather than denoting an integrated theory-based set of techniques, represents widely varied procedures whose nature and goals depend on the nature of the crisis-inducing stressor, its temporal relation to the individual experiencing it, and the setting in which the intervention is undertaken. In the foregoing, problems in defining and measuring the crisis construct will be considered first, followed by a discussion of the factors that seem to have influenced the growth of interest in crisis and crisis intervention in the mental health fields. The question of the validity of the major assumptions that have come to be associated with the crisis construct will then be considered in light of extant empirical evidence. These assumptions involve the time course and severity of effects of response to crisis-inducing stressors, and the role of individual differences and other moderators of the crisis response. Finally, an analysis of the range and types of procedures falling under the rubric crisis intervention will be presented. It will be argued that, from both procedural and evaluative standpoints, the most meaningful way to classify crisis intervention approaches is in terms of the temporal relation of the individual to the crisis-inducing stressor.

DEFINITION AND MEASUREMENT OF THE CRISIS CONSTRUCT

From a definitional standpoint, several major problems may be identified. First, though there is broad agreement as to the general meaning of the term crisis as it is used in literautre, the behavioral sciences, as well as in everyday language—a situation that is perceived as stressful and induces emotional disequilibrium, and one that impels a person toward decision making and therefore opportunity to change—the term is used differently across academic disciplines. In contrast to psychologists who focus on individuals facing aversive external events (primarily those posing threats to self-esteem and physical integrity), existential philosophers deal on a more internal level with threat of loss of individuality (*angst*), sociologists conceive of crisis in terms of the traditional structure of social systems being threatened (Wenger, 1978) and political scientists deal with threats to the integrity of nations in conflict (Hermann, 1972). Second, within psychology there is no well articulated, testable model. The most widely cited crisis "theory" is Caplan's (1964, 1974) conceptualization of crisis as a state of psychological disequilibrium brought about by a loss of "basic supplies" and subsequent breakdown in the hypothetical homeostatic problem-solving mechanism. As with most psychodynamically based approaches it is difficult to reduce to testable hypotheses, and thus has been widely accepted by clinicians as a self-evident truth without undergoing rigorous evaluation. Other clinically based theoretical models of crisis that have been proposed (Schulberg & Sheldon, 1968; Shontz, 1965; Taplin, 1971) have had little heuristic impact, and thus studies focused solely on theoretical questions relating to crisis have been rare. Much of the research that is available is narrowly conceived and contributes little to our understanding of the crisis construct (e.g., Smith, 1970). In one of few broadly conceived studies, Bloom (1963) addressed the question of what characteristics of life events are most influential in causing them to be classified as crises. He found simply that "expert judges" define situations as crises primarily based on knowledge of a precipitating stressful event with no identifiable reaction or a delayed resolution. In only one recent study (Lewis, 1982) has an attempt been made to explore the difference between the nature of the affective responses induced by what most would agree is a crisis-level stressor (surgery for cancer) versus a less severe stressor (surgery for serious but remedial problems). Lewis conjectured that crisis may be a qualitatively different state from that induced by a less severe stressor on the basis of crisis being characterized by sudden discontinuous changes in psychological functioning. In addition, based on his data and within the context of a multidimensional topographical model derived from catastrophe theory, he made explicit hypotheses regarding how level of depression, anxiety, and the passage of time may interact to influence the manifestation of the crisis response. Lewis's model stands out because it is empirically based, clinically relevant and testable, and represents the first serious step toward establishing discriminant and convergent validity for the crisis construct.

In addition to a lack of adequate theory, construct validity work has been hampered by the absence of a measure that reliably establishes the presence of a state of crisis. Most researchers assume a crisis-level reaction based on the presence of or proximity to a particular stressful event (e.g., death of a loved one, impending surgery) without obtaining an independent measure of emotional reaction. Lewis (1982) used the Halpern (1973) Crisis Scale as his independent measure, but this scale (which consists of items derived from the Minnesota Multiphasic Personality Inventory and the Community Adaptation Schedule) has poor face validity, only preliminary concurrent validity, and there is no evidence of discriminant validity.

No other scales attempt to provide a global measure of the crisis response. Much recent work has been done on the development of "stressful life event" scales such as the Social Readjustment Rating Scale (Holmes and Rahe, 1967) and the Life Experiences Survey (Sarason, Johnson, & Siegel, 1978), but these instruments by and large are used to evaluate the extent to which individuals have been exposed to a range of stressful events rather than emphasizing the subjective impact of events on the respondents. What is needed is a measure that evaluates the impact of stressful events along dimensions of subjective distress consistent with a theoretical formulation of crisis. The most promising measure currently available from this standpoint is the Impact of Event Scale (Horowitz, Wilner, & Alvarez, 1979; Zilberg, Weiss, & Horowitz, 1982).

CRISIS AND CRISIS INTERVENTION–GROWTH AND DEVELOPMENT

Crisis, more than any other concept (along with crisis intervention) has come to symbolize a discernible shift that has taken place in recent years in the mental health fields. Increasingly interest has moved away from the individual whose deviant behavior is long-standing and a product of "mental disease" to the everyday person confronted with untenable circumstances, from predisposing to precipitating factors (Bloom, 1980), from high-risk populations to high-risk situations (Price, Bader, & Ketterer, 1980), from long-term therapy designed to induce characterological change and modify traits to focused time-limited interventions designed to mitigate the effects of environmentally-induced stress. The factors accounting for this change are difficult to pinpoint; indeed, some are quite peripheral in their influence. Yet there clearly has been a convergence of events emanating from a range of sources. These include the growth and continuing development of the community mental health movement, the diminishing influence of the disease model of psychopathology and the trait approach in personality, disenchantment with traditional psychotherapy, and changes in the popular attitude toward mental health and self-help.

The single most tangible factor in effecting this transition has been the growth and development of the community mental health movement. Embedded in the spirit of social action and liberal legislation of the 1960s, the community approach has emphasized preventive procedures and other innovative intervention strategies vs. traditional long-term treatment, the use of paraprofessionals vs. total reliance on traditionally trained professionals, and has focused on stressors within the social environment as the primary agents of emotional disturbance vs. the traditional disease approach. All of these factors have become closely associated with that part of the crisis intervention movement that deals with provision of short-term emergency services via community-based agencies. A second specific thrust associated with community psychology has come from the suicide prevention movement and the development in 1958 of the Los Angeles Suicide Prevention Center (LASPC) (paralleled by the growth of the Samaritans in the United Kingdom). Community-based "hot lines" using paraprofessional service providers have continued to flourish, and many of them orient their training programs around the problem-oriented lethality detection and transfer and referral procedures developed at the LASPC.

The role of the federal government in establishing the crisis intervention movement and nurturing its growth is evident not only in the early funding for the LASPC and the 1963 Community Mental Health Centers Act (which mandated emergency mental health services as one of its five essential programs), but also the subsequent NIMH research and training monies provided through the Center for Studies of Suicide Prevention. In addition, there have been specialized programs such as the Federal Disaster Law of 1974 which authorizes NIMH to provide funds to alleviate mental health problems in victims of natural disasters (see Frederick, 1977), the National Center for the Prevention and Control of Rape which funds mental health programs to help rape victims, their families, and offenders, and monies recently provided through LEAA and other federal departments for crisis intervention services to victims of violent crime. In general, whereas there has been an overall dramatic decline in research monies available to study mental health related problems, there has been an increase in NIMH support for research dealing with prevention of psychological problems associated with exposure to stressful life events.

From a broader standpoint, within both psychology and psychiatry, there has been increasing emphasis on situationism and the role of transitory stressful experience in engendering psychopathology. In psychology, this is reflected in the fall from grace of the radical trait model of personality functioning and diminished confidence that we can measure broad personality dispositions which will effectively predict behavior over time and across situations (Mischel, 1968, 1973). Concomitantly, there has been an upsurge in research attempting to establish links between exposure to stressful life events and both pathological behavior and bodily conditions (cf. Rabkin & Struening, 1976), and in formulations such as catastrophe theory, which are geared toward accounting for sudden discontinuous behavioral transitions (Woodcock & Davis, 1978). Within the behavior change arena mental health professionals have begun to come out from under the highly credentialed cloak of long-term psychotherapy, and seriously question whether they can induce broad dispositional changes in people. As a result, psychotherapy has become increasingly situationally oriented and problem focused, emphasis is on producing observable short-term changes, and there is less of a feeling among therapists that they must adhere to the constraints of the classical patient-therapist face-to-face dyadic relationship.

Even that proverbial immovable object, psychiatry, has begun to move away from strict adherence to a stolid disease model and to recognize regularly occurring transitory stress reactions as meaningful categories of behavior. This is reflected in (a) acknowledgement in DSM-III of "severity of psychosocial stressors" as a major determinant of diagnostic status, (b) inclusion of new categories such as "panic disorder," "posttraumatic stress disorder," and "brief reactive psychosis," (c) a more delineated breakdown (vs. DSM-II) by predominant symptomatology of "transient situational disturbances" and inclusion of more problem areas for individuals who are considered "psychiatrically normal" (e.g., bereavement, marital problems). The statement that a problem "may be a focus of attention or treatment but . . . not attributable to a mental disorder (Diagnostic and Statistical Manual of Mental Disorders, 1980, p. 331)" indicates recognition of the need to deal with immediate short-term reactions which are primarily tied to environmental events rather than chronic maladaptive dispositions or disease states.

Finally, on a popular level there seems to be a heightened awareness in this country of individual vulnerability and susceptibility to being swept up in catastrophic circumstances ("It's crisis after crisis these days," Schaar, 1980, p. 15). Apprehensions about economic ruin and nuclear destruction have given rise to the "survivalism" movement, whose members hoard food and other essentials and prepare themselves militarily (and thus psychologically) for the ultimate confrontation or disaster. From another standpoint the public seems to be increasingly aware and supportive of the need to provide services to special victimized groups (e.g., battered wives, victims of sexual assault, disabling disease, natural disaster, captivity), to develop programs to deal with uncontrollable events that covary with advancing age (e.g., "empty nest," menopause, male mid-life crisis, relocation, institutionalization), and in general to make available a range of emergency services to individuals with situational difficulties. Having psychological problems is to a lesser degree viewed within a socially dishonorable and therefore disuseful context (cf. Szasz, 1966). There is in fact great popular concern with solving the problems and mini-crises that beset the everyday man, as reflected in the proliferation of crisis-oriented self-help books (e.g., Calhoun, Selby, & King, 1976; Ruben, 1976; Simons, 1972) and similar volumes geared to the professional (Aguilera & Messick, 1978; Burgess & Baldwin, 1981; Lieberman & Borman, 1979; France, 1982; Puryear, 1979; Specter & Claiborn, 1973; Whitlock, 1978). There seems to be a general sense that it is "okay" to have emotional problems. Undergoing and seeking aid for a stress reaction is viewed as a part of "normal" experience and is less associated with the stigma of mental illness.

In summary, there clearly has been an increased emphasis on stress-induced transient situational disturbances. It is tied into the popular self-help and self-protection movements, the continuing impact of the community psychology movement and the diminishing influence of traditional long-term psychotherapy, and the general thrust in psychology away from emphasis on traits and stable person variables as prime determinants of behavior, and toward a social learning reconceptualization emphasizing continuous interplay between the person and the situations he encounters. Thus, in the mental health fields, stressful life events and crisis intervention have become "hot" areas, with crisis intervention no longer reserved for counselors purportedly not equipped to deal with long-term mental disturbance, but indeed a legitimate concern of clinical psychologists and psychiatrists. In psychiatry, emergency and brief psychotherapy are now growth specialities, paralleling the general rise of emergency medicine.

With this growth of interest in stress and crisis intervention, there have developed a number of assumptions about the effects of life crises on functioning and the role and efficacy of crisis intervention procedures. In the next sections those assumptions will be explored in light of empirical data drawn from studies with humans and animals conducted in natural and laboratory settings.

CRISIS THEORY, RELATED ASSUMPTIONS, AND EMPIRICAL EVIDENCE

Time Course

It is generally presumed that reactions to stressful life events are inherently transient or temporally self-limiting, which is to say that "in the majority of cases symptoms disappear spontaneously within a limited time after termination of (an event)—even when a serious loss has been suffered" (Dohrenwend & Dohrenwend, 1969, p. 114). Specifically, it is widely assumed that crises are resolved within four to six weeks from point of onset (Baldwin, 1979; Bloom, 1977; Darbonne, 1967). The apparent empirical basis for this assumption is Lindemann's (1944) "classic" study of the bereaved relatives of the victims of a nightclub fire and others who had recently died, in which he observed that most bereaved individuals satisfactorily worked through their grief in this interval. Conceptually, the belief stems from Caplan's (1964; 1974) psychodynamic model describing crisis states as resulting from psychological disequilibrium and a break-down in the "homeostatic" problem-solving mechanism; it is purported that (within a few weeks) some resolution (which may be more or less adaptive) is established, equilibrium restored, and symptoms disappear.

Changes in "psychological equilibrium" cannot be directly observed. However, if one assumes that a stable equilibrium is reflected in coping, problem-solving ability and diminished emotional and motivational deficits, then the time course of such changes can be examined after termination of a stressful event. Though only a few investigators have systematically studied these variables in longitudinal fashion, a number have obtained postexposure data at a single time period.

Research with animals and humans indicates that the time course of response to stressful events differs greatly depending on a variety of circumstances. A number of early studies (e.g., Liddell, 1953; Maier, 1956) demonstrated that *chronic* behavior disorders readily develop in animals when they are placed in an insoluble problem-solving or avoidance situation. More recently, Seligman and associates have found that in dogs resumption of adaptive problem-solving following exposure to an inescapable aversive stimulus is related to the severity of the stressor. Overmier and Seligman (1967) and Overmier (1968) found that after exposure to *one session* of inescapable shock magnitude of interference with subsequent escape-avoidance learning dissipated rapidly in time and the dogs were apparently normal in this regard after 48 hours and 72 hours respectively. But after *multiple* sessions of inescapable shock, dogs were still unable to learn appropriate escape responses one week after initial exposure to shock (Seligman, Maier, & Geer, 1968; Seligman & Groves, 1970). No time course has been found in rats or other animal species (Miller, Rosellini, & Seligman, 1977).

A time course in humans is more difficult to trace because many investigators do long-term follow-ups at arbitrary intervals rather than at those intermediate stages likely to show a gradient of change. In general, duration of residual dis-turbance seems to be a function of the apparent stressfulness of the situation. For example, the experience of major surgery, especially when associated with cancer, results in severe emotional reactions in up to 40% of patients and continues at least one year and up to at least 5 years postsurgery (Maguire et al., 1978; Morris, Greer, & White, 1977; Ray, 1978). Lewis, Gottesman, and Gutstein (1979) studied the time course of dysphoric emotional reactions in a group of cancer surgery patients and another group about to undergo less severe general surgery. For the general surgery group, measures of anxiety, depression, externality, self-concept and "crisis" generally followed the predicted Lindemann duration, declining to well below preoperative levels at eight weeks postsurgery. The cancer surgery group, however, did not exhibit decreases on most measures until 28 weeks after surgery. Krouse and Krouse (1982) reported duration differences as a function of type of cancer surgery. They found that self-reported depression and negative perceptions regarding body image continued to increase in gynecological cancer surgery patients 20 months after surgery, whereas these measures declined to below pretreatment levels in breast biopsy and mastectomy patients by one month after surgery.

Dohrenwend and Dohrenwend (1969) review a number of earlier studies indicating that response to relatively less severe crisis situations has a more limited time course for most persons. For example, Fried (1963) found that only a minority of women (20%) relocated from a slum area reported feelings of sadness or depression two years later, with another 20% stating that the symptoms lasted between six months and two years. In Sheatsley and Feldman's (1964) study of reactions to President Kennedy's assassination, 89% of the sample reported experiencing physical and emotional symptoms during the first four days, but only 50% reported at least one symptom at the five- to nine-day post-assassination interview period. In contrast, more severe stressors have been found to produce longer term debilitation. Leopold and Dillon (1963) interviewed survivors of a maritime explosion 3½ to 4½ years later and concluded that appreciable psychological deterioration was present in 71% of the sample, and Henderson and Bostock (1977) found that among 7 men who survived a shipwreck and were not rescued until 13 days later, 5 had "developed substantial psychotic disorder," based on follow-up examination 12 to 24 months later (one was well and claimed to be enriched by the experience). In a recent study with former American POWs (Vietnam), Ursano, Boydstun, and Wheatley (1981) compared a group under "maximal stress"—POWs captured before October 1969 who had endured torture and complete separation from the outside world—and a group under "submaximal stress"—POWs captured after 1969 whose incarceration was more humane and whose total time of captivity averaged one-tenth the duration of the first group—and found significantly more MMPI scales above a T-score of 70 in the first group. In addition, though frequency of psychiatric diagnoses was about the same (23%) in the two groups at repatriation, the incidence had increased to about 27% in the maximal stress group and declined to less than 20% in the submaximal stress group at an 18-month follow-up period.

Recent research with rape victims in which repeated postrape measures have been obtained indicate that emotional and social adjustment levels increase and are similar to those of matched nonvictims by four to six months postrape (Atkeson, Calhoun, Resick, & Ellis, 1982; Kilpatric, Veronen, & Resick, 1979; Resick, Calhoun, Atkeson, & Ellis, 1981). But, as with repatriated POWs, severity of residual emotional disturbance at a given after the stress period appears to be directly proportional to the severity of the stress (Ellis, Atkeson, & Calhoun, 1981). Ellis et al. found that among women who had been raped, an average of three years previously, those who had been victims of sudden violent attacks by complete strangers showed the most severe reactions, being more depressed, fatigued, and fearful, and getting less satisfaction from activities than victims of other types of assaults.

Perhaps the most telling demonstration of the continuing disruptive effects of exposure to extreme stress comes from studies of victims of Nazi concentration camps. Studies of these survivors years after their incarceration present no evidence of a short-term "equilibrium" having been attained in any sense. Prevalent in the majority is a persistent continuing stress reaction, evidenced by a wide range of chronic emotional, motivational, sexual, interpersonal-social and family adaptation problems; a continuing "persecution syndrome" that persists in the absence of detectable neurological abnormalities in the majority (Eitinger, 1980). These conclusions are buttressed by interview (Niederland, 1968), and psychological test data (Dor Shav, 1978), as well as data indicating significantly higher psychiatric hospital admission rates for former prisoners than the population as a whole among Norwegians (Eitinger & Strom, 1981). In general, severity of behavioral disturbance increases as a function of severity and duration of captivity (Eitinger, 1963). Descriptive data suggest that not only are there anomalies in survivors, but that they often perpetuate dysfunctional behavior in their children, all of whom were born after the Holocaust yet who are ceaselessly exposed to the story of their parents' tribulations, and must live with the spectre of their experience and with the unspoken command that they must provide meaning for their parents' empty lives and vindicate their suffering (Davidson, 1980; Epstein, 1979; Trossman, 1968). Recent findings by Leon, Butcher, Kleinman, Goldberg, and Almagor (1981), however, indicate that this phenomenon may not be as widespread as suggested in earlier reports.

In summary, though many of the naturalistic investigations cited above lack methodological rigor and often involve subjective observation for crucial data, the evidence strongly points to the conclusion that the duration of the deleterious effects of extreme stress is related in roughly linear fashion to the degree of aversiveness of the stressor. Hence, there is no evidence at this time to support the traditional contention that emotional dysfunction or poor social adjustment in response to crisis follows a four- to six-week or any other uniform time course across stressors.

Severity of Effects

"If it moves, label it," is the approach of many mental health professionals to behaviors that occur in response to stressful life events. Thus we have the survivor syndrome (cf. Solkoff, 1981) and the KZ syndrome (Eitinger, 1963) of former concentration camp inmates, the apathy syndrome noted in World War II soldiers and Korean POWs (cf. Ursano, 1981), the post-Vietnam syndrome (Figley, 1978), the rape trauma syndrome (Burgess & Holstrom, 1974), the disaster syndrome and the counterdisaster syndrome (Wallace, 1956), the Stockholm syndrome (Strentz, 1980) which is said to afflict victims who have been taken hostage, the all-encompassing posttraumatic stress disorder syndrome recently formalized in DSM-III (1980), and most recently the herpes syndrome (Laskin, 1982), and somewhat facetiously, the "hip, Honda, and hirsute" syndrome of newly divorced males (Hetherington, 1983). Though the intent behind this nomenclature may be simply to provide descriptive lables for homogeneous groups of behaviors that seem to occur with some regularity in response to particular stressors, they in fact have more far reaching implications. They suggest that these behaviors are regularly manifested in most persons who are exposed to a given stress situation, and the syndrome labels indicate disease, thereby suggesting high-level disability from exposure to these stressors.

The "severity" issue has become most clearly polarized in the literature assessing psychological consequences of exposure to natural disaster. In contrast to the above researchers, sociologists seem bent on showing that there are no major breakdowns in human functioning; that organizations, institutions, and individuals continue to function, and therefore that disasters have only transitory effects that quickly dissipate, after which the orderly functioning of society resumes (cf. Taylor, Ross, & Quarantelli, 1976; Quarantelli & Dynes, 1977). They note that "mental illness . . . is not a major consequence of even massive disasters" (Taylor et al., 1976, p. 7) and point out that not only psychiatric disturbance but even panic is rare in the wake of natural disasters (e.g., Penick, Powell, & Sieck, 1976; Popovic & Petrovic, 1964; Taylor et al., 1976), and that psychiatric admissions show no change or actually decrease from predisaster levels (Perry & Lindell, 1978; Taylor et al., 1976). They argue that the "disaster syndrome"–in which the individual appears dazed and stunned, is hypersuggestible and virtually helpless in terms of self-care–is a short-term reaction (up to one-half hour after impact) and is rapidly replaced by euphoria and a surge of community participation (Wallace, 1956). In fact, the dominant short-term reactions are said to be helping-oriented activities, self-reliance and resource sharing (Perry & Lindell, 1978). They assert that families are often better off with respect to solidity and fluidity of relationships (Drabek, Key, Erickson, & Crowe, 1973), and long-term negative psychological reactions are said to be rare, if not nonexistent (Perry & Lindell, 1978).

Mental health professionals with an "illness" orientation, however, adduce studies that indicate high incidence of severe postdisaster emotional disturbance (e.g., Cobb & Lindemann, 1943; Leopold & Dillon, 1963; Moore & Friedsam, 1959), and press this point of view strongly. The strongest objective data in this regard comes from a study of 381 adult survivors of the 1972 Buffalo Creek Dam Disaster (Gleser, Green, & Winget, 1978). Standard interviews scaled for psychopathology on Spitzer, Endicott, Mesnikoff, & Cohen's (1968) Psychiatric Evaluation Form indicated that two years after the disaster survivors continued to experience disruption and maladaptive behaviors "of a severity comparable to that seen in the typical psychiatric outpatient" (Gleser et al., 1978, p. 216).

Whether simple exposure to severe stress can produce "mental illness" is of course a moot point since the behavioral referents of this hypothetical condition have not been established discriminantly.* It seems fair to conclude, however, that exposure to stressful life events produces responses ranging from the constructive and prosocial to the self-defeating and debilitating. The degree to which maladaptive behaviors are manifested as well as their extension in time appear to be largely a function of the degree of aversiveness of the stressor. Individual difference variables and other important moderators of this relationship are ·discussed presently.

Individual Differences and Other Moderator Variables

From one standpoint, consideration of the role of individual differences in crisis reaction and resolution is contradictory given the typical view of crises as focusing on "strong" situations which override dispositional differences and pro-

*From a practical standpoint in dealing with natural disaster victims, it should be noted that adoption of the psychiatric "mental illness" model has proved to be counterproductive. Very few disaster victims actively seek disaster-related mental health services (Baisden & Quarantelli, 1981), and the intervention of psychiatrists is actively resisted in the early postdisaster phases by other helpers, and in the last phases by the victims themselves who view negatively services offered under mental health labels. In fact, the bulk of mental health services are provided by newly emergent non psychiatrically oriented groups, rather than by formal mental health organizations (Taylor et al., 1976).

duce consistently high level stress responses [e.g., "the resolution of an emotional crisis is not necessarily determined by previous experience or character structure but rather shaped by current influences" (Baldwin, 1979, p. 46)]. Indeed, some phenomena to which people have been exposed are of such an extreme nature that dispositional factors have seemingly been neutralized by the brutality of the situation which pushed all exposed to the outer limits of coping capability and produced a relatively homogeneous set of behaviors. For example, in describing the survivors of the Buffalo Creek (W. Va.) mine disaster, Lifton and Olson (1976, p. 16) observed that "pre-existing pathology [became] buried under the unvaried likeness and monotony of the survivor syndrome." Similar observations have been made of concentration camp victims who regardless of previous history, personality, constitutional makeup, or social or cultural background displayed almost identical symptoms—"obsessions, nightmares, delusional and hallucinatory spells precipitated by auditory or visual perceptions reminiscent of the concentration camps" (Trautman, 1964, cited in Eitinger, 1980, p. 147).

But observational data such as these have been discounted by those who oppose claims of concentration camp survivors for reparations from Germany and who argue that "healthy persons should have the ability to endure nearly unlimited stress and indescribable difficulties without long-lasting psychic disturbances" (Eitinger, 1980). This naive extreme of the "trait" approach is supported by some psychoanalysts who hold that all maladaptive behaviors are ultimately traceable to early childhood experiences and cannot be understood as a response to trauma during adulthood, and by somatagenicists who insist that psychopathology primarily stems from biological inheritance differences (cf. Chodoff, 1980; Lifton, 1980).

There is, in fact, evidence that individual difference variables did make a difference in coping ability among camp prisoners. Gronvik and Lonnum (1962) found some relationship between premorbid history and severe psychiatric disturbance in survivors. In addition, while imprisoned, inmates who were able to apply coping styles (e.g., immersion in fantasy, total denial) that were appropriate to the situation more often survived than those whose predominant styles did not dovetail with the demands of the situation (total apathy and withdrawal) (Benner, Roskies, & Lazarus, 1980; Dimsdale, 1980). Also, recent data indicate that some camp survivors eventually adapted quite well to their postwar environment. Leon et al. (1981) found that a select group of hardy survivors who were still alive 33 years after the end of World War II, who had migrated to the United States, and who would participate in the study (less than 40% of those originally contacted) showed no significant psychopathology and were no different from a matched control group in this regard. Thus, even in the face of the brutal stress of the concentration camps individuals differed in coping ability and ultimate readjustment level. It should be noted that one had a chance to survive and cope in this setting only if uncontrollable factors (e.g., age, religion, physical condition) had not marked one for death or particularly brutal treatment. Thus, those who coped more successfully should be credited for their accomplishment, but those who failed to survive or cope successfully cannot be considered less competent people since chance situational factors played so great a role (Benner et al., 1980).

With stressors of lesser magnitude there is clear evidence that individual differences in self-reported trait anxiety and more situation-specific fears are good predictors of the level of anxiety individuals will experience in failure-threat and physical-harm-threat situations respectively (Auerbach, 1980; Mellstrom, Cicala, & Zuckerman, 1976; Spielberger, 1972). Locus of control orientation, which is usually conceptualized as a dispositional trait, has been found to be an important moderator of behaviors undertaken in response to natural disasters. Simpson-Housely (1979) found a positive relationship between internality as measured by Rotter's (1966) I-E scale and the degree to which individuals said they would take active preventive measures if confronted with the threat of an earthquake. This relationship has also been demonstrated behaviorally, and on a culture-wide basis. Sims and Baumann (1972) found that the disproportionately higher number of tornado deaths in the southern vs. northern portion of the United States was apparently due to differences in culturally-based attitudes; Alabama residents were found to be more fatalistic, passive, lacking in trust and inattentive to organized disaster warning systems, whereas Illinois residents were more accepting of technology, and more objective, rational, and action oriented in dealing with tornado disaster. Similarly, on Yap in the Western Caroline Islands, typhoons are viewed as uncontrollable and supernaturally determined, and despite clear warning and slow buildup time permitting anticipatory action, and clear knowledge of effective preventive measures, no anticipatory action is taken by the natives that could limit damages (Schneider, 1957). Historically, a similar "external" attitude was taken toward disasters such as plagues in the Middle Ages, when most individuals took catastrophe as an expression of God's wrath. The typical response included a range of dysfunctional superstitious behaviors such as upsurges of repentence in the form of flagellant processions, frenzied searches for scapegoats eventuating in large scale pogroms, and devotion to such good works as church repair and the founding of religious houses (Langer, 1958). At the other end of the continuum are "disaster subcultures," communities that have been repetitively exposed to a given disaster agent and which take extensive preventive measures such that the community is prepared psychologically, organizationally, and physically to deal with it. Underlying this goal-directed acitivity is an "attitude of defiance and pride in ability to 'take it' expressed in vehement refusal to 'flee before the winds' " (Moore, 1964, p. 195). An interesting and perhaps not unexpected by-product when community-wide preparatory procedures are repeatedly shown to be effective in these communities is a paradoxical kind of externality; individuals gradually become disinterested in and less knowledgeable about preventive procedures, apparently assuming that the amorphous "community" is now handling things (Hannigan & Kueneman, 1978).

One's perception of one's ability to manipulate and control a specific situation also clearly determines the meaning of a stressful situation and the degree to which coping behavior is initiated and persists. This perception is often related to specific competencies or situational variables rather than broad, generalized traits. Jumping off a highdiving board is pleasurable for the experienced diver and swimmer but may be perceived as a crisis with great harm potential for the nonswimmer, irrespective of differences in trait anxiety, coping style or any other dispositional variables. In disasters, those with relevant concrete coping skills show the lowest levels of maladaptive behavior (Barton, 1969) and usually emerge as leaders, rather than the proverbial "heroes" who seem somehow destined by an "enviable cast of personality" to take charge in all situations (Chapman, 1962). For example, in a disaster in which houses began to blow up as a result of a rush of illuminating gas, normally low status delivery truck drivers who could turn off house valves emerged as leaders. When crises begin to abate, however, social power and control redistribute in the direction of those who possess the more generalized reinforcers associated with wealth and high social standing (Wenger, 1978).

It seems clear then that, as with other stimuli, stressful events cannot be viewed in isolation, but need to be studied in their total context. Further, independent of dispositional traits, the way an event is construed, and its attendant elements, determine to a large extent how it is responded to. For example, for some concentration camp victims who were at the lowest status levels prior to internment and who were given "capo" (trustee) status as inmates and thus some degree of privilege and power over other inmaates, imprisonment may actually have had some positive elements. Similarly, pregnancy may be a strongly positive event for a woman who wants a child, but may be viewed as undesirable by an unwed teenager (Sarason et al., 1978). Even if such a teenager might on some level view pregnancy as a positive event, the complexities involved in coping with it often would make such a situation untenable. In disaster situations, the complexity of coping tasks for individuals often overrides specific problem-solving skills to put situations beyond the desired level of control. In natural disasters for example, individuals sometimes have responsibilities as a member of a formal rescue organization, as a member of a primary group (feed family, care for children, etc.), and as a community member engaged in voluntary activities. Sometimes formal organizations, families, and neighborhoods are in trouble at the same time, thus straining coping capability (cf. Barton, 1969).

The availability of supportive social relationships which may serve as a protective buffer is a contextual variable that is receiving growing recognition as an important mediator of degree of distress experienced by and coping ability of individuals confronted with stressful situations. Social support systems are said to provide emotional sustenance, tangible resources and aid, and information in times of need (Caplan, 1974). Numerous studies linking social support to good health and ability to withstand stress have validated this contention (e.g., Andrews, Tennant, Hewson, & Schonell, 1978; Cassel, 1976; Cobb, 1976; Gore, 1978; Holohan & Moos, 1978; Turner, 1981; Wilcox, 1981). For example, Gore found that unemployed men who felt unsupported (as assessed by a 13-item index) had higher serum cholesterol levels and more symptoms of illness, and experienced more depression regardless of employment status. Andrews et al. found that expectations of help in a crisis from friends, relatives, or neighbors were negatively correlated with psychological impairment. In the concentration camps if an inmate could not affiliate with a group within the first few days of internment, chances of survival were greatly diminished. Placement with inmates who spoke a different language was tantamount to a death sentence (Benner et al., 1980; Dimsdale, 1980). The results can be particularly devastating if a large gap between accustomed and actual levels of social support covaries with exposure to a crisis-level stressor. The 1972 Buffalo Creek dam disaster produced unusually severe levels of emotional disturbance in survivors, which in some persisted for many years (Gleser, Green, & Winget, 1981). The community affected, prior to the disaster, was unusually close-knit with much mutual support governed by long-standing traditions. As a result of the flood, "old bonds of kinship and neighborhood . . . were severed . . . people no longer related to each other in old and accustomed ways . . . the threads of the social fabric had snapped" (Erickson, 1976, pp. 302–305).

It should be noted that the data on the stress-buffering effects of social support are primarily correlational in nature. With the exception of subjective observations of the positive effects of peer-run social support groups (Ganikos et al., 1979; Silverman, 1974) few data have been reported evaluating the effects of actively providing social support to individuals in crisis. It could be argued that provision of support to a passive actor, without requiring independent activity on his part, would enhance his sense of dependency and do nothing to defuse a feeling of loss of control and inability to influence outcomes. In this regard, it has been observed that survivors of catastrophic events seem to fare best when they have the opportunity to have an *active* voice in community rebuilding. Hiroshima survivors benefitted from the knowledge that talking about the horror of their experience might help prevent future use of nuclear weapons; parents of leukemia victims by the same token derive solace from a "survivor mission" of supporting research that might prevent others from experiencing the same tragedy (Lifton & Olson, 1976). Eitinger (1980) similarly notes that many of the Jewish concentration camp survivors who showed the best adjustment were those who emigrated to Israel and became involved in an environment that was supportive but also made demands on them for cooperation, effort, and building the community.

In summary, though the term crisis generally implies an event that is disruptive in the extreme to all exposed, even highly aversive events such as concentration camp internment or exposure to a catastrophic natural disaster produce a range of response depending on a number of person and situational variables that might be operating at the moment. Thus the experience of psychological stress or at its extreme, crisis, and the ability to cope with same, is best conceptualized as a transactional process between person and environment, involving expectations of one's ability to manipulate a given situation (a function of perceived tangible and emotional resources), attitudinal and dispositional traits (which may be culturally conditioned), and contextual factors which help shape the cognitive and therefore affective impact of a stressor. Because the coping process is fluid and nonlinear it is very difficult to isolate single person or situational factors or even interaction terms as stable causative influences in the traditional deterministic sense (Coyne & Lazarus, 1979; Lazarus & Launier, 1978). Given this admonition, the single moderator variable that has been focused on in the clinical crisis literature as the most important determinant of coping ability is one's success in dealing with previous crisis situations. The validity of this notion will now be considered.

Previous Success in Coping with Crises

Obviously, we all experience stress. The psychoanalytic model holds that crises associated with psychosexual development in childhood are universal, and the manner in which they are resolved affects future functioning under stress. Recently, the notion that as adults we experience crises that automatically unfold as a function of events that covary with age (menopause, "empty nest," "midlife crisis") has been widely embraced, at least on a popular level (cf. Levinson, 1977; Neugarten, 1976). According to "crisis theory" how we deal with these "maturational" crises, as well as stressors that we are exposed to adventitiously, determines future coping ability. Successful resolution of crises is said to reduce the incidence of psychiatric disability and vice versa. Thus crises are said to represent opportunities for growth as well as for failure (Bloom, 1977). Depending on how they are resolved, the result may be increased problem-solving skills or reduced capacity to deal with problems (Caplan, 1964).

Experimental studies with animals generally support this formulation. Maier and Seligman (1976) and Miller, Rosellini, & Seligman (1977) cite a number of studies indicating that when organisms are exposed to uncontrollable aversive events (crises) their ability to function in future traumatic situations is adversely affected in a number of ways. Their motivation wanes (they do not subsequently initiate escape responses), their cognitive ability suffers (i.e., ability to perceive contingent relationships between behavior and outcomes), and dysphoric emotionality (depression, anxiety) is produced. For example, Braud, Wepmann, and Russo (1969) found that rats given inescapable shock were poorest in subsequently escaping from an alley flooded with water compared with yoked controls and rats previously given escapable shock. Brookshire, Littman, and Stewart (1961) found that when inescapable shocks were given to weaning rats their food-getting behavior was still disrupted as adults even under conditions of extreme hunger.

There is also evidence that successful dealing with an aversive event results in more persistent attempts to cope with new stress situations (Seligman & Maier, 1967) and more successful coping over an extended time interval (Hannum, Rosellini, & Seligman, 1976). Seligman and Maier found that dogs given escapable shocks in a shuttle box were much more persistent in attempting to escape shocks in another apparatus (the hammock) compared to naive dogs. Hannum et al. found that rats given escapable shock at weaning did not become helpless when given inescapable shock as adults; rats receiving inescapable shock were significantly poorer escapers than those previously given escapable shock or no shock.

Laboratory evidence from experiments with humans is less consclusive. Roth and Bootzin (1974) and Roth and Kubal (1975) obtained equivocal results in studies employing exposure to random positive reinforcement as the debilitating stimulus, Thornton and Jacobs (1972) found that subjects receiving inescapable shock on a button pressing task *increased* their pre-post scores on a mental ability test whereas subjects receiving avoidable shocks or no shock remained unchanged, and Cole and Coyne (1977) found that inescapable noise produced more debilitation in subsequent anagram solving performance than escapable noise only when performance was evaluated in the original noise exposure setting vs. a new setting. But positive findings were obtained by Thornton and Jacobs (1971), Gachtel, Paulus, and Maples (1975), and Hiroto and Seligman (1975). Thornton and Jacobs found that subjects who received unavoidable shock subsequently did more poorly on a different shock avoidance task than subjects who had received avoidable shock. In studies in which pretreatment with inescapable aversive tones served as the stressor, Gachtel et al. found that such exposure resulted in greatly debilitated subsequent performance on an anagram task relative to a group pretreated with escapable aversive tones, and Hiroto and Seligman found that this stressor as well as exposure to insoluble discrimination problems resulted in subsequent diminished ability to escape in a shuttle box task and to solve anagrams.

One might argue that though these studies with humans have the advantage of controlled experimental manipulations and objective assessment of outcomes while minimizing potentially relevant extraneous influences, the findings do not bear significantly on the quesiton of the role of "crisis" resolution on later functioning. Obviously random positive reinforcement or even exposure to aversive noise or unavoidable shock in a contrived situation from which the subject can exit at any moment do not produce cognitive, emotional, and physical dysfunction comparable to that wrought by an uncontrollable aversive life event. Yet three of the five studies employing clearly aversive stimuli (noise or shock) produced positive results, and the findings with animals are incontrovertible. In addition, ample data exist (reviewed above) that experience with uncontrollable events is debilitating and affects functioning in all types of situations, sometimes for extended periods. The questions that need answering at this point are: *How* do we learn from positive experience? *How* does successful coping in stress situations affect future coping ability? Is there a buildup in generalized ego strength that produces a more competent individual capable of coping with a wider and wider range of situations, or is it simply a function of learning specific instrumental responses via trial and error which may then be applied to new situations? How important are the nature of the causal attributions one makes to himself regarding why he was able to manipulate a situation; that is, does success in dealing with stress automatically breed more and more success in such situations or are there significant moderator variables to be considered?

Observational data suggest that the relationship between success in dealing with crises and future ability in similar situations is complex and dependent on how an event was coped with, how the individual construed the way he coped with it to himself (i.e., the causal attributions he made regarding the reason for his success or failure), and whether coping behaviors used successfully in a given stress situation were appropriately generalized to a new situation.

Findings with Nazi concentration camp victims best exemplify the role of some of these variables. If the relationship between successful coping with stress and future ability to deal with stress were simple and linear, then for those few who survived the extreme stress of the camps the comparatively milder stresses of everyday life should have been a "piece of cake." In fact, as noted above, the majority were greatly debilitated and continued to be so for extended periods. Most of the survivors, rather than attributing their success to superior ability to manipulate the environment, acknowledged the primary role of sheer chance (Benner et al., 1980). Thus what likely generalized was an "external" orientation rather than the more generally adaptive attitude that one is able to influence important outcomes through action. In addition, many survivors experienced severe debilitating guilt over compromises made to ensure their survival or the very fact of their survival while so many perished (Chodoff, 1975) rather than the heightened self-esteem we associate with triumph over a great obstacle.

The greater the extent to which a stressor is unusual and places atypical coping demands on an individual, the more likely are the coping mechanisms that were used and reinforced to be ineffective in other stress situations. This applies to both cognitive and instrumental coping mechanisms. Camp inmates used cognitive mechanisms such as depersonalization and intense vigilance adaptively in the camps but often were unable to give up these defenses outside that setting where they were no longer appropriate. Also, instrumental behaviors such as those pertaining to food getting and suppression of hunger cues, which were important for survival in the camps were inappropriately generalized to the postcamp environment (Benner et al., 1980). There is also evidence from laboratory and naturalistic studies with humans that coping strategies learned under more moderate and circumscribed stress situations (crowding, forced social interaction, noise) may be inappropriately maintained after termination of the stressor and employed ineffectively in other situations (Cohen, 1980).

Perhaps the grossest example of the disastrous consequences of misconstruing the appropriate mode for coping with a crisis involved the European Jews in the period preceding and during the Nazi holocaust. The Jews attempted to deal with Nazi aggression intellectually through written and oral appeals and petitions. This form of response was an established tradition. Jews had survived as a unit through 2000 years of repression in this fashion while making minimal use of physical retaliation. This well-learned response persisted despite its self-defeating nature and blatant lack of success (Hilberg, 1980). It may be conjectured that Israel's current militarism represents an over-generalized response on the other end of the continuum based on its recent successful use of force to deal with crises, and that a more effective response might include more of the elements of negotiation that historically were the hallmark of the Jewish response to aggression.

In summary, both laboratory studies with animals and humans and naturalistic observations of humans undergoing severe stress generally support the notion that failure experiences under stressful circumstances inhibit subsequent ability to function under stress. When the stress is severe as in the concentration camps or a devastating natural disaster, the debilitating effects may be pervasive and temporarily extensive. The relationship between successful resolution of crises and subsequent ability to deal with stress is more complex and appears to involve cognitive factors associated with induction of a generalized sense of self-efficacy as well as the learning of specific cognitive and instrumental skills and applying them appropriately to new settings. As evidenced by the camp survivors, performance attainment alone does not enhance self-efficacy. Attainment must take place under "conditions of perceived self-determination of outcomes" (Bandura, 1977, p. 201). Conditions that have been hypothesized to foster such a perception include success with minimal effort, success at tasks perceived to be difficult and challenging, a rate and pattern of attainments that enhance a perception of progress despite momentary setbacks, and success under varied circumstances in which threats are mastered independently (Bandura, 1977). Another important factor may be unsuccessful experience or at least experiences that require some expenditure of energy and effort. An individual who has confronted only easy successes will not develop the coping responses needed for failure situations and thus might be more debilitated when suddenly confronted with situations beyond his or her control.

Successful functioning under stress clearly requires not only a generalized sense of self-efficacy but a repertoire of concrete coping skills and the ability to apply them appropriately as situations arise. This notion is applicable to crisis intervention and the psychotherapy process in general. Many psychotherapists seem to assume that learning that occurs in therapy automatically transfers to the environment at large. In fact, in the large majority of therapeutic encounters, patient improvement neither persists nor generalizes to new settings (Goldstein, Lopez, & Greenleaf, 1979). As evidenced by the data on the camp survivors, coping mechanisms (cognitive and instrumental) learned in situations whose demands are atypical will be useless or even debilitating if rigidly applied to situations with new and different demands. In terms of the treatment setting, it follows then that in order to maximize the transferability of learned coping skills clients must be helped in choosing new living or treatment settings which allow for the maximization of new learning and which will provide contexts for continued growth.

The relationship between the assumptions discussed in this section and the development of crisis intervention procedures is a complex one. In the next section, issues in the implementation and evaluation of crisis intervention procedures will be considered in the context of these broad-based assumptions, other less pervasive assumptions associated with specific stressors, and assumptions directly associated with crisis intervention.

CRISIS INTERVENTION

Crisis intervention, neither in practice nor from an evaluative standpoint, has evolved in any coherent fashion from crisis theory or its attendant assumptions. Though often referred to as if they denoted widely acknowledged techniques applied in a prescribed manner at specific points in time and with agreed upon goals and outcome criteria, the procedures that have been subsumed under crisis intervention are more varied than in any other area of psychological treatment. Virtually every system of psychotherapy or behavior change includes crisis intervention in its domain, including existentially based approaches (May, 1958), psychoanalysis (Stricker, 1978), behavior modification (Eisler & Hersen, 1973), cognitive behavior modification (Kendall et al., 1979) and client-centered approaches (McGee, 1974a). Practitioners include professionals from every mental health subspecialty as well as specially-trained paraprofessionals who may be generalists or "peers" specializing in a particular problem area or population. Treatment may take place in the traditional office setting, over the phone, in the hospital emergency room, in community-based walk-in clinics or at the site of a crisis situation with the therapist sometimes involved in the patient's everyday work or living situation.

Telephone Hotlines and Walk-In Centers

The single intervention area whose development has been most consonant with prevalent notions of crisis theory is telephone hotlines and walk-in centers. Consistent with the hypothesis that crises follow a brief time course and intervention must therefore occur as early as possible to prevent serious pathology, hotlines provide anonymity and easy access to facilitate early client contact. In addition, consistent with the growing anti-traditional therapy zeitgeist, services are provided by specially trained nonprofessionals with professionals serving only in a consultant capacity, and services may involve such nontraditional activities as provision of shelter, transportation, and other ombudsmanlike activities on behalf of clients (McGee, 1974b). However, the research literature that has emerged has contributed little to our general understanding of the crisis construct or to the development of a general crisis intervention model. This is because of the great heterogeneity of the clientele (clients range from those in extreme distress about current, past or impending problems to those who are merely seeking information or calling for others), the tenuousness of client contact, and ethical considerations which minimize opportunity to systematically vary treatment procedures and make collection of certain kinds of outcome data difficult. Research in this area has thus been primarily atheoretical or program evaluative in nature, and the substantive findings relate to the development of measures and procedures for evaluating training, the process of counseling and adequacy of volunteer information and referral activities, and overall program impact on the community (see Auerbach, 1983; Auerbach & Kilmann, 1977).

Crisis-Oriented Psychotherapy

A second broad area of crisis intervention has its roots in traditional psycho-therapy. What has come to be called "crisis-oriented psychotherapy" is carried out by professionals in the traditional dyadic setting. It is geared toward patients in acute distress whose overall premorbid adjustment has been satisfactory and whose current emotional dysphoria seems to be largely a function of response to a specific stressor as opposed to a continuing psychiatric disorder. This setting does not have the inherent research limitations of telephone counseling in that the client is physically present and treatment ordinarily takes place in a relatively controlled professional environment. Thus one should more readily be able to systematically vary aspects of the treatment procedure, obtain individual difference and situational data on clients, evaluate structural aspects of the client-therapist interaction, and obtain outcome data. Nonetheless, the research literature that has accumulated provides little useful information on the parameters of the crisis construct, or generalizable information on the effectiveness of crisis intervention procedures. Methodological problems include failure to differentiate among heterogeneous clients on the basis of the stressors precipitating the need for treatment (Auerbach & Kilmann, 1977), high level client mobility resulting in a high attrition rate which inhibits collection of follow-up data, and negative (deterioration) effects of therapy which seem to be related to the experience level of therapists (Butcher & Koss, 1978).

In summary, though rather substantial research literatures have emerged in both the hot-line and crisis-oriented psychotherapy areas, neither have contributed significantly to the development of "science" of crisis intervention. The major difficulty common to both areas is client heterogeneity and thus a lack of anchor points (i.e., fairly delineated common stressors) around which to orient delivery and evaluation of treatment procedures. This difficulty is obviated, however, if one conceptualizes crisis intervention as treatment procedures designed to minimize emotional distress and behavioral dysfunction in individuals confronting specific aversive events. This is in a sense crisis intervention in its "pure" form, in that ideally treatment may be tailored to individuals to the degree to which the needs of the situation are known and there are established patterns of reaction to the stressor.

Crisis Intervention Programs Oriented around Specific Aversive Events

Virtually every form of crisis intervention involves preparing individuals for a stressor they are about to confront or helping them recover from the effects of one that has already impacted them. Thus it is meaningful to consider categorizing intervention procedures and evaluation criteria in terms of their commonality based on the temporal relationship of the individual to the stressor. From this standpoint four distinct types of intervention procedures may be distinguished. *Type 1* "distal prestress intervention" programs are designed to deal with individuals who have not yet been exposed to a stressor, yet for whom the stressor is sufficiently aversive, a reasonably high probability event, and for which it is thus reasonable to institute procedures that will minimize its likelihood of occurring or causing damage if it does occur. *Type 2* or "proximal prestress interventions" involve situations in which the crisis-inducing stressor has impacted the individual psychologically but is not yet a physical reality. The individual knows he is about to be confronted with a stressful event (e.g., surgery, natural disaster) but there is a period of waiting between knowledge of occurence and actual impact. Thus there is opportunity to intervene during the preimpact period and institute programmed treatment packages. *Type 3* or "proximal poststress interventions" involve situations in which the stressor has recently impacted the individual and he is attempting to adjust to the short-term effects of exposure. Finally, *Type 4* or "distal poststress interventions" occur with individuals who are having adjustment problems that are clearly associated with exposure to a stressor from which they have been divorced for an extended time period.*

This suggested formulation is roughly similar to the primary, secondary, tertiary prevention model used in public health and subsequently adopted by mental health practitioners (Caplan, 1964) but it is not oriented around the notion of decreasing vulnerability to or limiting damage associated with mental disease. Rather than starting with the fact of a disease (e.g., schizophrenia) or a major social problem (e.g., racism), making assumptions about its etiology and looking for ways to prevent it or reduce its incidence in the community, emphasis instead is on pinpointing specific stressors and isolating intervention procedures effective in limiting emotional distress and behavioral dysfunction associated with exposure to those stressors. As exemplified below, by taking a temporal perspective, similarities in procedures, goals, and outcome criteria can be identified so that a general model of crisis intervention, applicable across stressors, can begin to be developed.

Type 1 Interventions

Type 1 interventions involve prevention of possible misfortune and target individuals who do not currently perceive themselves to be in imminent danger, and who are thus not emotionally aroused. One of the tasks in Type 1 programming is therefore arousal of optimal fear levels to stimulate acceptance of communications and motivate preventive behaviors. Studies involving fear communications pertaining to dental hygiene practices, precautions to avert cancer, and the deleterious effects of smoking indicate that appeals producing low to intermediate levels of arousal most effectively stimulate optimal levels of preventive behavior; communications resulting in very high fear levels are less effective in producing acceptance of recommendations and seem to motivate minimization or denial of the importance of threats (Janis, 1969). In this regard, the current saturation of the public with fear arousing warning materials about potential crises (nuclear war, cancer, economic disruption), unmoderated by fear reducing reassurances, may be inhibiting receptivity to such input and diminishing the probability of individuals engaging in precautionary behavior.

The best motivator of preventive behavior may be previous experience with a given stressor, together with the conviction that it is manageable, and the knowledge that its recurrence is reasonably probable. This is best exemplified by the

---

*A fifth type of intervention, involving individuals who are currently being impacted by a crisis-inducing stimulus, may be identified. This area, which involves crisis intervention in the most literal sense, has, paradoxically, generated little research. It has been attended to most closely in the law enforcement fields where there is great concern with developing techniques to help police defuse hostage crises (Maher, 1977) and manage domestic disputes (Bard & Berkowitz, 1967; Driscoll, Meyer, & Schanie, 1973).

development of "disaster subcultures" where Type 1 programming is motivated by repetitive experience with natural hazards (e.g., floods, tornadoes, earthquakes). In such communities, since avoidance of the stressor is not possible, preparation is geared toward training individuals to take on specific roles and organizations to adopt specific functions in order to minimize the potential negative physical and psychological impact of the stressor (cf. Columbia Area Mental Health Center, 1974).

With some stressors, programs may be implemented that make the event less likely to occur. For example, if one assumes that the occurrence of sexually assaultive behavior is fostered by attitudes in our culture that encourage or justify rape (e.g., "women want to be raped," "only bad girls get raped"), then it is meaningful to implement programs targeted at potential offenders designed to change such attitudes (cf. Burt, 1966-1967). Similarly, intervention programs with chronic rapists geared toward diminishing their sexual arousal to rape-related stimuli and enhancing heterosexual arousal and heterosocial skills (Abel, Blanchard, & Becker, 1976) would also be expected to diminish rape incidence. From another standpoint, education programs geared toward potential victims, covering situations in which sexual attacks are likely to occur, myths and realities regarding behavior of sexual offenders, etc., would be hypothesized to stimulate appropriate avoidance behaviors and thus lower rape incidence among those exposed to the program; programs which teach instrumental behaviors effective in warding off attacks should similarly lower incidence of assaults or at least diminish their severity and therefore their physical and psychological impact.

Thus, cognitive changes, attitudinal changes, instrumental skill changes, self-reports of intent to engage in preventive behaviors, measures of actual preventive behaviors engaged in, or longer term follow-up measures of the degree to which individuals exposed to a program confronted the relevant stressor or experienced negative consequences if they did encounter it, are meaningful outcome criteria for Type 1 programs. Program effectiveness may be unambiguously evaluated, however, only if the research design is targeted toward specific relevant groups (e.g., individuals with a history of sexual assault; individuals who have been sexually assaulted or who reside in an area with a high incidence of sexual assault), and outcome is evaluated for the targeted group versus a matched control group not exposed to the program. Assessment of program impact becomes problematic if one attempts to infer that simple presence of an intervention program in a community has resulted in the lowering of the incidence of a given crisis event (e.g., sexual assault) in that community. This is best exemplified by research which has attempted to demonstrate that the presence of suicide prevention centers in particular communities results in lowering of suicide rates in those communities (Bagley, 1968; Lester, 1974; Walk, 1967; Weiner, 1969). In the best-controlled study Bagley found that in towns having Samaritan suicide prevention services average suicide rates declined from the pre-Samaritan to post-Samaritan years, whereas the average rate in a group of "ecologically similar" matched control towns having no suicide prevention services increased dramatically over the same period of time; he concluded that these differential changes in suicide rate were the result of the presence or absence of suicide prevention services in the respective sets of towns. His findings were not conclusive, however, since despite careful matching of experimental and control towns, reduction in suicide rate could as readily have been a function of those social changes in the community that prompted development of a Samaritan service as of the impact of the service itself. Consistent with this interpretation, Jennings, Barraclough and Moss (1978), using more recent suicide rate data than Bagley and more precisely matching experimental and control towns, found that despite continued growth in the number of Samaritan branches and a large increase in number of clients there were no significant pre-post differences in percentage change in suicide rate for the two sets of towns using any of four matching methods. Initially, when the Samaritans were new it is likely that only the most socially progressive towns developed branches, but as the organization became well established branches were established routinely and thus probably on a much less selective basis.

Type 2 Interventions

Type 2 interventions target emotionally aroused individuals who are exposed to crisis situations that are clearly imminent (e.g., natural disaster, surgery) and who have a limited period to prepare for the impact of the event. Two types of Type 2 situations are distinguishable: (a) those where the stressor may be avoided or its physical impact minimized if appropriate actions are taken, and (b) those where the stressor is unavoidable or where the individual has committed himself to confronting the stressor.

In avoidable situations, such as natural disasters or international crises, the individual has some time-limited opportunity to analyze warning cues and make decisions regarding the likelihood of a threatening event occurring and the effectiveness and potential cost of available coping measures, and to engage in instrumental behaviors designed to avoid or minimize the impact of the stressor. The factors influencing adaptive decision making in such situations are multiple and complex (cf. Janis & Mann, 1977). A persistent problem is a tendency for people to interpret warning cues in "normal" terms. For example, Fritz and Marks (1954) found that among those exposed to an Arkansas tornado who noted a roaring sound prior to actual impact less than one-third appraised it as implying a seriously threatening event, and many interpreted it as indicating a passing train. This situation is further complicated by the fact that many people become immune to warning signs such as tornado watches because they occur so frequently in particular areas without being followed by strikes, which is the result of inadequate technical capabilities of warning systems for several types of rapid onset of natural hazards including earthquakes and avalanches as well as tornadoes (White & Haas, 1975). Given that accurate warning information is available, there is still the question of how to transmit such information (in terms of mode of delivery, source, and message content) in order to maximize the probability that it will be acted on effectively. For example, in a study of responses to warnings about an impending flood, Drabek and Stephenson (1971) found that the source of the warning (from authorities but not from press or mass media) significantly influenced individual's perceptions of whether or not to take definitive evasive action (evacuation).

Information transmission is also an important technique with individuals about to confront unavoidable stressors. But its role, rather than imparting data to be acted on, is to induce a cognitive set which will in turn moderate dysphoric emotions and enhance subsequent adjustment to the stressor. This category includes preparation for such crisis events as the impending death of a spouse, an impending premature birth, or impending divorce proceedings. But the bulk of the systematic research has involved preparation of individuals for discrete medically related stressors such as surgery. Early studies in this area (e.g., Aiken & Henrichs, 1971; Field, 1974) attempted to enhance patient adjustment by directly minimizing anticipatory fear levels using techniques such as relaxation and hypnosis (with mixed results). More recently, the focus has been on inducing a sense of control and predictability in patients using pre-stress information packages or other cognitive-behavioral techniques such as reinforcement of coping imagery and coping self-statements.

Several important substantive findings have emerged from this literature which should be generalizable beyond the health care situation. First, individuals who are exposed during the anticipatory period to specific preparatory information or other coping strategies tend to respond more favorably than those who are given general, marginally relevant information or no special preparation (Auerbach, Martelli, & Mercuri, 1983; Johnson & Leventhal, 1974; Kendall et al., 1979; Langer, Janis, & Wolfer, 1975). Second, the nature of the interaction between information giver or health care provider and patient is important in affecting outcome. Patients who perceive providers as dominant and hostile during the prestress period tend to adjust more poorly while under stress than those who perceive the provider as friendly and cooperative (Auerbach et al., 1983). Third, mode of prestress intervention may be matched with particular patient types based on self-report measures of dispositional coping style (Goldstein, 1973; Shipley, Butt, & Horowitz, 1979; Shipley, Butt, Horowitz, & Farbry, 1978), locus of control orientation (Auerbach, Kendall, Cuttler, & Levitt, 1976; Pickett & Clum, 1982) and situation-specific measures of preference for information about impending health-related stressors (Auerbach et al., 1983) to maximize patient adjustment to the stressor. In addition, there are preliminary data suggesting it may be productive to reinforce particular modes of coping as a function of the nature of the stressor. Interventions geared at stimulating emotion-focused modes of coping (e.g., minimizing threat, seeking emotional support) may be more effective in influencing outcome in catastrophic situations involving low probability of manipulation (e.g., the Three Mile Island nuclear reactor disaster) or little hope for return to normality (e.g., disfiguring surgery, the dying patient) whereas problem-focused interventions geared at inducing a sense of cognitive control may be more effective in situations involving transitory stressors and thus the likelihood of full return to normal functioning (Auerbach et al., 1983; Collins, Baum, & Singer, 1983; Folkins, 1970; Folkman & Lazarus, 1980; Monat, Averill, & Lazarus, 1972).

In general, Type 2 situations involving unavoidable stressors provide an excellent opportunity to use experimental designs and investigate the effects of different modes of intervention in conjunction with such variables as individual differences in coping style and the nature of the stressor (along some relevant dimension such as controllability) as they affect outcome. Individual difference data may be obtained at a low stress period prior to instituting interventions, and assuming that one is assiduous in matching treatment and control groups, in eliminating confounds due to multiple component treatment packages (a problem with some surgical intervention studies; Auerbach & Kilmann, 1977), and in selecting outcome measures that are meaningfully related to the goals of treatment, there are no major stumbling blocks in setting up and evaluating such programs.

Type 3 Interventions

Type 3 programs provide interventions to individuals who have recently been impacted by a crisis situation. A number of investigations that fall in this category have been reported in the literature, including such diverse programs as studies of the effects of giving recovering heart attack patients different degrees of post-operative control over and participation in their own care (Cromwell, Butterfield, Brayfield, & Curry, 1977), of the effectiveness of imaginal flooding with a Vietnam veteran exhibiting posttraumatic stress disorder symptoms (Keane & Kaloupek, 1982), of nurses' effectiveness in delivering grief intervention to parents losing a baby because of Sudden Infant Death Syndrome (Lowman, 1979), comparing the differential effectiveness of behavioral techniques and individual peer counseling with recent rape victims (Kilpatrick & Veronen, 1977–1979), and descriptions of the use of desensitization (Church, 1974) and group counseling with natural disaster victims, and supportive intervention with family survivors of sudden death situations (Williams, Lee, & Polak, 1976), bereaved widows (Raphael, 1978), and children following a terrorist attack (Klingman & Ben-Eli, 1981). However, nothing close to a systematic body of research has emerged that would allow one to pinpoint useful Type 3 intervention techniques and target common outcome variables. This is because, in contrast to the immediate prestress situation, in which the salient emotional and cognitive states (anticipatory fear, perception of loss of control) are apparent, the immediate poststress situation is open-ended and its psychological parameters have not been determined. As noted above in the section on *Crisis Theory*, the duration and ultimate severity of emotional distress experienced in response to exposure to crisis-level stressors, though they seem to be linearly related to the aversiveness of the stressor, are not well established and are likely influenced by a number of moderator variables. Also unanswered is the question of the length of the interval between exposure to stress and the onset of emotional disturbance. It is widely accepted among clinicians ["traumatic stress disorder-delayed" (Diagnostic and Statistical Manual of Mental Disorders, 1980, p. 238)] that many victims such as combat veterans (Figley, 1978), repatriated prisoners of war (Figley & Sprenkle, 1978), and concentration camp survivors (Chodoff, 1963), after exposure to stress, experience a "latency period" of undefined length during which they seem to be coping adequately which is then followed by overt signs of emotional disturbance which purportedly stem from the previous contact with the stressor. One investigator claims, on the basis of "2000 case histories," that such time lags in stress reactions inevitably occur at multiples of the 12.4 hr. circadian half-wave (Bulkley, 1977; 1978), but there is no body of systematic research establishing the existence or parameters of a delayed stress response. From a qualitative standpoint, the nature of emotional responses to crisis-level events has also not been established. Many different models have been proposed asserting that particular response stages inevitably follow in sequential fashion after exposure to particular stressors. Some models suggest that the prescribed stages must be experienced in order to ultimately achieve a satisfactory level of adjustment. But Silver and Wortman (1980), in a comprehensive and well-documented review, conclude that there is "no body of methodologically sophisticated research that has systematically assessed changes in emotional reactions over time and reported the existence of stages" (p. 304).

Obviously, to the degree to which maladaptive stress reactions are predictable in terms of their latency, duration, and qualitative nature, appropriate intervention procedures may be targeted at particular points in time after exposure to a stressor. In contrast to models positing response latencies or complex stages, the classic "crisis theory" approach simply assumes that reactions to crises are of limited duration (four to six weeks), that individuals who have just been impacted are extremely anxious, their defenses are down, and therefore intervention must begin as soon as possible to be maximally effective (Bloom, 1977; Parad & Parad, 1968). This assumption is partially supported by findings that patients who are high in anxiety at the beginning of treatment are more likely to respond positively to psychotherapy in general (Luborsky, Chandler, Auerbach, Cohen, & Bachrach, 1971). But studies with crisis intervention clients in particular have found no relationship between outcome and timing of treatment in relation to the precipitating event (Calsyn, Pribyl, & Sunukjian, 1977; Parad & Parad, 1968). In addition, inconsistent with the assumption that crisis intervention should begin as soon as possible, observations of humans exposed to real-life crises such as rape (Thomas, 1977), natural disaster (Wallace, 1956), and widowhood (Blanchard, Blanchard, & Becker, 1976), suggest that for many there is an initial period of shock and relative psychological immobility that renders individuals unreceptive to any form of communication after which they gradually become more amenable to active rehabilitation attempts. Studies with dogs lend credence to this conclusion. Overmier & Seligman (1967) and Overmier (1968) found that in the initial 24 hours after exposure to a stressor the organisms, rather than being maximally receptive to input, were minimally able to learn responses necessary to extricate themselves from different stress situations. But magnitude of debilitation disappeared rapidly over time, leaving an apparently "normal" animal after 48 hours and 72 hours, respectively.

Such findings suggest that in the early stress impact period it may be more prudent to focus interventions on minimization of subjective distress and only gradually phase in more intensive, integrative approaches. Other observational data suggest that interveners might most productively invest their efforts in the initial poststress period with significant others or those on the periphery, rather than directly with victims. For example, husbands and boyfriends often react to a woman's rape maladaptively by either blaming the woman or by becoming enraged at the assailant, and thus they must be counseled to be supportive rather than overprotective of or reproachful toward the victim (Thomas, 1977). In bereavement situations, there is a tendency among family members not to discuss the death in order to protect each other, whereas a more functional approach would be to promote intrafamily support and sharing of grief in order to minimize the burden of the widowed individual (Kleiman, 1977). In the immediate aftermath of natural disasters, resources are used most effectively to reinforce the emergence of leaders who model altruistic and cooperative behaviors and thus draw community consensus away from counterproductive tendencies toward ascribing blame and scapegoating. Such indirect community-based intervention efforts have proved more useful than aggressive outreach programs by mental health workers geared directly toward disaster victims (Barton, 1969; Taylor et al., 1976).

Type 4 Interventions

Type 4 programs provide interventions to individuals who are experiencing long-term adjustment problems which are clearly traceable to exposure to a crisis-level stressor. The need for this form of intervention is based on the fact that many individuals experience extended periods of emotional distress after exposure to traumatic stressors, and even after dysphoric emotions have seemingly stabilized and gross indicants of behavioral dysfunction have diminished there is evidence that they "continually re-experience the crisis for the rest of their lives" (Silver & Wortman, 1980, p. 308).

Normative data are beginning to be collected on the duration of poststressor emotional responses for some crisis events (e.g., rape) but this is complicated by the influence of individual difference and situational moderators, and thus the dividing line between the end of the short-term response and the beginning of the longer-term readjustment phase is admittedly a gray one. However, though there is great variability in the pattern of short-term emotional responses, even within given stressors (Silver & Wortman, 1980), there seems to be more regularity and a confluence of needs after emotionality has stabilized. These needs seem to primarily involve learning instrumental skills and cognitive changes. The former area is most applicable to individuals for whom the stress experience has radically changed life demands, such as widows who depended on their husbands to manage financial matters, repairs, etc. and who in addition to these readjustments must also learn to relate socially as a single woman without a husband (Glick, Weiss, & Parkes, 1974).

The area of cognitive changes is more complex and seems to primarily involve (a) a need to conceptualize the experience and one's reaction to it as normal and rational and (b) reinstatement of the belief that one is generally in control of one's environment rather than subject to the whims of circumstance. The notion that a sense of normality might best be reestablished through the use of "peer" counselors who can share common reactions and experiences was pioneered by Silverman (1969) in her work with widows. Peers serve as a source of social support and appear to be effective in enhancing skill acquisition and in exemplifying successful recovery and return to normal functioning. However, though the use of peers is commonly accepted as a useful technique, its value has not been established empirically, nor have the circumstances under which or the outcomes for which peers might be particularly effective as compared with nonpeer interveners been explored.

Regarding the need for a sense of control, anecdotal evidence suggests that for many this may be achieved through involvement in rebuilding activities which might be construed as meaningful and contributory to a belief that there is morality in the world. In this way, parents whose children have died of leukemia seem to have benefitted from a "survivor mission" of supporting research that might prevent such tragedies in the future, antiwar Vietnam veterans "found their mission" in telling about the war (Lifton & Olson, 1976), and concentration camp survivors who "had lost all relation to life" and become completely isolated (Eitinger, 1980) emigrated to Israel and found a dynamic community to build on and seemed to find meaning and a sense of control. Unfortunately, though interventions based on such activities appear compelling there are no reports of research implementing and evaluating such programs.

Conclusions

Current thinking on crisis intervention is dominated by a medical model of prevention of psychopathology borrowed from public health, which assumes that exposure to a crisis-level stressor initiates a chain of responses that will eventuate in a disease process if not short-circuited at an early stage. The relevance of this model to schizophrenia and other psychiatric conditions is debatable. Its relevance to stress responses is at best unclear given that, except in extreme catastrophic situations, there is little evidence that exposure to aversive events eventuates in psychiatric symptomatology. Thus there is no more compelling rationale for conceptualizing crisis intervention under the prevention umbrella than other forms of psychotherapy or behavior change. But, whereas in psychotherapy research broad-based multiform outcome measures are rejected in favor of those specifically relevant to the treatments used (Bergin, 1971), the prevention model implicitly recognizes only one class of dependent variables—namely those associated with prevention of illness (e.g., incidence of psychiatric illness, length of hospitalization). Because there has been little evidence that crisis intervention programs reduce incidence of psychiatric illness or hospitalization the prevalent belief among clinicians, despite considerable outcome research on crisis intervention hotlines and crisis-oriented psychotherapy (Auerbach & Kilmann, 1977; Butcher & Koss, 1978) and an upsurge of studies associated with specific aversive events, is that there has been virtually no systematic research (Korchin, 1976) that has "tested the efficiency of crisis intervention as a technique or the ability of prevention programs to prevent" (Williams & Polak, 1979, p. 35).

Crisis intervention has not evolved as a coherent system based on clinical crisis theory or the associated prevention model. Procedures are often labeled as "crisis intervention" without any underlying theoretical conceptualization or rationale. The model outlined herein does not present a new theory. It is a research model specifying intervention procedures appropriate at different temporal stages in relation to the stressor, and outcome variables logically related to these procedures and to treatment goals at each stage. Clearly, much additional research is needed to fully answer questions about the effectiveness of crisis intervention procedures. Very little research has been reported assessing the effectiveness of Type 1 programming. A substantive research literature is beginning to emerge on the role of Type 2 interventions in effecting changes in behavioral measures of coping and poststress adjustment. But lack of basic information on the quantitative (latency and duration of response) and qualitative (patterns of response) nature of short-term poststress reactions has inhibited systematic Type 3 research. In particular, regarding Type 2 and Type 3 research, problems arise when signs of emotional distress are construed as indicants of poor poststress adjustment. There are insufficient data on what constitutes the normative pattern of emotional response to given stressors, and contrary to the assumption of many researchers, there are data indicating that under some circumstances emotional dysphoria may play a positive role in motivating individuals to engage in coping behaviors and thus can be an indicant of good adjustment (Silver & Wortman, 1980). In general, the role of emotional status in influencing outcome across the temporal spectrum needs further investigation. In prestress situations it has been theorized (Janis, 1958; 1969) that intermediate levels of arousal facilitate adaptation to stress, but the weight of recent evidence indicates an inverse linear relationship between prestress arousal level and poststress adjustment (Auerbach et al., 1983). Type 4 situations are conceived of as periods of relative emotional stability, but for many survivors of catastrophic stressors resolution of guilt feelings over having survived (which are sometimes reinforced by others—"second victimization:" Symonds, 1980) may be essential for long-term adjustment. For others, the readjustment process is integrally entwined with "learning to feel" again after extensive use of "psychic numbing" as a survival mechanism (Lifton, 1980). In general, though there seems to be great current interest in enhancing the long-term adjustment of widows, victims of crime, medically related disabilities, and catastrophic events such as the Holocaust and the Hiroshima A-bomb, Type 4 interventions have received virtually no systematic evaluation.

SUMMARY AND CONCLUSIONS

"Crisis theory" reifies crisis as a dynamic entity, induced by undefined levels of situational stress, which generates an inferred response state (emotional disequilibrium) that is independent of observable behavior. It is referred to as if it represents a state with special properties, but at present there is no compelling evidence that it is meaningful to differentiate crisis from high-level stress, anxiety, fear or other related constructs. Assumptions about the purported uniform effects of exposure to crisis-inducing events persist because of the lack of an integrated, testable theoretical model and validated operational measures of the crisis construct. In positing that exposure to crises exerts uniform effects on behavior, traditional crisis theory takes an extreme situationist view that paradoxically parallels the unidimensional approach of radical personality trait theory. In both quarters, behavioral uniformities are causally attributed to a single class of variables and insufficient attention is paid to the influence of interacting, moderating variables.

It is generally accepted that reactions to crises follow a uniform delimited (four to six weeks) time course, that successfully dealing with crises invariable results in an individual more capable of dealing with future stresses, and it is implicitly assumed that in the absence of preventive intervention exposure to extreme stress eventuates in behavioral dysfunction of "mental illness" proportions. But available data are largely at variance with these assumptions. Rather than following a regular time course or invariably resulting in high levels of disturbance, duration and severity of response to stressful events in humans is related in roughly linear fashion to the aversiveness of the stressor. Individual appraisals of stressfulness and ability to cope with given stressors is in turn influenced by predispositional differences (which may be culturally conditioned), and a range of situational moderator variables including perceived social supports, material resources, and covarying major stressors and chronic background stressors (Baum, Singer, & Baum, 1981).

Previous experience with uncontrollable aversive events adversely affects future ability to function effectively in both similar and dissimilar stress situations. But rather than resulting in a blanket strengthening in coping ability, the effect of successful coping on future ability to deal with stress is a function of the degree to which performance attainment has induced a generalized sense of self-efficacy, as well as the degree to which learned cognitive and/or instrumental coping skills are appropriately generalized to new settings.

The prevention of psychopathology model is viewed as inappropriate as applied to crisis intervention. The proposed psychological model shifts the focus from modification of a hypothetical disease state to observable behaviors. Thus, meaningless conjecture as to whether crisis intervention is "really" a form of primary or secondary prevention is obviated. The greatest obstacle at present to evaluating crisis intervention research is the lack of normative data on the parameters of the stress response during the short-term poststress period (within and across major classes of stressors). Under what circumstances and to what extent is there a latency period between stress exposure and onset of debilitating stress effects? To what degree are there predictable patterns of emotional response during the poststress period and what is the relationship between poststress emotionality and tangible measures of coping and adjustment? Answers to these questions will help guide selection and timing of poststress intervention procedures, and also provide a baseline against which to evaluate the impact of pre- and poststress interventions.

REFERENCES

Abel, G. G., Blanchard, E. B., & Becker, J. V. (1976). An integrated treatment program for rapists. In R. Rada (Ed.), *Clinical aspects of the rapist.* New York: Grune & Stratton.

Aguilera, D. C., & Messick, J. M. (1978). *Crisis intervention: Theory and methodology.* St. Louis: Mosby.

Aiken, L. H., & Henrichs, T. F. (1971). Systematic relaxation as a nursing intervention technique with open heart surgery patients. *Nursing Research, 20,* 212-217.

American Psychiatric Association. (1980). *Diagnostic and statistical manual of mental disorders* (3rd ed.). (DSM-III). Washington, DC: Author.

Andrews, G., Tennant, C., Hewson, D., & Schonell, M. (1979). The relation of social factors to physical and psychiatric illness. *American Journal of Epidemiology, 109,* 186-204.

Atkeson, B. M., Calhoun, K. S., Resick, P., & Ellis, E. M. (1982). Victims of rape: Repeated assessment of depressive symptoms. *Journal of Consulting and Clinical Psychology, 50,* 96-102.

Auerbach, S. M. (1983). Crisis intervention research: Methodological considerations and some recent findings. In L. H. Cohen, W. L. Claiborn, & G. A. Specter (Eds.), *Crisis intervention* (2nd ed.). New York: Human Sciences Press.

Auerbach, S. M. (1980). Surgery-induced stress. In R. H. Woody (Ed.), *Encyclopedia of clinical assessment.* San Francisco: Jossey-Bass.

Auerbach, S. M., Kendall, P. C., Cuttler, H. F., & Levitt, N. R. (1976). Anxiety, locus of control, type of preparatory information, and adjustment to dental surgery. *Journal of Consulting and Clinical Psychology, 44,* 808-818.

Auerbach, S. M., & Kilmann, P. R. (1977). Crisis intervention: A review of outcome research. *Psychological Bulletin, 84,* 1189-1217.

Auerbach, S. M., Martelli, M. F., & Mercuri, L. (1983). Anxiety, information, interpersonal impacts, and adjustment to a stressful health care situation. *Journal of Personality and Social Psychology, 44,* 1284-1296.

Bagley, C. (1968). The evaluation of a suicide prevention schema by an ecological method. *Social Science and Medicine, 2,* 1-14.

Baisden, B., & Quarantelli, E. L. (1981). The delivery of mental health services in community disasters: An outline of research findings. *Journal of Community Psychology, 9,* 195-203.

Baldwin, B. (1979). Crisis intervention: An overview of theory and practice. *Counseling Psychologist, 8,* 43-52.

Bandura, A. (1977). Self-efficacy: Toward a unifying theory of behavioral change. *Psychological Review, 84,* 191-215.

Bard, M., & Berkowitz, B. (1967). Training police as specialists in family crisis intervention: A community psychology action program. *Community Mental Health Journal, 3,* 315-317.

Barton, A. H. (1969). *Communities in disaster.* New York: Doubleday.

Baum, A., Singer, S. E., & Baum, C. S. (1981). Stress and the environment. *Journal of Social Issues, 37,* 4-35.

Benner, P., Roskies, E., & Lazarus, R. S. (1980). Stress and coping under extreme conditions. In J. E. Dimsdale (Ed.), *Survivors, victims, and perpetrators: Essays on the Nazi holocaust.* Washington, DC: Hemisphere.

Bergin, A. (1971). The evaluation of therapeutic outcomes. In A. E. Bergin & S. L. Garfield (Eds.), *Handbook of psychotherapy and behavior change.* New York: Wiley.

Blanchard, C. G., Blanchard, E. B., & Becker, J. V. (1976). The young widow: Depressive symptomatology throughout the grief process. *Psychiatry, 39,* 394-399.

Bloom, B. L. (1979). *Community mental health: A general introduction.* Monterey, CA: Brooks/Cole.

Bloom, B. L. (1963). Definitional aspects of the crisis concept. *Journal of Consulting Psychology, 27,* 498-502.

Bloom, B. L. (1980). Social and community interventions. *Annual Review of Psychology, 31,* 111–142.

Braud, W., Wepman, B., & Russo, D. (1969). Task and species generality of the "helplessness" phenomenon. *Psychonomic Science, 16,* 154–155.

Brookshire, K. H., Littman, R. A., & Stewart, C. (1961). Residue of shock trauma in the white rat: A three factor theory. *Psychological Monographs, 75,* (10, Whole No. 514).

Bulkley, D. H. (1978). *Circadian time-lags in stress reactions.* Paper presented at American Association for Advancement of Science Annual Meeting, Seattle, WA.

Bulkley, D. H. (1977). A 37-hour time-lag for accidental and psychosomatic responses to stress incidents? *Psychological Reports, 40,* 1022.

Burgess, A. W., & Baldwin, B. (1981). *Crisis intervention theory and practice: A clinical handbook.* Englewood Cliffs, NJ: Prentice-Hall.

Burgess, A. W., & Holstrom, L. (1974). The rape trauma syndrome. *American Journal of Psychiatry, 131,* 981–986.

Burt, M. R. (1976-1977). *Attitudes supportive of rape in American culture.* Research grant No. 1 R01 MH29023-01, National Center for Prevention and Control of Rape/National Institute of Mental Health.

Butcher, J. N., & Koss, M. P. (1978). Research on brief and crisis-oriented therapies. In S. Garfield & A. Bergin (Eds.), *Handbook of psychotherapy and behavior change: An empirical analysis.* New York: Wiley.

Calhoun, L. G., Selby, J. W., & King. H. E. (1976). *Dealing with crisis.* Englewood Cliffs, NJ: Prentice-Hall.

Calsyn, R. J., Pribyl, J. F., & Sunukjian, H. (1977). Successful outcome in crisis intervention therapy. *American Journal of Community Psychology, 5,* 111–119.

Caplan, G. (1964). *Principles of preventive psychiatry.* New York: Basic Books.

Caplan, G. (1974). *Support systems and community mental health.* New York: Behavioral Publications.

Cassel, J. (1976). The contribution of social environment to host resistance. *American Journal of Epidemiology, 104,* 107–123.

Chapman, D. W. (1962). A brief introduction to contemporary disaster research. In G. W. Baker & D. W. Chapman (Eds.), *Man and society in disaster.* New York: Basic Books.

Chodoff, P. (1963). Late effects of the concentration camp syndrome. *Archives of General Psychiatry, 8,* 323–342.

Chodoff, P. (1975). Psychiatric aspects of Nazi persecution. In S. Arieti (ed.), *American handbook of psychiatry,* Vol. VI (2nd ed.). New York: Basic Books.

Chodoff, P. (1980). Psychotherapy of the survivor. In J. E. Dimsdale (Ed.), *Survivors, victims, and perpetrators: Essays on the Nazi holocaust.* Washington, DC: Hemisphere.

Church, J. S. (1974). The Buffalo Creek disaster: Extent and range of emotional and/or behavioral problems. *Omega, 5,* 61–63.

Cobb, S. (1976). Social support as a moderator of stress. *Psychosomatic Medicine, 38,* 300–314.

Cobb, S., & Lindemann, E. (1943). Neuropsychiatric observations. *Annals of Surgery, 117,* 814–824.

Cohen, S. (1980). Aftereffects of stress on human performance and social behavior. A review of research and theory. *Psychological Bulletin, 88,* 82–108.

Cole, C. S., & Coyne, J. C. (1977). Situational specificity of learned helplessness. *Journal of Abnormal Psychology, 86,* 615–623.

Collins, D. L., Baum, A., & Singer, J.E. (1983). Coping with chronic stress at Three Mile Island: Psychological and biochemical evidence. *Health Psychology, 2,* 149–166.

Columbia Area Mental Health Center. (1974). Plan for minimizing psychiatric casualties in a disaster. *Hospital and Community Psychiatry, 25,* 665–668.

Coyne, J. C., & Lazarus, R. (1979). *The ipsative-normative framework for the longitudinal study of stress.* Paper presented at Annual Convention of the American Psychological Association, New York, NY.

Cromwell, R. L., Butterfield, E. C., Brayfield, F. M., & Curry, J. J. (1977). *Acute myocardial infarction: Reaction and recovery.* St. Louis: C. V. Mosby.

Darbonne, A. (1967). Crisis: A review of theory, practice and research. *Psychotherapy: Theory, research, and practice, 4,* 49–56.

Davidson, S. (1980). Transgenerational transmission in the families of Holocaust survivors. *International Journal of Family Psychiatry,* 95–112.

Dimsdale, J. E. (1980). The coping behavior of Nazi concentration camp survivors. In J. E. Dimsdale (Ed.), *Survivors, victims, and perpetrators: Essays on the Nazi holocaust*. Washington, DC: Hemisphere.

Dohrenwend, B. P., & Dohrenwend, B. S. (1969). *Social status and psychological disorder:* A causal inquiry. New York: Wiley.

Dor Shav, N. K. (1978). On the long range effects of concentration camp internment on Nazi victims: 25 years later. *Journal of Consulting and Clinical Psychology, 46,* 1–11.

Drabek, T. E., Key, W. H., Erickson, P. E., & Crowe, J. L. (1973). *Longitudinal impact of disaster on family functioning*. Denver, CO: University of Denver, Department of Sociology.

Drabek, T. E., & Stephenson, J. S. (1971). When disaster strikes. *Journal of Applied Social Psychology, 1,* 187–203.

Driscoll, J. M., Meyer, R. G., & Schanie, C. F. (1973). Training police in family crisis intervention. *Journal of Applied Behavioral Science, 9,* 62–82.

Eisler, R. M., & Hersen, M. (1973). Behavioral techniques in family-oriented crisis intervention. *Archives of General Psychiatry, 28,* 111–116.

Eitinger, L. (1980). The concentration camp syndrome and its late sequelae. In J. E. Dimsdale (Ed.), *Survivors, Victims, and perpetrators: Essays on the Nazi holocaust*. Washington, DC: Hemisphere.

Eitinger, L. (1963). Preliminary notes on a study of concentration camp survivors in Norway. *Israeli Annals of Psychiatry, 1,* 56–67.

Eitinger, L., & Strom, A. (1981). New investigations on the mortality and morbidity of Norwegian ex-concentration camp prisoners. *Israeli Journal of Psychiatry and Related Sciences, 18,* 173–195.

Ellis, E. M., Atkeson, B. M., & Calhoun, K. S. (1981). An assessment of long-term reaction to rape. *Journal of Abnormal Psychology, 90,* 263–266.

Epstein, H. (1979). *Children of the Holocaust*. New York: Putnam.

Erickson, K. (1976). Loss of communality at Buffalo Creek. *American Journal of Psychiatry, 133,* 302–305.

Field, P. (1974). Effects of tape-recorded hypnotic preparation for surgery. *International Journal of Clinical and Experimental Hypnosis, 22,* 54–61.

Figley, C. R. (Ed.) (1978). *Stress disorders among Viet Nam veterans*. New York: Brunner/Mazel.

Figley, C. R., & Sprenkle, D. H. (1978). Delayed stress response syndrome: Family therapy implications. *Journal of Marriage and Family Counseling, 1,* 53–60.

Folkins, C. (1970). Temporal factors and the cognitive mediators of stress reactions. *Journal of Personality and Social Psychology, 14,* 173–184.

Folkman, S., & Lazarus, R. S. (1980). An analysis of coping in a middle-aged community sample. *Journal of Health and Social Behavior, 21,* 219–239.

France, K. (1982). *Crisis intervention: A handbook of immediate person-to-person help.* Springfield, IL: Charles C Thomas.

Frederick, C. J. (1977). Current thinking about crisis or psychological intervention in United States disasters. *Mass Emergencies, 2,* 43–50.

Fried, M. (1963). Grieving for a lost home. In L. J. Duhl (Ed.), *The urban condition*. New York: Basic Books.

Fritz, C. E., & Marks, E. S. (1954). The NORC studies of human behavior in disaster. *Journal of Social Issues, 10,* 26–41.

Gachtel, R. S., Paulus, P. B., & Maples, C. W. (1975). Learned helplessness and self-reported affect. *Journal of Abnormal Psychology, 84,* 732–734.

Ganikos, M. L., Grady, K. A., & Olson, J. D. (1979). *Counseling the aged: A training syllabus for educators*. Washington, DC: American Personnel and Guidance Association.

Gleser, G. C., Green, B. L., & Winget, C. (1981). *Prolonged psychosocial effects of disaster: A study of Buffalo Creek*. NewYork: Academic Press.

Gleser, G. C., Green, B. L., & Winget, C.M. (1978). Quantifying interview data on psychic impairment of disaster survivors. *Journal of Nervous and Mental Disease, 166,* 209–216.

Glick, I. O., Weiss, R. S., & Parkes, C. M. (1974). *First year of bereavement*. New York: Wiley.

Goldstein, A., Lopez, M., & Greenleaf, D. O. (1979). Introduction. In A. Goldstein and F. Kanfer (Eds.), *Maximizing treatment gains: Transfer enhancement in psychotherapy*. New York: Academic Press.

Goldstein, M. J. (1973). Individual differences in response to stress. American *Journal of Community Psychology, 1,* 113–137.

Gore, S. (1978). The effect of social support in moderating the health consequences of unemployment. *Journal of Health and Social Behavior, 19,* 157–165.

Gronvik, O., & Lonnum, A. (1962). Neurological conditions in former concentration camp inmates. *Journal of Neuropsychiatry, 4,* 50–54.

Halpern, H. (1973). Crisis theory: A definitional study. *Community Mental Health Journal, 9,* 342–349.

Hannigan, J. A., & Kueneman, R. M. (1978). Anticipating flood emergencies: A case study of a Canadian disaster subculture. In E. L. Quarantelli (Ed.), *Disasters: Theory and research.* Beverly Hills, CA: Sage Press.

Hannum, R. D., Rosellini, R. A., & Seligman, M. E. P. (1976). Learned helplessness in the rat. *Developmental Psychology, 12,* 449–454.

Henderson, S., & Bostock, T. (1977). Coping behavior after shipwreck. *British Journal of Psychiatry, 131,* 15–20.

Hermann, C. F. (Ed.), (1972). *International crises: Insights from behavioral research.* New York: Free Press.

Hetherington, E. M. (1983, April). *Stress and coping in family transition.* Paper presented at Conference on Children's Life Crisis Events and Preventive Intervention Strategies, Virginia Commonwealth University, Richmond, VA.

Hilberg, R. (1980). The nature of the process. In J. E. Dimsdale (Ed.), *Survivors, victims, and perpetrators: Essays on the Nazi holocaust.* Washington, DC: Hemisphere.

Hiroto, D. S., & Seligman, M. E. P. (1975) Generality of learned helplessness in man. *Journal of Personality and Social Psychology, 31,* 311–327.

Holmes, T. H., & Rahe, R. H. (1967). The social readjustment rating scale. *Journal of Psychosomatic Research, 11,* 213–218.

Holohan, C., & Moos, R. (1981). Social support and psychological distress: A longitudinal analysis. *Journal of Abnormal Psychology, 90,* 365–370.

Horowitz, M. J., Wilner, N., & Alvarez, W. (1979). Impact of event scale: A measure of subjective stress. *Psychosomatic Medicine, 41,* 209–218.

Janis, I. L. (1958). *Psychological stress.* New York: Wiley.

Janis, I. L. (1969). Some implications of recent research on the dynamics of fear and stress tolerance. *Social Psychiatry, 47,* 86–100.

Janis, I. L., & Mann, L. (1977). Emergency decision making: A theoretical analysis of responses to disaster warnings. *Journal of Human Stress, 3,* 35–48.

Jennings, C., Barraclough, B. M., & Moss, J. R. (1978). Have the Samaritans lowered the suicide rate? A controlled study. *Psychological Medicine, 8,* 413–422.

Johnson, J. F., & Leventhal, H. (1974). Effects of accurate expectations and behavioral instructions on reactions during a noxious medical examination. *Journal of Personality and Social Psychology, 29,* 710–718.

Keane, T. M., & Kaloupek, D. G. (1982). Imaginal flooding in the treatment of posttraumatic stress disorder. *Journal of Consulting and Clinical Psychology, 50,* 138–140.

Kendall, P. C., Williams, L., Pechacek, T. F., Graham, L. E., Shisslak, C., & Herzoff, N. (1979). Cognitive-behavioral and patient education interventions in cardiac catheterization procedures: The Palo Alto medical psychology project. *Journal of Consulting and Clinical Psychology, 47,* 49–58.

Kilpatrick, D., & Veronen, L. (1977–1979). *Treatment of fear and anxiety in victims of rape.* Research grant No. R01 MH29602, National Center for Prevention and Control of Rape/National Institute of Mental Health.

Kilpatrick, D. G., Veronen, L. J., & Resick, P. A. (1979). The aftermath of rape: Recent empirical findings. *American Journal of Orthopsychiatry, 49,* 658–669.

Kleiman, R. (1977). The bereavement crisis: A review of the literature with implications for intervention. *Crisis Intervention, 8,* 126–145.

Klingman, A., & Ben-Eli, Z. (1981). A school community in disaster: Primary and secondary prevention in situational crisis. *Professional Psychology, 12,* 523–533.

Korchin, S. J. (1976). *Modern clinical psychology: Principles of intervention in the clinic and community.* New York: Basic Books.

Krouse, H. J., & Krouse, J. H. (1982). Cancer as crisis: The critical elements of adjustment. *Nursing Research, 31,* 96–101.

Langer, E. J., Janis, I., & Wolfer, J. (1975). Reduction of psychological stress in surgical patients. *Journal of Experimental Social Psychology, 11,* 155–165.

Langer, W. L. (1958). The next assignment. *American Historical Review, 63,* 283–304.

Laskin, D. (1982). The herpes syndrome. *New York Times Magazine,* February 21, 94–98, 108.

Lazarus, R. S., & Launier, R. (1978). Stress-related transactions between person and environment. In L. A. Pervin & M. Lewis (Eds.), *Perspectives in interactional psychology.* New York: Plenum.

Leon, G. R., Butcher, J. N., Kleinman, M., Goldberg, A., & Almagor, M. (1981). Survivors of the Holocaust and their children: Current status and adjustment. *Journal of Personality and Social Psychology, 41,* 503–516.

Leopold, R., & Dillon, H. (1963). Psycho-anatomy of a disaster: A long-term study of post-traumatic neuroses in survivors of a marine explosion. *American Journal of Psychiatry, 119,* 913–921.

Lester, D. (1974). Effect of suicide prevention centers on suicide rates in the United States. *Public Health Reports, 89,* 37–39.

Levinson, D. J. (1977). The mid-life transition: A period in adult psychosocial development. *Psychiatry, 40,* 99–112.

Lewis, M. S. (1982). Topological relationships among crisis variables. *Psychotherapy: Theory, Research, and Practice, 19,* 289–296.

Lewis, M. S., Gottesman, D., & Gutstein, S. (1979). The course and duration of crisis. *Journal of Consulting and Clinical Psychology, 47,* 128–134.

Liddell, H. S. (1953). A comparative approach to the dynamics of experimental neurosis. *Annals of the New York Academy of Sciences, 56,* 164–170.

Lieberman, M. A., & Borman, L. D. (Eds.) (1979). *Self-help groups for coping with crisis.* San Francisco: Jossey-Bass.

Lifton, R. J. (1980). The concept of the survivor. In J. E. Dimsdale (Ed.), *Survivors, victims, and perpetrators: Essays on the Nazi holocaust.* Washington, DC: Hemisphere.

Lifton, R. J., & Olson, E. (1976). Human meaning of total disaster. *Psychiatry, 39,* 1–18.

Lindemann, E. (1944). Symptomatology and the management of acute grief. *American Journal of Psychiatry, 101,* 141–148.

Lowman, J. (1979). Grief intervention and sudden infant death syndrome. *American Journal of Community Psychology, 7,* 665–677.

Luborsky, L., Chandler, M., Auerbach, A. H., Cohen, S., & Bachrach, H. M. (1971). Factors influencing the outcome of psychotherapy: A review of quantitative research. *Psychological Bulletin, 75,* 145–185.

Maguire, G. P., Lee, E. G., Bevington, D. J., Kuchemann, C. S., Crabtree, R. J., & Cornell, C. E. (1978). Psychiatric problems in the first year after mastectomy. *British Medical Journal, 1,* 963–965.

Maher, G. F. (1977). *Hostage: A police approach to a contemporary crisis.* Springfield, IL: Charles C Thomas.

Maier, N. R. F. (1956). Frustration theory: Restatement and extension. *Psychological Review, 63,* 370–388.

Maier, S. F., & Seligman, M. E. P. (1976). Learned helplessness: Theory and evidence. *Journal of Experimental Psychology: General, 105,* 3–46.

May, R. (1958). The origins and significance of the existential movement in psychology. In R. May (Ed.), *Existence.* New York: Simon & Schuster.

McGee, R. K. (Ed.). (1974a). *An evaluation of the volunteer in suicide prevention* (Final Project Report, Research Grant MH-16861, National Institute of Mental Health). Gainesville: University of Florida, Department of Clinical Psychology, Center for Crisis Intervention Research.

McGee, R. K. (1974b). *Crisis intervention in the community.* Baltimore: University Park Press.

Mellstrom, M., Cicala, G. A., & Zuckerman, M. (1976). General versus specific trait anxiety measures in the prediction of fear of snakes, heights, and darkness. *Journal of Consulting and Clinical Psychology, 44,* 83–91.

Miller, W. R., Rosellini, R. A., & Seligman, M. E. P. (1977). Learned helplessness and depression. In J. D. Maser and M. E. P. Seligman (Eds.), *Psychopathology: Experimental models.* San Francisco: Freeman.

Mischel, W. (1968). *Personality and assessment.* New York: Wiley.

Mischel, W. (1973). Toward a cognitive social learning reconceptualization of personality. *Psychological Review, 80,* 252–283.

Monat, A., Averill, J. R., & Lazarus, R. S. (1972). Anticipatory stress and coping reactions under various conditions of uncertainty. *Journal of Personality and Social Psychology, 24,* 237–253.

Moore, H. E. (1964). *And the winds blew*. Austin: The Hogg Foundation for Mental Health.

Moore, H. E., & Friedsam, H. J. (1959). Reported emotional stress following a disaster. *Social Forces, 38,* 135–139.

Morris, T., Greer, H. S., & White, P. (1977). Psychological and social adjustment to mastectomy: A two-year follow-up study. *Cancer, 40,* 2381–2387.

Neugarten, B. L. (1976). Adaptation and the life cycle. *Counseling Psychologist, 6,* 16–20.

Niederland, W. G. (1968). Clinical observations on the survivor syndrome. *International Journal of Psychoanalysis, 49,* 313–315.

Overmier, J. B. (1968). Interference with avoidance behavior: Failure to avoid traumatic shock. *Journal of Experimental Psychology, 78,* 340–343.

Overmier, J. B., & Seligman, M. E. P. (1967). Effects of inescapable shock upon subsequent escape and avoidance responding. *Journal of Comparative and Physiological Psychology, 63,* 28–33.

Parad, L. G., & Parad, H. (1968). A study of crisis-oriented planned short-term treatment: Part II. *Social Casework, 49,* 418–426.

Penick, E. C., Powell, B. J., & Sieck, W. A. (1976). Mental health problems and natural disaster: Tornado victims. *Journal of Community Psychology, 4,* 64–67.

Perry, R. W., & Lindell, M. K. (1978). The psychological consequences of natural disaster: A review of research on American communities. *Mass Emergencies, 3,* 105–115.

Pickett, C., & Clum, G. A. (1982). Comparative treatment strategies and their interaction with locus of control. *Journal of Consulting and Clinical Psychology, 50,* 439–441.

Popovic, M., & Petrovic, D. (1964). After the earthquake. *Lancet, 2,* 1169.

Price, R. H., Bader, B. C., & Ketterer, R. F. (1980). Prevention in community mental health: The state of the art. In R. H. Price, R. F. Ketterer, B. C. Bader, and J. Monahan (Eds.), *Prevention in mental health: Research, policy, and practice.* Beverly Hills, CA: Sage Publications.

Puryear, D. A. (1979). *Helping people in crisis*. San Francisco: Jossey-Bass.

Quarantelli, E. L., Dynes, R. R. (1977). Response to social crisis and disaster. *Annual Review of Sociology, 49,* 3–23.

Rabkin, J. G., & Struening, E. L. (1976). Life events, stress, and illness. *Science, 194,* 1013–1020.

Raphael, B. (1978). Mourning and the prevention of melancholia. *British Journal of Medical Psychology, 51,* 303–310.

Ray, C. (1978). Adjustment to mastectomy. The psychological impact of disfigurement. In P. C. Brand & P. A. van Keep (Eds.), *Breast cancer: Psychosocial aspects of early detection and treatment.* Baltimore: University Park Press.

Resick, P., Calhoun, K. S., Atkeson, B. M., & Ellis, E. M. (1981). Social adjustment in victims of sexual assault. *Journal of Consulting and Clinical Psychology, 49,* 705–712.

Roth, S., & Bootzin, R. R. (1974). Effects of experimentally induced expectancies of external control: An investigation of learned helplessness. *Journal of Personality and Social Psychology, 29,* 253.

Roth, S., & Kubal, L. (1975). Effects of noncontingent reinforcement on tasks of differing importance: Facilitation and learned helplessness. *Journal of Personality and Social Psychology, 32,* 680–691.

Rotter, J. B. (1966). General expectancies for internal versus external control of reinforcement. *Psychological Monographs: General and Applied, 80,* (1, Whole No. 609).

Ruben, H. L. (1976). *Crisis intervention*. New York: Popular Library.

Sarason, I. G., Johnson, J. H., & Siegel, J. M. (1978). Assessing the impact of life changes: Development of the Life Experiences Survey. *Journal of Consulting and Clinical Psychology, 46,* 932–946.

Schaar, K. (1980). Crisis. *APA Monitor, 11* (9+10), 14–15.

Schneider, D. M. (1957). Typhoons on Yap. *Human Organization, 16,* 10–15.

Schulberg, H. C., & Sheldon, A. (1968). The probability of crisis and strategies for preventive intervention. *Archives of General Psychiatry, 18,* 553–558.

Seligman, M. E. P., & Groves, D. P. (1970). Nontransient learned helplessness. *Psychonomic Science, 19,* 191–192.

Seligman, M. E. P., & Maier, S. F. (1967). Failure to escape traumatic shock. *Journal of Experimental Psychology, 74,* 1–9.

Seligman, M. E. P., Maier, S. F., & Geer, J. H. (1968). Alleviation of learned helplessness in the dog. *Journal of Abnormal Psychology, 73,* 256–262.

Sheatsley, P. B., & Feldman, J. (1964). The assassination of President Kennedy: Public reaction. *Public Opinion Quarterly, 28,* 189–215.

Shipley, R. H., Butt, J. H., Horowitz, B., & Farbry, J. E. (1978). Preparation for a stressful medical procedure: Effect of amount of stimulus preexposure and coping style. *Journal of Consulting and Clinical Psychology, 46,* 499-507.

Shipley, R. H., Butt, J. H., & Horowitz, E. A. (1979). Preparation to reexperience a stressful medical examination: Effects of repetitious videotape exposure and coping style. *Journal of Consulting and Clinical Psychology, 47,* 485-492.

Shontz, F. C. (1965). Reactions to crisis. *Volta Review, 67,* 364-370.

Silver, R. L., & Wortman, C. B. (1980). Coping with undesirable life events. In J. Garber & M. E. P. Seligman (Eds.), *Human helplessness.* New York: Academic Press.

Silverman, P. (1974). *Helping each other in widowhood.* New York: Health Sciences Press.

Silverman, P. (1969). The widow-to-widow program: An experiment in preventive intervention. *Mental Hygiene, 53,* 333-337.

Simons, G. (1972). *Coping with crisis.* New York: Macmillan.

Simpson-Housely, P. (1979). Locus of control, repression-sensitization and perception of earthquake hazard. Natural Hazard Research Paper No. 36, Institute of Behavioral Science, University of Colorado, Boulder, CO.

Sims, J. H., & Baumann, D. D. (1972). The tornado threat: Coping styles of north and south. *Science, 176,* 1386-1391.

Smith, R. E. (1970). Changes in locus of control as a function of life crisis resolution. *Journal of Abnormal Psychology,* 328-332.

Solkoff, N. (1981). Children of survivors of the Nazi holocaust: A critical review of the literature. *American Journal of Orthpsychiatry, 51,* 29-42.

Specter, G. A., & Claiborn, W. L. (Eds.) (1973). *Crisis intervention.* New York: Behavioral Publications.

Spielberger, C. D. (1972). Anxiety as an emotional state. In C. D. Spielberger (Ed.), *Anxiety: Current trends in theory and research.* New York: Academic Press.

Spitzer, R. L., Endicott, J., Mesnikoff, A. M., & Cohen, G. M. (1968). *Psychiatric Evaluation Form.* New York: Biometrics Research, New York State Department of Mental Hygiene.

Strentz, T. (1980). The Stockholm Syndrome: Law enforcement policy and ego defenses of the hostage. *Annals of the New York Academy of Sciences, 347,* 137-150.

Stricker, G. (1978). Therapeutic crises. In G. D. Goldman & D. S. Milman (Eds.), *Psychoanalytic psychotherapy.* Reading, MA: Addison-Wesley.

Symonds, M. (1980). Victim responses to terror. *Annals of New York Academy of Sciences, 347,* 129-136.

Szasz, T. (1966). The uses of naming and the origin of the myth of mental illness. In J. R. Braun (Ed.), *Clinical psychology in transition.* Cleveland, OH: World Publishing Company.

Taplin, J. R. (1971). Crisis theory: Critique and reformulation. *Community Mental Health Journal, 7,* 13-23.

Taylor, V. A., Ross, G. A., & Quarantelli, E. L. (1976). *Delivery of mental health services in disasters: The Xenia tornado and some implications.* Disaster Research Center, Ohio State University, Book and Monograph Series No. 11.

Thomas, R. M. (1977). The crisis of rape and implications for counseling: A review of the literature. Part I. *Crisis Intervention, 8,* 105-116.

Thornton, J. W., & Jacobs, P. D. (1972). The facilitating effects of prior inescapable/unavoidable stress on intellectual performance. *Psychonomic Science, 26,* 185-187.

Thornton, J. W., & Jacobs, P. D. (1971). Learned helplessness in human subjects. *Journal of Experimental Psychology, 87,* 367-372.

Trautman, E. C. (1964). Fear and panic in Nazi concentration camps. *International Journal of Social Psychiatry, 10,* 134-141.

Trossman, B. (1968). Adolescent children of concentration camp survivors. *Canadian Psychiatric Association Journal, 13.*

Turner, R. J. (1981). Social support as a contingency in psychological well-being. *Journal of Health and Social Behavior, 22,* 357-367.

Ursano, R. J. (1981). The Viet Nam era prisoner of war: Precaptivity personality and the development of psychiatric illness. *American Journal of Psychiatry, 138,* 315-318.

Ursano, R. J., Boydstun, J. A., & Wheatley, R. D. (1981). Psychiatric illness in U. S. Air Force Viet Nam prisoners of war: A five-year follow-up. *American Journal of Psychiatry, 138,* 310-314.

Walk, D. (1967). Suicide and community care. *British Journal of Psychiatry, 113,* 1381-1391.

Wallace, A. F. C. (1956). An exploratory study of individual and community behavior in an extreme situation: Tornado in Worcester. Disaster Study Number 3, Publication 392, National Academy of Sciences–National Research Council, Washington, DC.

Weiner, I. (1969). The effectiveness of a suicide prevention program. *Mental Hygiene, 53,* 357–373.

Wenger, D. E. (1978). Community response to disaster: Functional and structural alterations. In E. L. Quarantelli (Ed.), *Disasters: Theory and research.* Beverly Hills, CA: Sage Press.

White, G. F., & Haas, J. E. (1975). *Assessment of research on natural hazards.* Cambridge, MA: MIT Press.

Whitlock, G. E. (1978). *Understanding and coping with real-life crises.* Monterey, CA: Brooks/Cole.

Wilcox, B. L. (1981). Social support, life stress and psychological adjustment. A test of the buffering hypothesis. *American Journal of Community Psychology, 9,* 371–385.

Williams, W. V., Lee, J., & Polak, P. (1976). Crisis intervention: Effects of crisis intervention on family survivors of sudden death situations. *Community Mental Health Journal, 12,* 128–136.

Williams, W. V., & Polak, P. R. (1979). Follow-up research in primary prevention: A model of adjustment in acute grief. *Journal of Clinical Psychology, 35,* 35–45.

Woodcock, A., & Davis, D. (1978). *Catastrophe theory.* New York: Avon.

Zilberg, N. J., Weiss, D. S., & Horowitz, M. J. (1982). Impact of Event Scale: A cross-validation study and some empirical evidence supporting a conceptual model of stress response syndromes. *Journal of Consulting and Clinical Psychology, 50,* 407–414.

2

Unraveling the Gordian Knot in Life Change Inquiry

A Critical Examination of Crisis, Stress, and Transitional Frameworks for Prevention

Robert D. Felner, Richard T. Rowlison, and Lisa Terre
Auburn University

Currently life events occupy a place of prominence in the search for potential psychosocial pathogens and are thought to be optimal points for intervention by those in a wide array of health-related disciplines (Felner, Jason, Moritsugu and Farber, 1983). As prevention and early intervention have increasingly been stressed by health professionals and policymakers, there has been a concomitant proliferation of theory and research on the nature of life events and life changes, their role in the etiology of mental and physical disorders, and their potential as focal points for intervention. Medicine, sociology, psychology, public health, psychiatry, social work, and numerous other fields have all been represented in the quest for clarification of these issues. This intense scrutiny from such a broad array of fields has resulted in substantial gains in our understanding of life events as well as their implications for physical and emotional well-being. However, despite the obvious benefits of such interdisciplinary enthusiasm, this broad-based interest in life events may actually jeopardize the further development of a knowledge base to inform preventive efforts in this area. That is, this rather unplanned and uncoordinated interdisciplinary union has led us inadvertently (but in retrospect quite predictably) to overlook a critical point. Namely, that individuals from different disciplines bring to a problem quite different professional socialization experiences, goals, and assumptions. These differences may have a profound effect not only on the questions asked but also on the nature of the data drawn upon or developed to answer them, and the interpretation given to that data (Sarason, 1981). The failure to consider the ways in which the involvement of individuals from disparate disciplinary contexts may shape the process of inquiry may have relatively little impact in the study of issues that are relatively circumscribed or discipline specific. However, in an area such as life events which is the focus of individuals representing so many disciplines and such a wide array of concerns the problem may be severe, resulting in the development and application of theoretical frameworks and empirical findings to the solution of problems for which they are ill suited.

Let us now make the above issues more specific to the focus of this chapter. An examination of the literature on life events reveals that an almost bewildering array of terms and concepts has been used to refer to life events and life changes. The terms life crisis, stressful life events, crisis events, transitions, stress, life change events, milestones, and proximal and distal stressors all have been used to refer to sets or subsets of significant occurrences in an individual's life, often in ways which imply that these concepts are roughly equivalent or that differences are insignificant. This may have indeed been the case in some instances given a particular author's idiosyncratic usage of the terms and the particular argument or issue he or she was addressing. However, obscured by this frequent virtually synonymous usage of these terms has been the quite distinct view of life events and their adaptive significance that each at least initially represented, and the importance of maintaining this distinctness for heuristic and intervention reasons. Are, for example, a crisis, a stressful life event, a distal stressor and a transition all the same thing? The answer is a resounding "YES and NO"! Based on the theoretical models from which the concepts derive the answer may be "yes" if the question is whether the same environmental occurrence (e.g., the death of a spouse, job loss, divorce, marriage) may, at times, be "loosely defined" using any or all of these terms. On the other hand, the answer is "no" when the questions are: "Does each of these terms refer to essentially similar views of the adaptive significance of the occurrence for the individual? Do the conceptual frameworks from which each term evolved view the significant elements of the coping process similarly? Were the issues which led to the initial emphasis on life events as focal points the same? And, finally, are the implications of each for the design and development of preventive programs the same?" The essential point here is that each term initially represented a view of life events that developed within a particular line of inquiry. These diverse contexts may act to make certain "facts" more relevant than others, resulting in quite dramatic differences in the organization and interpretation of the observed data, depending on the framework employed. As Sameroff (1983) states, "There is a reciprocal relationship between theory and facts in which both have an inseparable role . . . . What the scientist observes is strongly influenced by what theory is held and at the same time what theory is held is strongly influenced by what facts are observed" (p. 243).

If we are to advance in our understanding of the process by which individuals and families adapt to life events a necessary step that must be taken is the unraveling of the "Gordian Knot" that has resulted from the haphazard intertwining of the lines of thought and inquiry that has characterized this area. In the remainder of this chapter we will try to move us closer to the accomplishment of this task. First, in order to restore some of the conceptual clarity we have lost, we will attempt to sort out the distinct processes that underlie what may be the three most widely used terms that have been applied to significant life events and that have the clearest theoretical referents: "crises," "stressful life events," and "transitions." Here particular attention will be paid to the theoretical, practical, and empirical issues that provided the unique intellectual contexts in which each concept has evolved. Next, we will consider how the application of one model rather than another may lead to similarities or differences in which events are of concern and how the adaptive process is viewed. Finally, the implications of each of the different viewpoints for the shape of preventive programming will be discussed.

CRISES AND CRISIS EVENTS

There are two primary theoretical roots to modern crisis theory and, hence, most current conceptualizations of life crises or crisis events. The first of these, whose origins are detectable early in the psychodynamic movement, is primarily concerned with the periods of flux and reorganization during which individuals move from one phase of personality development to the next. Termed "developmental crises" by Erikson (1959), these are relatively short periods during which individuals must confront and attempt to master new developmental tasks that then become integrated with prior patterns of functioning. With slight variations most analytic or ego analytic theorists see these developmental crises as precipitated by either biological maturation (e.g., puberty) or by normative developmental shifts in the demands the social environment places on the individual (e.g., toilet training, school entry, retirement). The degree to which the individual successfully resolves the central tasks of the particular crisis is thought to determine whether the person will remain mired in the intrapsychic conflict precipitated by these challenges or, alternatively, whether the individual will move forward in their development of new competencies and strengths (Erikson, 1959; Rapoport, 1965a).

The second and perhaps more salient path for prevention which led to modern crisis theory has its origin in the work of Lindemann (1944) and Caplan (1964). Lindemann's work on the grief reaction of survivors of the tragic Coconut Grove Night Club fire in the winter of 1942 served to set out many of the basic formulations and ideas which shaped early crisis theory (Lindemann, 1944; Lindemann & Cobb, 1943). Caplan further refined and developed crisis theory drawing heavily from both Erikson and Lindemann. He proposed a model to guide primary prevention which had as its core organizing focus the impact of life crises and the importance of their successful resolution for emotional well-being. Of particular concern was the extension of crisis theory to include both developmental or normative crises (Datan & Ginsberg, 1975) as well as what have come to be called accidental (Erikson, 1959) or situational, nonnormative crises (Callahan & McCluskey, 1983, Rapoport, 1965a, 1965b). This more general formulation of crisis theory views the individual as a system which is generally in a state of homeostatic balance on both interpersonal and intrapsychic levels with long-term developmental changes typically occurring in a slow, orderly manner. Sudden discontinuities in the process of development are seen as reflecting times of crises. These discontinuities are precipitated by a life problem or situation that disrupts the homeostatic equilibrium of the individual's system. For our discussion a critical often overlooked point here is that not all life problems or life stresses result in homeostatic imbalance and, hence, a crisis reaction in an individual. Rather, crisis theory requires that there be an imbalance between the difficulty and importance of the problem and the coping resources and problem-solving abilities of the individual (Caplan, 1964; Parad & Caplan, 1965). That is, to precipitate a crisis the problem has to be of sufficient importance to the individual so that it cannot simply be denied or avoided without causing the person to experience extreme conflict or distress. Further, it has to be of sufficient adaptive difficulty so that the individual's normal coping resources and mechanisms cannot adequately resolve the challenge posed by the problem.

The homeostatic balance model of crisis theory has direct implications for defining the nature of a crisis. From it we can see that crises are not events. Instead, the concept of crisis refers to the internal state of an individual who is reacting to a problem stimulus that has overwhelmed their coping capabilities and resources. Thus, it is the individual's response which determines whether a crisis has occurred, not the mere occurrence of an event. That is, not all people faced by the same event will experience a state of crisis which, in its simplest definition, is "an upset in a steady state" (Caplan, 1964; Rapoport, 1965a; Felner, Stolberg, & Cowen, 1975). Although some events may precipitate crisis reactions in a majority of individuals who experience them, such as the loss of a significant other (Klein & Lindemann, 1961), no single event automatically produces crises for all people (Felner et al., 1975). Similarly, some events which may be well within the capacities of most individuals to manage with the experience of only transitory stress (e.g., a deadline at work) may precipitate a crisis reaction either because of their history, additional stresses, or deficits in their coping resources.

Once it is clear that crisis theory views a crisis as a state and not an event we need to turn to the characteristics of that state and their implications for the coping process. Coping efforts are seen to follow a definite pattern with the level of strain experienced by the individual differing during each phase of the evolution of the crisis reaction (Bloom, 1975; Taplin, 1971). In the face of a potentially crisis-precipitating stressor habitual problem-solving mechanisms are called upon. In the relatively short period prior to the solution, the organism experiences heightened tension and anxiety, which is tolerated by drawing upon problem-solutions and expectations they have developed in previous experiences with similar circumstances. A crisis occurs if and when these processes fail. Such failure results in a further rise in tension and in efforts to resolve the problem through redefinition or other avoidance strategies and, ultimately, in a loss of homeostatic balance and a state of crisis (Caplan, 1964; Taplin, 1971).

Another important defining feature of the state of crisis is its temporal qualities. Crises are seen as having relatively short durations, generally from about "one to four or five weeks" (Caplan, 1964, p. 35). However, in these brief periods rapid significant modifications in people's adaptative styles and adjustments which have pronounced and enduring consequences may occur (Caplan, 1964; Felner et al., 1975). For prevention, the importance of the long-term impact of crisis resolution and the brief period involved cannot be overemphasized. Caplan states, "The significance of a crisis is in its temporal telescoping of development. Major alterations in pattern may occur in a relatively short period and may subsequently remain stable for a long time" (p. 39). In addition to underscoring the significance of the temporal qualities of crises and their potential importance for intervention efforts, this statement also raises another key characteristic of the state of crisis that makes crises important targets for prevention. That is, crises are not always, nor even generally, associated with maladaptive outcomes. Indeed, they may result in an enhanced level of adaptation and the development of new coping mechanisms and resources (Felner et al., 1975; Lindemann, 1956; Morley, 1964; Stein, 1970; Waldfogel & Gardner, 1961).

Proponents of crisis theory have outlined a number of factors which are believed to relate to crisis resolution and outcomes. Among those factors brought to the situation by the individual, the symbolic relationship of the current problem to prior ones, the degree of efficacy with which the earlier situations were handled, and their appraisal of the situation as problematic or stressful are each thought to play a central role in the process of coping. In this latter view it has been argued that a crisis "must be perceived as a loss of or a threat to need satisfaction, and, like all perceptions, this depends on culture and personality" (Caplan, 1964, p. 42). Based on this statement it may be seen that although we may not be able to predict which events will predispose particular individuals to a crisis reaction, it may be possible to predict, at least in a given culture, the probability that certain circumstances may be hazardous or engender crisis in significant percentages of populations (Caplan, 1964; Darbonne, 1967).

Situational factors are also seen to play a role in the resolution of crises. Among the most critical of these may be the availability and intervention of significant others or formal helpers. According to crisis theory when the individual is in a crisis state they may be particularly receptive to and desirous of help from others (Bloom, 1975; Rapoport, 1965a; Taplin, 1971). Lindemann has suggested that caregivers wishing to help the individual resolve the crisis adaptively should focus on "the mastery of attending emotions, the review of possible suitable responses and the rehearsal of feasible role patterns . . . ." (Lindemann, 1979, p. 174).

STRESSFUL LIFE EVENTS

The current intense interest in single or multiple life events, and the personal and situational variables that relate to their "stressfulness," has its primary origin in the fields of public health and epidemiology. In addition, it also owes some debt to the development of crisis theory which, in large part, preceded it (Dohrenwend, 1979; Felner, Farber, & Primavera, 1980). As the term "stressful life event" implies, this line of inquiry views life events as sources of significant environmental demands or "stress." According to the model, these demands may tax the individual's psychological resources, activate internal biological response patterns and, ultimately, play a role in the onset of disorder or disease (Neufeld, 1982).

In keeping with the traditional goals of epidemiology, early research in this area was interested in the prediction of physical or emotional disorders and, more importantly, in the identification of the etiological factors that might contribute to such disorders. Cannon's early work on the association between strong emotions and bodily changes pointed toward life events as sources of these emotions and, hence, as possible factors in disease onset (Cannon, 1929). Meyer (1951) further contributed to the notion of life events as potential antecedents of illness through the use of the life chart as an adjunct to medical diagnosis.

Although these issues received further attention through the following two decades (c.f. Appley & Trumbull, 1967), it was not until the work of Holmes and Rahe (1967) that the concept of stressful life events captured the attention of investigators in the form and to the extent that it enjoys today. As part of their efforts to identify antecedents or precipitants of disease onset these authors published the Social Readjustment Rating Scale (SRRS). With this scale they sought to both identify whether or not an individual had recently experienced one of 43 different life events and to quantify the cumulative stressfulness of these events to predict risk for disorder.

A central assumption made by Holmes and Rahe (1967) in the development of their scale scores was that life events produce changes in an individual's life and consequent demands for readjustment and, further, that these changes and demands, in effect, define the level of stress the individual experiences. Subsequent work by Holmes and Rahe and their colleagues (Masuda & Holmes, 1967; Komaroff, Masuda, & Holmes, 1968; de Araujo, Van Arsdel, Holmes, & Dudley, 1973; Rahe, Mahan, & Arthur, 1979) has given rise to numerous attempts to develop and further refine life events scales that are better predictors of emotional or physical symptomatology for both children and adults (e.g., Coddington, 1972; Dohrenwend, Krasnoff, Askenasy, & Dohrenwend, 1978; Johnson, 1982; Hough, Fairbank, & Garcia, 1976; Monaghan, Robinson, & Dodge, 1979; Sarason, Johnson, & Siegel, 1978). A major focus of the work with these scales has been the identification of factors that, when used to inform the construction of the scales themselves, their scoring, and/or the weightings or significance assigned to life events that are included as items, enhance our ability to predict dysfunction (Dohrenwend & Dohrenwend, 1978, 1984; Felner et al., 1983; Monroe, 1982; Johnson & Sarason, 1978; Perkins, 1982). It is not our intent in this work to once again review this frequently tilled ground. Indeed reviews of this work discussing the above issues have become almost as plentiful as the empirical studies themselves. What is of concern for this discussion is the general direction this work has taken and the conclusions about life events which have been drawn from it. Hence, the ensuing discussion shall refer to this work only insofar as it proves instructive for our consideration of differences among life event models and/or research traditions and their implications for intervention.

As should be clear by now most of the work on "stressful life events" has been guided not by an interest in life events per se nor in their general significance for the full range of human functioning and development (Felner et al., 1983). Instead, this work may be better characterized as a special core segment of more general investigations into the nature and consequences of stress. While a primary goal in this area work has continued to be the development of markers and instruments which facilitate the prediction of the development of disorder, a second major focus of research in this area has been on the further elaboration of models of life stress which allow for the testing of hypotheses about specific aspects of stress and dysfunction or disease (Dohrenwend & Dohrenwend, 1984). Notice that both of these goals are primarily focused on pathology or pathogenic factors. Nowhere in them is there a concern with life events or changes for their own sake. Hence, the questions that underlie the models and instruments developed in this area are "what is a stressful life event" and "what makes it stressful." The search for answers to these questions have generally fallen into three broad categories: (a) the examination of the properties of events themselves; (b) efforts to identify psychological characteristics or personal disposition of the individuals experiencing the event that influence the degree to which it is appraised as stressful; and (c) environmental-contextual factors that may influence the individual's appraisal of the event, the demands it places on them, and the resources they have available to cope with the stress it engenders.

The life events with which researchers in this area are primarily concerned involve those which occur in close temporal proximity to the onset of disorder (Dohrenwend & Dohrenwend, 1984). For example, the focus would be on the relatively recent divorce of an individual but not with losses they had suffered as a child. Dohrenwend and Dohrenwend argue that the latter circumstance "is not irrelevant to life stress but is subsumed under personal dispositions since we assume that the earlier event ... can affect an adult's behavior only insofar as its impact was internalized" (pp. 2-3). The first step then in delineating what constitutes a stressful life event is to identify events that are associated with adverse mental or physical health outcomes for significant numbers of individuals (Bloom, 1979; Felner et al., 1983). Evidence that the event is associated with the onset of pathology in previously healthy individuals is seen as an a priori indication that the event is both stressful and important (Dohrenwend, 1979).

Once an event has been identified as a significant source of stress the next issue to be addressed relates to what the dimensions or qualities of the event are which make it stressful and the degree to which it differs on these dimensions from other stressful life events. Here investigators have identified a number of properties of events and proposed a range of alternative weighting strategies that they feel may be salient. The selection of the properties of events to use in arriving at the weightings assigned to the event is particularly critical in that it defines our view of what is stressful about these events (Stone & Neale, 1982). As noted above Holmes and Rahe (1967) used the degree of change associated with an event to define the level of stress associated with it. This is a view that is quite similar to Selye's (1978) position that stress is defined by environmental change. This viewpoint has not, however, been well supported. Change associated with positive or desirable events has not been found to be consistently associated with symptoms of psychological or physical dysfunction (c.f. Dohrenwend & Dohrenwend, 1984; Felner et al., 1983; Johnson & Sarason, 1978; Miller, Ingram, & Davidson, 1976; Paykel, 1974; Vinokur & Selzer, 1975; Zimmerman, 1983). Lending further support for a move away from change as the defining characteristic of stress that accompanies life events is the fact that on many life events scales which purport to assess such stress a number of items may, in fact, relate to circumstances which are not necessarily associated with changes in the circumstances of the individual's life. Illustratively, Sandler, Wolchik, Braver, and Fogas in Chapter 3 in this volume note that 25% or more of the items on life events scales may actually refer to events where change is not necessarily a property of the item.

Other properties of events that have been used to define the level of stress associated with them or to distinguish among them are their desirability (Dohrenwend, 1979; Gersten, Langner, Eisenberg, & Orzeck, 1974; Johnson, 1982; Sarason et al., 1978; Stone & Neale, 1982; Zautra & Simons, 1979) their upsettingness (Dohrenwend & Dohrenwend, 1984; Sandler et al., this volume; Stone & Neale, 1982), the degree of control people have over their occurrence (Brown, Sklair, Harris, & Birley, 1973; Dohrenwend & Martin, 1979), the degree to which they can be anticipated (Dohrenwend & Martin, 1979; Felner, Primavera, & Cauce, 1981), the area of life they affect (Chiroboga & Dean, 1978), the level of threat they represent (Brown & Harris, 1978) and their perceived stressfulness (Stone & Neale, 1982). The strength of the association between the life events scores yielded or a set of particular discrete events and health outcomes appears to be a function both of which of these dimensions are used and the criterion variables selected (Stone & Neale, 1982). Building on such findings both Hurst (1979) and Sandler and Lakey (1982), after reviewing studies in this area have suggested that future work which focuses on qualitative differences among events in addition to qualitative ones may be helpful for identifying events with common effects on individuals and thus help to clarify the nature of the stress which contributes to disorder in the specific samples of interest.

The properties of life events used to determine their relative weightings have also served as focal points for discussions of which events may be rightly categorized as stressful life events and included on such inventories. Here questions have also been raised about whether events should be a priori identified as stressful using either the consensus ratings of those who have experienced them or of expert raters, or whether more individually tailored determinations should be made (Dohrenwend, 1979; Felner et al., 1983). These discussions have resulted in several conclusions about the nature of events which are of most interest to life stress researchers as well as a number of alternative hypotheses about ways in which life events may interact with personal coping styles and contextual factors to influence health outcomes. The central characteristics of life events that stress researchers have been able to agree upon as most salient for affecting adaptation and health are the degree to which an event is negative, aversive or undesirable, the potential threat it holds in terms of loss or harm, and the degree to which its outcome is under the control of the individual (Dohrenwend & Dohrenwend, 1984; Felner et al., 1983; Lazarus & Folkman, 1984; Sandler et al., this volume). Further, in terms of health outcomes, it has been emphasized that it may not be the objective characteristics of the events on these dimensions as determined by consensus weightings that are the most critical. Instead, the critical factor seems to be the degree to which the individual appraises the event as possessing more or less of the above characteristics and the extent to which the person, in turn, reacts physiologically in a way that characterizes stress response patterns (Lazarus & Folkman, 1984; Felner et al., 1983; Stone & Neale, 1982).

Dohrenwend and Dohrenwend (1984) have recently articulated six different hypotheses, each of which has at least some data at present to support them, which attempt to explain the ways in which life events may interact with personal dispositions and the environment of the individual to describe the life-stress process. The first of these, the "victimization" hypothesis, underlies the original work of Holmes and Rahe (1967). This view holds that the unfortunate occurrence of a significant number of life events over which the individual has little control, in a relatively brief period of time (i.e., one to two years) may lead to physical and emotional exhaustion and concomitant disorder.

A second hypothesis posits that it is the extent and type of psychophysiological strain that results from the life events which determines their health consequences. The third view, labeled as the "vulnerability hypothesis," has received a great deal of attention from life events researchers and it, or a variation of it, tempered by the "proneness model" to be discussed shortly, is perhaps the most widely accepted currently. Dohrenwend and Dohrenwend (1984) note that this "hypothesis indicates that stressful life events, moderated by existing personal dispositions and social conditions . . . make the individual vulnerable to the impact of life events, and cause adverse health outcomes" (p. 21). They go on to point out that this is the position that is reflected most strongly in certain conceptions of coping ability (e.g., Hamberg & Adams, 1967) and social support (e.g., Caplan & Killilea, 1976; Cobb, 1976).

The next two hypotheses, the "additive burden" and "chronic burden" views, are variations of each other. In the first of these personal and environmental factors are seen to add to the impact of life events rather than moderating the stress associated with them. In the second, existing personal dispositions and contextual factors *rather than life events* are seen as the causative agents in negative health outcomes. Finally, the "proneness" hypothesis suggests that it is the presence of existing disorder which leads to the occurrence of a high frequency of life events, particularly negative ones, which then lead to further disorder.

As noted all of these models attempt to account for the relationship between the occurrence of major life events and the onset of disorder. What of the strength of the relationship that is the focus of so much attention? Although generally these associations have been statistically significant, particularly when the focus of attention has been on those events which have the characteristics that are seen to increase their "stressfulness" (e.g., negative, not predictable, etc.), it has generally been in the vicinity of .30 (Rabkin & Struening, 1976) and accounted for less of the variance than researchers in the area feel is necessary to be a viable way of assessing stress (DeLongis, Coyne, Dakof, Folkman, & Lazarus, 1982; Stone & Neale, 1982). Illustratively, in discussing this association and the method-ological difficulties that plague the area, DeLongis et al. conclude, "Those con-cerned with the impact of stress on health status must search for alternative and more promising ways of assessing stress and the processes mediating health out-comes" (p. 120). Here they are building on Lazarus' (c.f. Lazarus & Folkman, 1984) conceptualization of stress which posits that stress is best viewed in terms of person-environment transactions that tax or exceed the resources of the person. From this model stress is not thought to be located solely in either the person or in environmental conditions, instead; it is believed to arise from the relationship between them, with a reciprocal interaction occurring such that each, in turn, affects the other. In keeping with this model they and other workers in this area (e.g., Stone & Neale, 1982, 1984; Sandler et al., this volume; Wolchik, Fogas, & Sandler, in press) have sought potential environmental contributors to stress that are, to a greater degree, part of the individual's daily experiences. This has led to a shift in attention from major life events to more minor events that occur with greater frequency and are part of the more immediate social environment of the individual than are major events (DeLongis et al., 1982). When these events are negative and, as a result, potentially stress associated, they have been labelled as "hassles" (Kanner, Coyne, Schaefer & Lazarus, 1981). Lazarus and his colleagues (DeLongis et al., 1982) argue that such events may have a stronger association to both perceived stress and health outcomes than major life events since they are "proximal" measures of stress while life events scores are "distal." That is, hassles may describe the actual person-environment transactions being demanded by the individual's circumstances while major life events may not adequately describe the ongoing demands for coping that they require. Finally, it should be noted that in addition to arguing for the need to focus on negative daily experiences, Kanner et al. also pointed to the potential importance of small, positive daily events, which they termed "uplifts."

Several other research groups have also sought to develop procedures for assessing elements of daily experience. This work has resulted in Lewinsohn's Pleasant Events Schedule (MacPhillamy & Lewinsohn, 1971; Lewinsohn & Libet, 1972) and the Unpleasant Events Schedule (Lewinsohn, 1974, 1975) as well as Assessment of Daily Experience process developed by Stone and Neale (1982) which assesses not only daily experiences but moods and symptoms as well. Taken together the results of studies of the association between daily experiences and either health status and/or disorder have generally been mixed. A number of studies have found unpleasant experiences or hassles to be associated with a range of difficulties, including poorer somatic health (DeLongis et al., 1982; Kanner et al., 1981), and depression and lowered mood (Lewinsohn & Talkington, 1979; Stone & Neale, 1982). More recent work by Stone and Neale (1984) however, has failed to support the view that severe daily experiences are associated with enduring mood shifts and studies of desirable daily events and adaptational outcomes have yielded even less consistent findings (DeLongis et al., 1982). It should be noted, however, that in the one study to date of the relative contribution of life events, hassles, and uplifts scores to health outcomes hassles were found to share most of the variance in health that could be attributed to major life events and that the significant association between health status and hassles remained even when the variance attributable to major life events was removed. Uplifts were found to have little association to health status (DeLongis et al., 1982).

The above findings lend support to the notion that the assessment of smaller, more proximal events may be helpful for refining our understanding of the relationship between environmental stress and emotional or physical disorder. This support is, nonetheless, not as clear-cut as advocates of this approach might wish. Findings have been somewhat inconsistent and perhaps even more importantly, some of the methodological problems which have been the source of criticism of studies which employ life events inventories are now increasingly recognized as being present in the study of daily experiences as well (Dohrenwend, Dohrenwend, Dodson, & Shrout, 1984). For example, Stone and Neale (1982) argue that they "chose to assess daily experiences because they are not subject to some of the methodological shortcomings of previous life-event work and would allow us to examine the life events illness relationship over time" (p. 53). However, recent work by Dohrenwend et al. (1984) nicely illustrates one of the most serious limitations of work that has sought to establish the potentially detrimental effects of major life events and shows how this methodological problem may also shape the findings of studies of both daily experiences or other mediators of the life events/stress-illness process. These authors note that conceptual and operational distinctions among measures of life events, mediators of the impact of life events or the life-stress process (e.g., social support, hassles) and disorder may not be sufficiently developed to permit causal models to be developed based on interrelationships observed among these factors. The problem of the confounding of the measurement of stress with the assessment of health outcome is underscored by these authors who state that not only may many of the events which appear on life stress scales also be symptoms of mental or physical disorder but, "There are indications that these problems of confounded measurement are present in measures of social support and hassles as well" (p. 223). To explore this issue further Dohrenwend et al. (1984) asked expert raters to indicate the degree to which items on the Holmes & Rahe (1967) scale examining life events, the Kanner et al. (1981) "Hassles" scale, and a measure of social support developed by Lin, Dean, and Ensel (1981) could be indicative of psychological disorder. Overall their results indicated that for all three measures there were serious difficulties in this regard, with over three-fourths of the items on the "Hassles Scale," two-thirds of the items on the social support measure, and nearly half the items on the Holmes and Rahe scale being seen as frequently providing evidence for the presence of psychological disorder. They also note that on the Holmes and Rahe scale the items that were most likely to be judged as symptoms were those that were negative or undesirable.

TRANSITIONAL EVENTS

In recent work Felner and his colleagues (Felner, 1984; Felner, Farber, & Primavera, 1980; Felner, Ginter, & Primavera, 1982) have proposed a model for considering the adaptive significance of life events and the organizing of preventive programs targeted to them, which places the focus on the changes such events may engender and the adaptive tasks these changes may pose for the individual. By contrast to those who are primarily interested in the stressful and pathological properties of life events and who have argued for a move away from a focus on the degree of change as the salient property of life events (e.g., Dohrenwend & Dohrenwend, 1984; Sandler et al., this volume) what Felner terms a "Transitional Events" model would reemphasize the importance of the changes associated with life events as central to understanding their adaptive significance.

Further, of particular importance is that the transitional event perspective puts a far greater emphasis on the period that precedes this transitional event and the one that follows it as being critical in the determination of the adaptive outcomes associated with the event per se. Indeed, as we shall attempt to demonstrate below, a view of the event with which the individual is "coping," as "unitary," such as that which characterizes the two earlier models, is not a central element of the transitional events perspective. Rather, "transitional events" are seen to actually consist of a collection of smaller changes and stressors to which the individual is attempting to adapt, and it is the sum of the collective experiences in this process which defines the way in which they evaluate their experience of the significant marker event in the transitional process.

In contrast to the preceding models, this model is seen to be more congruent with the dual emphasis of primary prevention on both the enhancement of well-being and adaptive functioning as well as the avoidance of pathology than are prior models. While drawing from both of the views of life events discussed thus far, it also has its roots in developmental models of transitions. However, a unique focus is that that transitional events framework was developed specifically with the goal of enhancing and informing the development of preventive interventions. Before proceeding with our discussion of this perspective we will turn to a brief consideration of prior views of life transitions which help in understanding the Transitional Events model that follows.

Caplan (1964) and Lindemann (1943, 1944) frequently used the terms "crises" and "transitions" interchangeably, with the characteristics of the former seen as synonymous with latter. This equivalent usage is nicely demonstrated in a series of quotes from Caplan. When discussing the state of crisis he argues, "These transitional points in (the individual's) history have usually been characterized by acute psychological upset, lasting from one to four or five weeks" (Caplan, 1964, p. 35). Later, in comparing his model of crisis to earlier trauma perspectives he begins by saying, "This view of crisis as a transitional period presents the individual both with an opportunity for personal growth and the danger of increased vulnerability to mental disorder" (Caplan, 1964, p. 36).

Two other variations on the term "transition" are found in the works of Tyhurst (1958) and Parkes (1971). Tyhurst's model is actually not that different from a crisis perspective in that it emphasizes transition states that characterize an individual's reaction to change, and this change is thought to be precipitated by a disequilibrating event (Felner et al., 1983). By contrast, Parkes (1971) views a transition as a process which requires an interaction between the individual and his environment. Summarizing across these and a number of other efforts to define transitions, Golan (1981) states that a good summary definition would be "a period of moving from one state of certainly to another, with an interval of uncertainty and change in between" (p. 12). And, similarly, a common element of typologies of transitions is that they all share the view that, "a period of adaptation is involved, not only by the individual undergoing the change, but by (his/her) interacting social environment as well" (p. 14).

The Transitional Events model proposed by the senior author of this chapter builds on these views of transitions as well as the two life events models discussed earlier. In so doing, it has a number of points of overlap but also differs in certain important ways. The three primary areas of divergence relate to (1) what are viewed as the crucial aspects of life events that impact adaptive outcome, (2) the types of life events which are of concern, and (3) the processes related to the success or failure of the individual's coping efforts. Let us now turn to a more detailed consideration of this model.

The term Transitional Event, much like the term Community Psychology, combines two ideas that are often viewed as not being complementary. However, this juxtaposition was chosen with the intent of capturing the unique nature of the phenomenon we seek to explain. On the one hand, the inclusion of the term "transition" is meant to underscore our concern with a process that involves change and the ways in which individuals adapt to it. Here, the change process and accompanying adaptive demands and challenges may extend temporally, for long distances on either side of the central "marker" event. That is, we are not only concerned with the event proper but also the adaptive efforts which lead up to and follow it. The word "event" is nonetheless included as it needs to be recognized that we are dealing with both a particular type of transition as well as a particular type of event. Before turning to a consideration of the adaptive process we will begin with the latter point.

Among life transitions a broad dichotomy may be drawn between those due primarily to normative maturational changes in the organism and those characterized by fundamental and clearly identifiable shifts in the organism's environment. The movement between the stages of personality development postulated by Erikson, Sullivan, or Levinson, the shift from one level of Piagetian development to another, the onset of adolescence, or the beginning of the process of physical decline which accompanies aging are all examples of maturationally keyed "developmental" transitions. By contrast, there are those transitions marked by identifiable events in the life history where the event signals that the individual is in the midst of or at one of the end points of a profound and extensive reorganization of their place in the social environment. It is with these "transitional events" that we are concerned. Examples of such transitional events include retirement, entering the work force, getting married or divorced, changing jobs or schools, having a first child, death of a family member, the onset of a chronic illness, the development of a disability either by the individual or a significant other, residential relocation, or being promoted at work or school. Certainly, at times, this latter type of transition may occur, at least in part, as a function of the individual's movement through the life course. But it may also occur non-normatively at times that are not anticipable based on development. For these transitions the keys are that there are identifiable and observable changes in the relationship between the organism and the elements of the social system in which they live and that these changes are marked by clear environmental events. As should be obvious, such changes may involve not only the restructuring of the individual's cognitive representations of reality but also the reorganization and restructuring of the environmental systems involved.

Transitional events are not only different from other transitions they are also very different from other types of life events (Felner et al., 1983). For example, some of the events on life events inventories are truly events in the sense that they are highly circumscribed and limited both in their direction and in their repercussions for the individual's life (e.g., a family quarrel). By contrast, transitional events serve as "markers" of extensive and enduring changes in an individual's life which may precipitate further challenges and changes and, thus, demand significant adaptive efforts for some time to come (e.g., divorce, retirement, marriage) (Felner et al., 1980, 1983). Evidence to support this position comes from a number of recent studies on such diverse transitional events as school change, divorce, birth of a first child, and the onset of a life threatening illness (Cowan & Cowan, 1981, 1983; Felner, Ginter, Primavera, 1982; Gottesman & Lewis, 1982; Hetherington, 1979; Lewis, Gottesman, & Gutstein, 1979). This work has shown that adaptation to the changes and resultant adaptive tasks that follow these transitional events may extend for several years and, indeed, in some cases, may begin before the event itself (e.g., preparation for or anticipation of child birth, divorce, retirement). Thus, given a transitional events rather than a stressful life events or crisis perspective, we may ask: What is the nature of the adaptive process and what are the key elements relating to its successful resolution? rather than How does one cope with a particular "event"?

The differences in the duration of the adaptive processes that are of concern to each of these perspectives is a central point of departure. For transitional events, as noted, the researcher or intervenor is concerned with a fairly long process that may extend for several years. For the other two perspectives, the point of focus is temporally far more limited (e.g., Caplan's statements about crises or transitions being resolved in a four- to eight-week period). A second and equally important distinction is that the transitional model proposed by Felner and his colleagues shifts the focus from stress and its pathogenic effects or the re-establishment of organismic homeostatic balance following a threat as the predominant concerns to the nature of the changes which accompany such transitions and the factors which influence the process of adapting to them. As Felner et al. (1983) state, "Here the stress involved is but one element of a larger process which includes mastery of the range of adaptive tasks engendered by the life change (transitional event)" (p. 209).

A transitional events perspective then places the primary emphasis on what people must do behaviorally and/or cognitively to adapt to the new or changing circumstances in their lives, rather than on their efforts to cope with affective responses to the changes. These changes are hypothesized to be accompanied by or precipitants of a number of "adaptive tasks" (Felner et al., 1983) and the affective responses an individual experiences following or during life changes may, in large part, be understood to result from the extent and difficulty of these tasks and the success they have in mastering them. This perspective also postulates that although the specific content or nature of the transitional event may vary, there are certain adaptive tasks that are characteristic across transitions. Felner et al.,

(1983) in considering the literature to date, identified five domains of adaptive tasks that may be confronted by individuals going through a transitional event and the process of change that accompanies it. These include:

1. The need for the individual to reorganize his or her "assumptive world" (Parkes, 1971),
2. The need for the person to redefine and reshape social roles,
3. The reorganization and/or reconstruction of their social networks and social support systems,
4. The re-establishment and/or reorganization of daily routines and patterns of behavior, and
5. Adjusting to shifts in material circumstances and resources.

A sixth common task domain is identified for those individuals living in a house-hold where other family members are present, that is, the restructuring of family interaction patterns. It should be noted here that we have referred to domains of adaptive tasks rather than simply discussing each set of tasks as though they were unitary. The reason for this is that, clearly, each of these task domains may include a number of more discrete tasks (e.g., an individual may have a number of social roles or be involved in multiple social networks that are fairly independent with the degree of success they have in reorganizing or restructuring one not necessarily bearing on the outcome achieved with the others).

A final point on the process of adaptation from a transitional events perspective: such a model does not ignore the role of stress nor its sources (Felner et al., 1983). Indeed, it may be more able to incorporate recent findings and emergent directions in the stressful life events area than could a model in which the emphasis was still on relatively infrequently occurring significant stressful life events. DeLongis et al. (1982) have drawn a distinction between major life events and the residual day-to-day stressors they may engender or exacerbate. The former are classified as distal stressors while the latter are proximal stressors. Distal stressors are those which do not describe directly the demands that result from them nor the adaptive process they require. Proximal stressors are those daily person-environment transitions that the person sees as a threat. A life transition perspective with its emphasis on the changes that are part of the transitional process and the delineation of the major tasks that characterize it can certainly easily accommodate a focus on daily stressors and help to delineate their specific relationship to the more distal event than can the more static stressful life events models that have been used previously. For a more extensive discussion and examples of how this may be accomplished see Chapter 3 by Sandler and his colleagues.

This then, very briefly, outlines some of the major components of a transitional life events framework (for a more extended discussion see Felner et al., 1983; Felner, 1985). The further elaboration of this framework, its implications for viewing the process by which individuals cope with such life changes, and its utility for informing the design and development of preventive interventions (the purpose of this paper) is perhaps best accomplished by a discussion of the commonalities and differences between the crisis, stressful life events and transitional events models, particularly as they pertain to the latter two issues.

SIMILARITIES AND DIFFERENCES AMONG LIFE EVENTS PERSPECTIVES

There are several key dimensions of life events and the coping process they require that each of the above models addresses, and it is to these that we shall now turn to help clarify how the application of one model rather than another may lead to quite different points of emphasis as well as the ways in which they may complement one another. Our discussion shall focus primarily, although not exclusively, on:

1. Nature of the "events" that are of concern,
2. Process of adaptation and the significant elements of it, and
3. Outcomes that are of concern.

Target "Events"

The life events with which the crisis and stressful event perspectives are concerned are quite different than those emphasized by the transitional events view. Both of the former are primarily concerned with events which, although having the potential for positive developmental outcomes (see below) are at the time of their occurrence negative, at least as appraised by the individual experiencing them. Specifically, the crisis perspective emphasizes that crisis events are those which pose a threat to the organism that is sufficiently beyond its abilities to deal with it given their current resources. These events are thought to stress the organismic system and produce a state of homeostatic disequilibrium which renders the system vulnerable. Similarly, a stressful life events perspective is concerned with those events in an individual's life which are associated with increased risk for adverse physical and mental health outcomes (Dohrenwend & Dohrenwend, 1984). Indeed, as noted above, research in this area has relegated positive life events to the status of having little adaptive significance. By contrast to these positions the transitional events model emphasizes the individual's need to master the adaptive tasks associated with significant changes in the nature of the patterns of person-environment transactions that characterize their lives. Thus it is concerned not only with negative changes in an individual's life but also with positive ones. Here is is recognized that although such occurrences may not be highly correlated with the onset of disorder they may nonetheless be of great significance for the long-term adaptation and well-being of the organism (Felner et al., 1983). For us this is a key point, and it should be clear that for those concerned with the enhancement of functioning that a concern with adaptation to such "positive" transitions as marriage, a job or school promotion, or the birth of a child may be as important, if not more so, than a concern with mastery of negative life changes. Indeed, it may be the failure to adequately adapt to one or more positive transitions which leads to the occurrence of negative changes and poor health outcomes (e.g., a "happy couple's" failure to cope adaptively with the birth of a child or increased professional status of one spouse resulting, ultimately, in a significant increase in daily hassles and/or, eventually, divorce).

The Adaptive Process

Viewing life events from one model rather than another also has quite dramatic implications for the answers to the questions of what it is that is the primary focus of the person's coping efforts, what the key elements of the coping process are and what factors influence the relative success or failure of such efforts. Of course, they also significantly influence the perspective taken on the duration of the adaptive process of concern. In crisis formulations the emphasis is on the restoration of the integrity of the organismic system as well as homeostatic balance and a stable state of intra-organismic functioning. Although precipitated by an inability to deal with a problem or situation that may signal that the individual's ability to continue to satisfy a fundamental need is in danger (Caplan, 1964), the management of affective responses (e.g., the increase in tension, feelings of ineffectuality, and personal strain) is, along with seeking a resolution to the problem, of primary concern. That is, that while resolution of some environmentally based problem or threat may be part of crisis resolution such problem solving may also take place without a crisis occurring. Thus when compared to other situations or events that require problem-solving responses a crisis is distinguished by:

1. Nature of the affective response of the organism,
2. Internal state that results, and
3. Potential for producing profound alterations in the basic personality structure of the organism (i.e., "telescoping of development").

The individual's appraisal of the situation and the affective response which results are also the central focus of what stressful life events formulations emphasize as needing to be dealt with by intervention efforts. Indeed, this is even more the case for this conceptualization of the adaptive significance of life events than for crisis theory. While in the latter case the degree to which the individual sucessfully solves the problem that precipitates a crisis is an important determinant of its long-term adaptive consequences, in the former case the actual resolution of the stress-producing situation is of far less importance than the management of the stress that accompanies it, as it is the stressfulness of the situation that seems to have the most direct impact on the resulting health outcomes. By contrast to both transitional event and crisis perspectives, the emphasis of stressful life events formulations is not on the salience of the situation for extensive shifts in the organism's overall functioning and reordering of the person-environment transitions. Rather, the emphasis is placed on the degree to which the situation leads to stress and pathogenic health outcomes. Further, the transitional events framework focuses on the active mastery of the adaptive tasks that arise as a function of changes in circumstances that are taking place in the individual's life and environment. Attention is not, as in the other two models, predominantly on the affective responses of the individuals experiencing the life change to the particular event. Rather, the central concern is with what it is that people must actively do, cognitively and behaviorally, to satisfactorily adapt to the new circumstances in their lives that result from the changes and tasks they engender. Recall that the crisis model is also concerned, at least to some extent, with problem solving. However, from a crisis perspective the problems are significant only insofar as they involve certain negative affective components. Further, the focal change process is of far briefer duration. As should be clear, a transitional events perspective makes no demand that the changes being dealt with are either positively or negatively affectively valenced nor time limited but merely that they require significant reorganization and readjustment in a number of spheres of the individual's life.

The differences in positions among the various models of life events about what "events" are the central focus of the individual's coping efforts have direct consequences for what is seen to be the nature and key elements of the coping process. From a stressful life events framework the coping process is seen to be one in which the potentially pathogenic stress stemming from a unitary life event (Felner et al., 1980) is what must be dealt with and the stressfulness of the event is mediated by a combination of personal and situational factors that exist at the time. With the exception of the individual's active involvement in shaping their personal appraisal of the event they are seen to be relatively passive with respect to the nature and availability of other mediating or "stress buffering" factors (Dohrenwend, 1979; Wilcox, 1981). For example, social support is viewed as having a "protective effect" and a major focus of research is on "situational factors that may mediate the effects of these (life) events" (Dohrenwend & Dohrenwend, 1984, pp. 98–99).

Adoption of a crisis perspective provides for a bit more of an active-process view of what is called for in coping with a life event. As for the stressful life events view the individual's cognitive appraisal of the situation is seen to be an important element of the coping process. Further, given the somewhat clinical/psychodynamic roots of this model, the experiences with similar problems the person has had and, particularly, the symbolic conscious or unconscious links between the current circumstances and prior ones are viewed as critical in shaping the appraisal of the situation. The primary role of the environment is in the degree to which it may help or hinder the reestablishment of homeostatic equilibrium, by providing either affective support or information that may aid in the resolution of the problem situation. Indeed, as the individual's tension rises she or he may not only solicit help from others but, given their state of disequilibrium, may be particularly susceptible to outside forces (Caplan, 1964). However, given the origins of this model the role of environmental factors is either limited to (a) that of being the source of the threat to need satisfaction that has given rise to the crisis or (b) the location of "therapeutic agents."

A transitional events position views the coping process and its significant elements very differently than does either of the other two frameworks, although elements of each are incorporated. Indeed, this position owes much to the perspective on how individuals cope with ongoing stress in their lives (e.g., Lazarus & Folkman, 1984; Coyne & Holroyd, 1982). This latter influence is perhaps best reflected in the transactional nature of the model in which the individual actively interacts with the environment to adapt to the challenges that the process of change poses. However, by contrast to stress positions the emphasis is not on the stressor or, in the particular case under discussion, the stressful event, but on the more prolonged adaptive process which may both precede and follow it. Rather than simply focusing on the event or specific change, what is of central concern is the further changes, tasks, and stressors that may accompany the event. A transitional events perspective also emphasizes that the individual is actively involved in shaping both his/her internal representations of the world and the place they have in it, as well as the characteristics of the environment which may place adaptive demands on them. It also considers that the degree to which the individual may successfully master these adaptive tasks may be enhanced or constrained by characteristics of the environment, their current functioning, and their problem-solving styles and skills. Several examples of how this perspective leads to quite different consequences for understanding the adaptive process that crisis or stressful life events models may help to clarify these points.

Rather than viewing the person's cognitive appraisal of the situation as a factor that is salient primarily because of its association with the level of threat or stress that is experienced, from a transitional perspective two of the more important adaptive tasks confronted by an individual going through a transition involve the alteration and reorganization of major components of how they view the world. Transitions are seen to necessitate both the reorganization of the assumptive world of the individual and shifts in the role definitions they hold for themselves (Felner et al., 1983; Parkes, 1971; Pearlin, Menaghan, Lieberman, & Mullen, 1981). In addition, the degree to which these tasks are mastered in ways that complement the individual's changed circumstances and enhance the efficacy with which they conduct transactions with their environment is an indicator of adaptive success in its own right rather than being only indirectly important, as they influence cognitive appraisal and the experience of stress.

A second example: Few variables in life events research have received as much attention as social support. From a stress viewpoint, as noted in preceding sections of this chapter, social support is often conceptualized moderator or buffers the effects of stress. Significant, yet ofttimes weak, improvements in the degree to which life events predict dysfunction that occur when social support is considered as a factor are the primary source of evidence for these arguments (Barrerra, Sandler, & Ramsey, 1981; Sandler & Lakey, 1982; Wilcox, 1981). However, these studies have tended to overlook the fact that social support does not remain static as an individual goes through a transition. From a transitional events perspective however, individuals going through major life change face the task of reorganizing and reconstructing their social networks and social support. The degree of difficulty of this task may be influenced by the nature of the changes the individual is experiencing and the environmental context in which the changes are taking place. Similarly, personal factors such as problem-solving abilities and social skills may also have some bearing on and resolution of this task. Thus, while the quality and quantity of the social support available to an individual may influence adjustive outcomes, so too may the individual's levels of adjustment and functioning influence the type and extent of support received. From this perspective it may be seen that the consistent associations found between adjustment following life events and level of social support may, at least in part, be accounted for by the fact that social support levels can be viewed as another index of "outcome." Similarly, as recent work on depression makes clear (Doerfler & Chaplin, 1985) poorer adjustment may make the task of obtaining new sources of support more difficult. Thus, the relationship found between adjustment and social support that have been interpreted as supporting a "buffering" hypothesis (i.e., more social support following life events leading to lower levels of depression) may be seen as also supporting an alternative "main effect" explanation. That is, that level of adjustment prior to and following a life change may directly influence the level of support an individual receives. This is not to deny that social support may have important stress-reducing and protective features. Rather it is merely to make clear that the relationship between social support and adjustment found for individuals who are experiencing life events is a reciprocal one, with at least part of the shared variance stemming from assessing the same factor, that is, the adequacy of the individual's coping skills and/or level of social adjustment.

Implications for Preventive Intervention

Once the various models are specified and their differences highlighted we can see that the adoption of one perspective over another may lead to perhaps equally valid but quite different intervention efforts. Moreover, as should by now be clear, the criteria that may be appropriate for use in the evaluation of a program based on one model may be far less appropriate for use in evaluation of one derived from a different stance. In the ambiguity that has surrounded the usage of these terms, this is a point that has been generally overlooked. Nevertheless, this issue is essential for developing and refining our intervention efforts. Now to some brief specifics on these issues.

Intervention based on crisis theory should have as its targets those individuals who identify themselves as "in crisis," since a priori identification of such individuals is not, as we have seen, possible based merely on the knowledge of an individual's having experienced a particular event. Of course, one caveat here is that there may be a few situations that are sufficiently traumatic and disruptive (e.g., the loss of a loved one) for which the "base rate" occurrence of crisis reactions that follow them is sufficiently high as to warrant crisis intervention programs being targeted to them. Interventions based on a crisis model would have as their primary point of intervention the individual rather than the environment. A major program goal that derives directly from this model and is appropriate to it is the restoration of homeostatic equilibrium in the organization of the individual's personality structure at a level equal to or better than that prior to their experience of the crisis. The primary mechanism for achieving such outcomes would be the affective resolution of the upset, anxiety, and turmoil that characterize crises. The optimal duration of a crisis intervention is quite clearly delineated by crisis theory as ranging from one to eight weeks. Although evaluations of crisis program effects may concern themselves with changes in the behavior of the person, if we are to remain consistent with the overall model then such changes should only be viewed as secondary outcome criteria with the primary emphasis being on the internal well-being and affective state of the person.

Interventions based on stressful life events conceptualizations of the adaptive significance of life events may be targeted at individuals experiencing life events or stressors that have been identified through epidemiological procedures to be associated with heightened risk for the development of emotional or physical disorder. The primary focus of intervention efforts based on stress models is, as for crisis-based efforts, the management of the person's affective state. Behavioral shifts associated with stressful events again are seen as secondary outcomes that result from the failure to adequately manage the "stress." The central goal of the intervention from this perspective would be the enhancement of the individual's ability to cope with the stress precipitant and on factors that influence the appraisal of the situation. For the sake of clarity we should note here that we are adopting a definition of coping which comes from the Lazarus group. That is, "Problem-oriented coping involves efforts to deal with the source of stress, whether by changing one's own problem-maintaining behavior or by changing environmental circumstances. Emotion regulation involves coping efforts aimed at reducing emotional distress and maintaining a satsifactory internal (i.e., hormonal) state for processing information and actions" (Coyne & Holroyd, 1982, p. 109). Generally, given the circumscribed event notion embodied by this model, interventions would be fairly short term and administered in a single set of sessions that occurred fairly close together in time. Some program efforts may be aimed at modifying the environment in ways that increase their coping abilities or influence their appraisal of the event (e.g., increasing the level and availability of social support). However, even when such steps are taken the predominant emphasis is the alteration of those processes occurring in the individual. Appropriate outcome measures for programs based on this model are ones concerned with shifts in subjectively perceived stress, physiological arousal, and the development of new cases or symptoms of emotional or physical disorder.

A transitional life events perspective views as potentially important intervention "targets" all individuals confronting major life changes whether the changes are positive and desirable or negative and undesirable. The primary goal is not, as in the prior models, on the management of affective states of the individual but on enhancing the adequacy with which certain adaptive tasks that are major elements of the transitional process are mastered. Internal states, key component of person-environment transitions, and environmental conditions are all seen to require active restructuring or shaping during such transitions, and both the person's problem-solving and/or coping abilities as well as characteristics of the environment in which the transition is taking place may be critical for influencing the efficacy with which the tasks are mastered. Thus, interventions may be person focused, aimed at enhancing the skills and competencies of the individual, as in training for entering a new school or becoming a parent, or as in more generic transitions training for helping individual's identify tasks and develop problem-solving solutions in a wide array of situations. Interventions may also be environmentally focused. Indeed, this framework may have the most direct implications for facilitating the design and implementation of environment-focused interventions. Here, elements of the environment that may facilitate the individual's efforts to master the task confronting them may be modified to reduce the difficulty of the tasks and, in so doing, decrease the "threshold level of competency" necessary for mastering. Such actions would result in an increase in the number of individuals who are able to adequately adapt to transitions without special help (e.g., reducing flux in the environment confronted by adolescents making the transition to high school; Felner et al., 1982) and reduce the need for individually focused intervention efforts. Appropriate outcome measures for interventions guided by this framework would focus on the adequacy of the individual's general adaptation and well-being as well as the adequacy with which the major adaptive tasks have been dealt with. Stress still plays a role in this process but now it is seen to arise from difficulties the individual experiences in mastering the adaptive tasks and changes they confront. The level of proximal stressors and hassles experienced by the individual are seen to result directly from this process. The duration of interventions aimed at facilitating adaptation to a transition from this model may be significantly longer than those that derive from the prior models, since different tasks may arise at different points in the transition, the same task may be different in form and degree later in the process than it was earlier, or it may require continued attention throughout. Further, given the emphasis on the additional changes and stressors that may result from the transitional event and, depending on the specific concerns of the intervention agent, the length and form of the intervention may also be influenced by these factors. Indeed, it might well be the case that we would want to develop programs which intervened at several points in the process with temporal gaps between them.

CONCLUDING COMMENTS

Clearly, the preceding models are in no way mutually exclusive and may in fact be employed in a complementary fashion to shape intervention efforts. For example, we might want to do crisis intervention with an individual who has experienced a traumatic life event, follow it with stress management procedures to keep the person from again lapsing into crisis while the person is trying to deal with the changes in his or her life precipitated by the event, and attempt training in problem-solving or environmental modifications to enhance the person's ability to develop adaptive solutions to these changes and tasks. Such an intervention would provide a comprehensive program dealing with the full range of affective, cognitive, and behavioral concerns. What is important to recognize is that each different model leads to quite different conceptualizations of the issues of concern, what is to be dealt with, and how it may be done. Clear, intentional, and systematic use of these positions either singly or in combination may prove valuable both for the design of intervention strategies as a means of further clarifying the strength and limitations of each, and for facilitating the development of a knowledge base for prevention. Application and overlapping of these concepts and the models they represent without such systematic attention may, however, result in a failure to make progress in the development of effective intervention efforts for individuals experiencing crises, stress, or transitions, and, ultimately may reduce the utility of any of these concepts to the point where statements such as "the term of life crisis is hardly a theoretical concept or indeed even a term with any precise empirical reference" (Proshansky, Nelson-Shulman, & Kaminoff, 1979) may be accurately applied to all of them. As we hope we have demonstrated this statement is not yet true for either the term "life crisis," or for the terms "stressful life events" or "transitional events." From the foregoing it seems as if the maintenance they derive may serve us well in the pursuit of models to inform and guide preventive efforts. We hope that this chapter has served both to reduce some of the ambiguity that has surrounded them and to help to achieve prevention's goals.

REFERENCES

Appley, M. H., & Trumbull, R. (1967). On the concept of psychological stress. In M. H. Appley & R. Trumbull (Eds.), *Psychological stress.* New York: Appleton.

Barrerra, M., Sandler, I. N., & Ramsey, T. B. (1981). Preliminary development of a scale of social support: Studies on college students. *American Journal of Community Psychology, 9*, 435–448.

Bloom, B. L. (1975). *Community mental health: A general introduction.* Monterey, CA: Brooks/Cole.

Bloom, B. L. (1979). Prevention of mental disorders: Recent advances in theory and practice. *Community Mental Health Journal, 15,* 179–191.

Brown, G. W., & Harris, T. (1978). *Social origins of depression.* New York: Free Press.

Brown, G. W., Sklair, F., Harris, T. O., & Birley, J. L. T. (1973). Life-events and psychiatric disorder (Part I): Some methodological issues. *Psychological Medicine, 3,* 74–87.

Callahan, E. J., & McCluskey, K. A. (1983). *Life-span developmental psychology: Nonnormative life events.* New York: Academic Press.

Cannon, W. B. (1929). *Bodily changes in pain, hunger, fear, and rage.* New York: D. Appleton and Co.

Caplan, G. (1964). *Principles of preventive psychiatry.* New York: Basic Books.

Caplan, R. D., & Killilea, M. (Eds.), (1976). *Support systems and marital help: Multidisciplinary explorations.* New York: Grune & Stratton.

Chiroboga, D. A., & Dean, H. (1978). *Journal of Psychosomatic Research, 22,* 47–55.

Cobb, S. (1976). Social support as a moderator of life stress. *Psychosomatic Medicine, 38,* 300–313.

Coddington, R. D. (1972). The significance of life events as etiological factors in the disease of children. A survey of professional workers. *Journal of Psychosomatic Research, 16,* 7–18.

Cowan, C., & Cowan, P. (1981). Becoming a family: Couple relationships during family formation. Symposium presented at the American Psychological Association Meeting, Los Angeles, CA.

Cowan, C., & Cowan, P. (1983). Individual and couple satisfaction during family formation: A longitudinal study. Symposium presented at the American Psychological Association Meeting, Anaheim, CA.

Coyne, J., & Holroyd, K. (1982). Stress, coping and illness: A transactional perspective. In T. Millon, C. Green, & R. Meagner (Eds.), *Handbook of clinical health psychology* (pp. 103–126). New York: Plenum.

Darbonne, A. R. (1967). Crises: A review of theory, practice, and research. *Psychotherapy: Theory, Research and Practice, 4,* 49–56.

Datan, N., & Ginsberg, L. H. (Eds.), (1975). *Life-span developmental psychology: Normative life crises.* New York: Academic Press.

de Araujo, G., Van Arsdel, P. P., Holmes, T. H., & Dudley, D. L. (1973). Life change, coping ability and chronic intrinsic asthma. *Journal of Psychosomatic Research, 17,* 359–363.

DeLongis, A., Coyne, J. C., Dakof, G., Folkman, S., & Lazarus, R. S. (1982). Relationships of hassles, uplifts, and major life events to health status. *Health Psychology, 1,* 119–136.

Doerfler, L. A., & Chaplin, W. F. (1985). Type III error in research on interpersonal models of depression. *Journal of Abnormal Psychology, 9,* 227–230.

Dohrenwend, B. P. (1979). Stressful life events and psychopathology: Some issues of theory and method. In J. E. Barrett (Ed.), *Stress and mental disorder.* New York: Raven Press.

Dohrenwend, B. S., & Dohrenwend, B. P. (1978). Some issues in research on stressful life events. *Journal of Nervous and Mental Disease, 166,* 7–15.

Dohrenwend, B. S., & Dohrenwend, B. P. (1984). Life stress and illness: Formulations of the issues. In B. S. Dohrenwend & B. P. Dohrenwend (Eds.), *Stressful life events and their contexts* (pp. 1–27). New Brunswick, NJ: Rutgers University Press.

Dohrenwend, B. S., & Dohrenwend, B. P., Dodson, M., & Shrout, P. E. (1984). Symptoms, hassles, social supports and life events: Problem of confounded measures. *Journal of Abnormal Psychology, 93,* 222–230.

Dohrenwend, B. S., Krasnoff, L., Askenasy, A. R., & Dohrenwend, B. P. (1978). Exemplification of a method for scaling life events: The PERI life events scale. *Journal of Health & Social Behavior, 19,* 205–229.

Dohrenwend, B. S., Martin, J. L. (1979). Personal versus intentional determination of anticipation and control of occurrence of stressful life events. *American Journal of Community Psychology, 7,* 453–468.

Erikson, E. H. (1959). Identity and the life cycle. *Psychological Issues Monographs, 1.* New York: International Universities Press.

Felner, R. D. (1985). Vulnerability in childhood: A preventive framework for understanding children's efforts to cope with life stress and transitions. In M. C. Roberts and L. Peterson (Eds.), *Prevention of problems in childhood: Psychological research and applications.* New York: Wiley-Interscience.

Felner, R. D., Farber, S. S., & Primavera, J. (1980). *Transitions and stressful life events: A model for primary prevention.* In R. H. Price, R. F. Ketterer, B. C. Bader, & J. Monahan (Eds.), Prevention in mental health: Research, policy and practice. Beverly Hills, CA: Sage Publications.

Felner, R. D., Ginter, M. A., & Primavera, J. (1982). Primary prevention during school transitions: Social support and environmental structure. *American Journal of Community Psychology, 10,* 227–290.

Felner, R. D., Jason, L. A., Moritsugu, J. N., & Farber, S. S. (1983). Preventive psychology: Evolution and current status. In R. D. Felner, L. A. Jason, J. N. Moritsugu, & S. S. Farber (Eds.), *Preventive Psychology: Theory, research & practice* (pp. 3–10). New York: Pergamon.

Felner, R. D., Primavera, J., & Cauce, A. M. (1981). The impact of school transitions: A focus for preventive efforts. *American Journal of Community Psychology, 9,* 449–459.

Felner, R. D., Stolberg, A. L., & Cowen, E. L. (1975). Crisis events and school mental health referral patterns of young children. *Journal of Consulting and Clinical Psychology, 43,* 302–310.

Gersten, J. C., Langner, T. S., Eisenberg, J. G., & Orzeck, L. (1974). Child behavior and life events: Undesirable change or changes per se. In B. S. Dohrenwend & B. P. Dohrenwend (Eds.), *Stressful life events: Their nature and effects* (pp. 159–170). New York: Wiley.

Golan, N. (1981). *Passing through transitions: A guide for practioners.* New York: Free Press.

Gottesman, D., & Lewis, M. (1982). Differences in crisis reactions among cancer and surgery patients. *Journal of Consulting and Clinical Psychology, 3,* 381–388.

Hamberg, D., & Adams, J. (1967). A perspective on coping behavior: Seeking and utilizing information in major transitions. *Archives of General Psychiatry, 17,* 277–284.

Hetherington, E. (1979). Divorce: A child's perspective. *American Psychologist, 34,* 851–858.

Holmes, T. H., & Rahe, R. H. (1967). The social readjustment rating scale. *Journal of Psychosomatic Research, 11,* 213–218.

Hough, R. L., Fairbank, D. T., & Garcia, A. M. (1976). Problems in the ratio measurement of life stress. *Journal of Health and Social Behavior, 17,* 70–82.

Hurst, M. W. (1979). Life changes and psychiatric symptom development: Issues of content, scoring, and clustering. In J. E. Barrett (Ed.), *Stress and mental order.* New York: Raven Press.

Johnson, J. H. (1982). Life events as stressors in childhood and adolescence. In B. B. Lahey & A. E. Kazdin (Eds.), *Advances in clinical child psychology.* New York: Plenum.

Johnson, J. H., & Sarason, I. G. (1978). Life stress, depression and anxiety: Internal and external locus of control as a moderator variable. *Journal of Psychosomatic Research, 22,* 205–208.

Kanner, A. D., Coyne, J. C., Schaefer, C., & Lazarus, R. S. (1981). Comparisons of two models of stress measurement: Daily hassles and uplifts versus major life events. *Journal of Behavioral Medicine, 4,* 1–39.

Klein, D. C., & Lindemann, E. (1961). Preventive intervention in individual and family crisis situations. In G. Caplan (Ed.), *Prevention of mental disorders in children.* New York: Basic Books.

Komaroff, A. L., Masuda, M., & Holmes, T. H. (1968). The social readjustment rating scale: A comparative study of Negro, Mexican, and White Americans. *Journal of Psychosomatic Research, 12,* 121–128.

Lazarus, R. S., & Folkman, S. (1984). *Stress, appraisal and coping.* New York: Springer.

Lewinsohn, P. M. (1974). A behavioral approach to depression. In R. M. Friedman & M. M. Katz (Eds.), *The psychology of depression: Contemporary theory and research.* Washington, DC: Winston-Wiley.

Lewinsohn, P. M. (1975). *The unpleasant events schedule.* Unpublished manuscript, University of Oregon.

Lewinsohn, P. M., & Libet, J. (1972). Pleasant events, activity schedules, and depression. *Journal of Abnormal Psychology, 79,* 291–295.

Lewinsohn, P. M., & Talkington, J. (1979). Studies of the measurement of unpleasant events and relations. *Applied Psychological Measurement, 3,* 83–101.

Lewis, M. S., Gottesman, D., & Gutstein, S. (1979). The course and duration of crisis. *Journal of Consulting and Clinical Psychology, 47,* 128–134.

Lin, N., Dean, A., & Ensel, W. M. (1981). Social support scales: A methodological note. *Schizophrenia Bulletin, 7,* 73–87.

Lindemann, E. (1944). Symptomatology and management of acute grief. *American Journal of Psychiatry, 101,* 141–148.

Lindemann, E. (1956). The meaning of crisis in individual and family living. *Teachers College Record, 57,* 310–315.

Lindemann, E. (1979). Beyond grief: Studies in crisis intervention. New York: Jason Aronson.

Lindemann, E., & Cobb, S. (1943). Neuropsychiatric observations after the Coconut Grove fire. *Annals of Surgery, 117,* 814–824.

MacPhillamy, D., & Lewinsohn, P. M. (1971). *The pleasant events schedule.* Unpublished manuscript, University of Oregon.

Masuda, M., & Holmes, T. H. (1967). The social readjustment rating scale: A cross-cultural study of Japanese and Americans. *Journal of Psychosomatic Research, 11,* 221–237.

Meyer, A. (1951). The life chart and obligation of specifying positive data in psychopathological diagnosis. In E. E. Winters (Ed.), *The collected papers of Adolf Meter: Vol. III. Medical teaching* (pp. 52–56). Baltimore: Johns Hopkins University Press.

Miller, P. M., Ingram, J. G., & Davidson, S. (1976). Life events, symptoms and social support. *Journal of Psychosomatic Resarch, 20,* 515–522.

Monaghan, J. H., Robinson, J. O., & Dodge, J. A. (1979). The Children's Life Events Inventory. *Journal of Psychosomatic Research, 23,* 63–68.

Monroe, S. M. (1982). Life events assessment: Current practices, emerging trends. *Clinical Psychology Review, 2,* 435–454.

Morley, W. (1964). Treatment of the patient in crisis. Unpublished manuscript, Los Angeles Psychiatric Service.

Neufeld, R. J. (1982). *Psychological stress and psychopathology.* New York: McGraw-Hill.

Parad, H. J., & Caplan, G. (1965). A framework for studying families in crisis. In H. J. Parad (Ed.), *Crisis intervention: Selected readings* (pp. 53–72). New York: Family Service Association of America.

Parkes, C. M. (1971). Psycho-social transactions: A field for study. *Social Science and Medicine, 5,* 101–115.

Paykel, E. S. (1974). Life stress and psychiatric disorder: Applications of the clinical approach. In B. S. Dohrenwend & B. P. Dohrenwend (Eds.), *Stressful life events: Their nature and effects* (pp. 136–150). New York: Wiley.

Pearlin, L. I., Menaghan, E. G., Lieberman, M. A., & Mullen, J. T. (1981). The stress process. *Journal of Health and Social Behavior, 22,* 337–356.

Perkins, D. V. (1982). The assessment of stress using life events scales. In L. Goldberger & S. Breznitz (Eds.), *Handbook of stress* (pp. 320–331). New York: Free Press.

Proshansky, H. M., Nelson-Shulman, Y., & Kaminoff, R. D. (1979). The role of physical settings in life-crisis experiences. In I. G. Sarason & C. D. Spielberger (Eds.), *Stress and anxiety, Vol. 6* (pp. 3–26). Washington, DC: Hemisphere.

Rabkin, J. G., & Struening, E. L. (1976). Life events, stress, and illness. *Science, 194,* 1013–1020.

Rahe, R. H., Mahan, J. L., & Arthur, R. J. (1979). Prediction of near-future health changes from subjects preceding life changes. *Journal of Psychosomatic Research, 14,* 401–406.

Rapoport, L. (1965a). The state of crisis: Some theoretical considerations. In H. J. Parad (Ed.), *Crisis intervention. Selected readings* (pp. 23–31). New York: Family Service Association of America.

Rapoport, L. (1965b). Working with families in crisis: An exploration in preventive intervention. In H. J. Parad (Ed.), *Crisis intervention. Selected readings* (pp. 129–139). New York: Family Service Association of America.

Sameroff, A. J. (1983). Developmental systems: Contexts and evolution. In P. H. Mussen (Ed.), Handbook of child psychology (4th ed.). Volume I. W. Kessen (Ed.), *History, theory and methods* (pp. 237–294). New York: Wiley.

Sandler, I. N., & Lakey, B. (1982). Locus of control as a stress moderator: The role of control perceptions and social support. *American Journal of Community Psychology, 10,* 65–81.

Sarason, I. G., Johnson, J. H., & Siegel, J. M. (1978). Assessing the impact of life changes: Development of the Life Experiences Survey. *Journal of Consulting and Clinical Psychology, 46,* 932–46.

Sarason, S. B. (1981). *Psychology misdirected.* New York: Free Press.

Selye, H. (1978). *The stress of life* (2nd ed.). New York: McGraw-Hill.

Stein, K. A. (1970). A challenge to the role of the crisis concept in emergency psychotherapy. *Dissertation Abstracts International, 30,* 5045B.

Stone, A. A., & Neale, J. M. (1982). Development of a methodology for assessing daily experiences. In A. Baum & J. Singer (Eds.), *Advances in environmental psychology: Environment and health* (Vol. 4, pp. 49–83). Hillsdale, NJ: Erlbaum.

Stone, A. A., & Neale, J. M. (1984). The effects of "severe" daily events on mood. *Journal of Personality and Social Psychology, 46,* 137–144.

Taplin, J. R. (1971). Crisis theory: Critique and reformulation. *Community Mental Health Journal, 7,* 13–23.

Tyhurst, J. S. (1958). The role of transition states–including disaster–in mental illness. *Symposium on Preventive and Social Psychiatry.* Washington, DC: U. S. Government Printing Office.

Vinokur, A., & Selzer, M. L. (1975). Desirable versus undesirable life events: The relationship to stress and mental distress. *Journal of Personality and Social Psychology, 32,* 329–337.

Waldfogel, S., & Gardner, G. E. (1961). Intervention in crises as a method of primary prevention. In G. Caplan (Ed.), *Prevention of mental disorders in children.* New York: Basic Books.

Wilcox, B. L. (1981). Social support, life stress, and psychological adjustments: A test of the buffering hypothesis. *American Journal of Community Psychology, 9,* 371–386.

Wolchik, S. A., Fogas, B. S., & Sandler, I. N. (in press). Environmental change and children of divorce. In J. H. Hamphrey (Ed.), *Stress in childhood.* New York: AMS Press.

Zautra, A., & Simons, L. S. (1979). Some effects of positive life events on individual and community mental health. *American Journal of Community Psychology.*

Zimmerman, M. (1983). Methodological issues in the assessment of life events: A review of issues and research. *Clinical Psychology Review, 3,* 339–370.

3

Significant Events of Children of Divorce

Toward the Assessment of Risky Situations

Irwin N. Sandler, Sharlene A. Wolchik, Sanford L. Braver,
and Bruce S. Fogas
Arizona State University

In order to plan interventions that prevent psychological disorder, it is useful to know (1) what factors increase people's risk for disorder and (2) the processes by which these factors lead to disorder. Often risk factors are identified as difficult life situations (e.g., poverty, family disruption) on the basis of an empirical association between the situation and disorder. The next step is rarely taken: carefully assessing what occurs in these risky situations and how these occurrences impact on the development of disorder. The problem of assessment of risky situations is the subject of this chapter.

In the first section we briefly examine those risk factors consistently associated with psychological disorder for children. This will be followed by a discussion of a framework in which risk factors are conceptualized as life situations in which multiple specific stressful events occur to children. We will then discuss the conceptual and methodological issues involved in identifying those stress events. Implementation of this approach will then be illustrated using research we are conducting on the significant events that happen to children following the divorce of their parents. More specifically, the development of a life events schedule for children of divorce will be discussed and research addressing such questions as the relation between the frequency of occurrence of specific events and age, gender, income level, and time since separation will be presented.

HIGH RISK SITUATIONS AND LIFE EVENTS RESEARCH

Situations Associated with Increased Mental Health Risk for Children

Although the primary focus of child psychiatric epidemiological research to date has been to establish the prevalence rates for various disorders, several studies have also identified factors related to higher rates of disorder. Links (1983) reviewed community survey research in this area and identified the risk factors that

Support for this research was provided by a grant from the National Institute of Mental Health (#1R03MH38474-01) awarded to the first three authors. Partial support for writing the manuscript was also awarded by a Preventive Intervention Research Center grant (#1P50MH39246-01) from the Center for Prevention Research at NIMH.

have consistently been associated with psychological disorder for children. We will focus on the particular risk factors that involve situations to which the child is exposed, rather than unmodifiable characteristics of the children per se, such as age or gender.

The two situational risk factors cited by Links (1983) that have been most studied by researchers are socioeconomic status and family instability, including marital separations and broken homes. Ten studies were reported that examined socioeconomic status (SES). In five of those studies researchers found a significant relation between SES and pathology, while in five others no significant relation was found. There is more consistent evidence concerning the relation between the group of variables included as family instability and child psychopathology. Eight of ten studies found a significant relationship between family instability and deviance, while two failed to obtain this relationship.

Other variables cited by Links (1983) include large family size, poorly educated mothers, crowded living conditions, and parental psychiatric or physical illness. Large families was found to be significantly correlated with pathology in five of eight studies, poorly educated mothers was related in two of four studies, crowded living conditions in three of three studies, and parental illness in three of four studies. Upon examination of this last set of variables, one can easily see the potential overlap with SES and family instability, so that identifying the independent contribution of any one variable is complicated.

Along with family and demographic variables some researchers have also examined school variables. Douglas, Ross, and Simpson (1968) and Shepherd, Oppenheim, and Mitchell (1971) have documented the relationship between school progress and psychological deviance. Rutter et al. (1975) identified several school variables that have been associated with higher rates of psychological disorder (e.g., pupil turnover, teacher turnover, absenteeism, pupil/staff ratio).

Significant Events of High Risk Situations

Although the epidemiological evidence consistently points to the association of several risk situations with psychological disorders in children, it tells us little about how these situations lead to disorder. One's approach to this question depends on the model of development employed. Sameroff and Seifer (1983) propose an active transactional model in which "both the child and the environment are seen as actively engaged with each other, changing while being changed by their interactions" (p. 1264). One important implication of this model is that research on the development of disorder requires sophisticated assessment both of the individual characteristics of the child and the impacting social environment.

In epidemiological research, risk is usually assessed as a broad category such as poverty, psychiatrically ill parent, or family conflict, for example. These categories represent situations that may include a range of experiences that impact on the child. For example, the Rochester Longitudinal Study finds that the risk factor of maternal schizophrenia often overlaps with an environment that is low social status, and in which the parent is incompetent and impaired in her performance of life tasks. Furthermore, the life conditions that this creates for the children are similar to those experienced by children whose parents have other psychiatric diagnoses (depression, personality disorders), and these conditions are better predictors of child impairment than parent diagnosis per se (Sameroff & Seifer, 1983).

Researchers in the area of parental separation/divorce (Felner, Farber, & Prima-vera, 1980; Hetherington, 1979; Kurdek, 1981) have pointed out that this life transition needs to be considered a series of experiences involving changes in relationships between child and parents, between the parents, in the physical environment, in economic conditions, and so on. Furthermore, there is evidence that the effect of parental divorce/separation on children is significantly affected by which of these changes occur (e.g., Hetherington, Cox, & Cox, 1978).

Two studies have examined the cumulative effect of such changes on the child's functioning. Stolberg and Anker (1984) examined the changes in family income, time spent with father, time spent with mother, and residence subsequent to separation. High scores on this scale were associated with perceptions of being less able to control one's world. Kurdek and Blisk (1983) also studied the relationship between child adjustment and changes in the following areas: number of people living in the home, monthly income, hours each parent spends with the child, waking hours each parent spends in the home where the child lives, and monthly rent or mortgage. High levels of change were related to children's social and psychological maladjustment. While these studies are promising, they are limited because very few environmental changes were assessed and we cannot determine whether the assessed changes are indeed the most significant experiences for children of divorce.

One research methodology that may be helpful to obtain a more thorough assessment of the high risk social environment is life events methodology. This methodology was first developed by Holmes and Rahe (1967) to assess events that cause significant changes in people's lives. It was proposed that such life changes caused individual stress, an excess of which caused a wide range of psychological and physical disorders. Thus, for example, divorce, parental death, and moving are significant events because they mark major changes in people's lives.

These major life change events are sometimes contrasted with the ongoing life situations that are described by social risk factors such as poverty, marital disharmony, and so on. The risk factors are seen as continuous situations (e.g., having a mentally ill parent) while life events are seen as temporally circumscribed occurrences (e.g., parent hospitalized for mental illness). Gersten, Langner, Eisen-berg, and Simcha-Fagan (1977) contrasted these two approaches in a five-year prospective longitudinal study of the development of psychological disorder in children ages 6 to 18. They posed the question of whether life change events make any incremental contributions to the prediction of the development of childhood disorder (over a 5-year period) after the effects of the ongoing stressful situations are accounted for. They found that life events did not add any meaningful con-tribution to the prediction of disorder and concluded that life changes do not add to our understanding of the etiology of disorder beyond our knowledge of the risky sociofamilial milieu per se. However, what do we know about these ongoing situations? What are the experiences that lead to psychological disorder for children with psychiatrically disturbed parents, divorcing parents, or conflicted homes? We propose that the life event methodology can be employed to study this question.

ASSESSING THE SIGNIFICANT EVENTS OF RISKY SITUATIONS

Steps in Assessing the Significant Events

In order to use life event methodology to study risky situations one must

1. Define what will be considered an event,
2. Identify a representative sample of events (which impact on children in the situations),
3. Develop a system to score the events so that their cumulative effect can be assessed,
4. Assess the psychometric properties of the event measures, and
5. Place the construct within a larger theoretical and ecological context so that the occurrence and effects of events can be predicted and understood.

In this paper these issues will be discussed as they were approached to develop a life event scale for children of divorce.

Definition of an Event

Surprisingly little attention has been explicitly paid to the issue of defining an event in the life events literature. This is in part reflected by the variety of terms used to refer to events: stressful life events, life change events, life experiences, and others (e.g., Holmes & Rahe, 1967; Sarason, Johnson, & Siegel 1978). Dohrenwend and Dohrenwend (1980) suggest that most definitions of events allude to one of three factors: (1) change in the life pattern of individuals for better or worse, (2) undesirability, or (3) upsettingness. Because of the central role of environmental change in the seminal work of Holmes and Rahe (1967) this concept is most often identified as the conceptually unique feature of life events. Actually, the life events literature is operationally inconsistent on whether change is a necessary condition of life events. It is not unusual for over 25 percent of the events on major life event scale to *not* specify change as an event property. On Holmes and Rahe's original 43-item scale, 8 of the items (18%) are not necessarily changes (e.g., trouble with in-laws, trouble with boss, minor violations of the law). Twelve of the 34 events used by Gersten et al. (1977) to assess life change events were not necessarily changes (e.g., sibling in trouble because of drugs, family had serious financial troubles). In Johnson and McCutcheon's (1980) newly developed child life event scale, 28 percent (13 out of 46) of the items do not specify change (e.g., special recognition for good grades, trouble with teachers, failing a grade). A further reason not to define events in terms of change per se is that despite considerable research there is sparse evidence that change is the property of events that leads to psychological or physical disorder (Zimmerman, 1983).

The major characteristic that has been proposed as an alternative to the change concept of life events is that of aversiveness (e.g., undesirability and upsettingness). Numerous studies report that it is primarily negative events and not positive events that have a stressful impact on people (Gersten, Langner, Eisenberg, & Orzek, 1974; Sandler & Block, 1979; Vinokur & Selzer, 1975). Thus it could be proposed that the focus of life events research be placed squarely on negative events.

There are good reasons, however, not to restrict life event scales in this way. Felner, Farber, and Primavera (1983) suggest the need to study positive as well as negative events in order to develop an empirical base for the development of prevention programs. They point out that prevention is interested in positive psychological development (e.g., development of cognitive and interpersonal competencies) as well as the reduction of adverse outcomes. Since there is evidence that positive events contribute to the development of competence and life satisfaction (Harter, 1982; Zautra & Sandler, 1983), they have implications for prevention.

For those who are solely interested in negative outcomes there is also empirical evidence that positive events are important. Two studies (Cohen & Hoberman, 1983; Reich & Zautra, 1981) report an interaction effect of positive and negative events on psychological symptomatology.

Since neither of the major defining characteristics of events are warranted, how should an event be defined? We propose that events be defined as objectively verifiable occurrences in an individual's environment or transactions between the individual and the environment of which the individual is aware and which have a significant impact on the individual. This definition excludes events that are primarily internal to the subject and that are not potentially verifiable by outside observers. The definition does not assume the mechanism by which good or bad outcomes are caused by events (e.g., change, aversiveness, etc.), but instead utilizes a response-based definition of stress in which events are identified because of their impact. The property of events that is responsible for the impact is an issue that can be addressed by different methods of scaling and analyzing event data as it relates to the outcomes of concern.

Sampling Life Events

The next step is to develop a representative sample of events for the risk situation. It is assumed that each situation is manifest via an identifiable population of events from which it is necessary to identify a representative sample. Dohrenwend, Krasnoff, Askenasy, and Dohrenwend (1978) have advocated generating events from those which occur to a random sample of subjects in the situation of concern. Although it is appealing, one practical shortcoming of this method is that it is expensive. Also, particularly when subjects are difficult to obtain (e.g., people in high risk situations such as divorce, death of a parent or spouse, child of a schizophrenic parent) this approach may not be practically feasible.

An alternative is to obtain event nominations from knowledgeable informants. These informants may include people who have experienced the situation themselves or people who have had close contact with and knowledge of the experiences of people in this situation. For example, if one were interested in significant events for the unemployed it would be appropriate to interview the unemployed themselves, their spouses, their friends, colleagues, union leaders, and mental health personnel who work with them. The purpose at this stage is to obtain as broad a list of events as possible, so informants should be asked to describe all the events they know of that have an important impact on the adjustment of people in this situation.

While it may not be feasible to obtain a random sample of nominees, it is important to avoid systematic biases in event nomination that could result from interviewing a restricted set of nominees. For example, the representativeness of the Holmes and Rahe SRE has been criticized because the items were derived from medical patients in the Seattle, Washington area. Knowledge of the nominee characteristics on which it is important to obtain heterogeneity will to a large extent be a function of one's understanding of the risk situation; however, it should usually be assumed that major demographic characteristics such as gender, age, and social class of the subject are important.

A final item sampling question is how to judge when a sufficient number of nominees have been queried and a sufficiently representative sample of events obtained. This question is particularly difficult because there is no objective way to identify the population of events. While it is not very precise, one useful criterion for making this judgment is a subjective judgment of redundancy, that the same events are being generated as previously and that additional sampling does not yield new events.

Scoring Events

The issue of how to score life event scales has two major components: (1) what dimensions or characteristics should be used to score the events, and (2) who should rate the events on these dimensions.

Numerous dimensions or characteristics of events have been identified in the life events literature, such as change, negativeness, positiveness, loss, entrance, meaningfulness, upsettingness, and control. The dimensions used to rate events have theoretical significance in that one can use the event score on a dimension to assess the amount of this kind of experience the individual has had and thereby study the effects of this kind of experience. For example, the issue of whether change or aversiveness is the critical stressful property of events has been argued using empirical evidence on the correlates of the scales score using these different scoring schemes (Gersten, Langner, Eisenberg, & Orzek, 1974; Vinokur & Selzer, 1975). While this theoretical controversy is still lively, the weight of evidence seems to be that a simple (unit-weighted) count of negative events yields the best predictor of psychological distress (Ross & Mirowsky, 1979) while both positive and negative events predict measures of satisfaction, although in opposite directions (Reich & Zautra, 1981). Life events scales provide considerable opportunity for the investigator to derive scores on different dimensions, and in light of the current limitations in our knowledge of what makes an event impactful (in either a positive or negative direction), the investigator has considerable latitude in the choice of event dimensions.

Two distinct approaches to the issue of who is to rate events are the nomothetic and idiographic approaches. The nomothetic approach uses the judgments of a group of subjects to derive normative event weightings on dimensions. Use of nomothetically derived weights avoids the use of the subject's own judgment of the event characteristics (Dohrenwend et al., 1978). Thus the confound between these judgments and subject's psychological state is avoided, an advantage that is particularly important in cross-sectional, correlational studies. The idiographic approach uses the subject's own rating of the event characteristics. The advantage of the idiographic approach is that it is consistent with most cognitive theories of stress (e.g., Lazarus & Launier, 1978) in which the individual's own appraisal of the stressor is viewed as the critical mediating step leading from the transaction (event) to the stress response. A third, less frequently used approach is to have trained independent judges rate the events based on a contextual knowledge of the person's life at the time the event occurs. Brown and Harris (1978) have argued for this approach and report that one particular event dimension "long term threat" accounts for the relationship between events and depression.

ASSESSING THE EVENTS OF PARENTAL DIVORCE

To illustrate the process of developing a life events schedule that includes the specific events occurring in risk situations, we will outline the steps we have taken in the development of the Divorce Events Schedule for Children.

Selection of Events

In order to obtain a representative list of significant event that happen to children of divorce, we used a group of knowledgeable informants. More specifically, approximately 40 children, 40 parents and 20 lawyers and psychologists involved in working with families in this life transition participated in this initial step. Subjects were asked to identify those events that they believed had a significant positive or negative impact on the lives of children of divorce. After the subjects had completed their lists the interviewer asked them to think about and to list additional events in each of the following areas: parent-child relationships, relationships with friends and relatives, changes in parents' lives, economic changes, and legal concerns. Approximately 210 events were nominated using this process. Although there was considerable overlap among the events nominated by professionals, parents, and children, a few items were mentioned only by one group. For example, only the children mentioned giving up a pet as a negative event.

The research team used this list to write nonoverlapping items that described the events in an unambiguous way. Inclusion of events was decided on the basis of the following criteria. First, the event could not involve a symptom of psychological disorder or physical problem. Thus, items such as "decrease in grades" or "worsening of relationships with Mom" were eliminated. This criterion was used to avoid confounding of events with outcomes of interest (e.g., mental health problems; Zimmerman, 1983). Second in a further effort to eliminate event outcome confounding, we attempted to only include events that were primarily beyond the child's control. This criterion was difficult to implement, however, and could not be completely accomplished. Since many critical post-divorce events involve transactions between the child and his/her environment, some of these items may reflect the response of the social environment to the child's behavior (e.g., "Mom gets mad at you or tells you that you're bad"). These items were retained because although their occurrence may be affected by the child they may also reflect important effects of the divorce on the child's environment. The final step involved pilot testing of the 62 items that resulted from discussion among the research staff. After administering the schedule to 10 children of divorce, we made several minor modifications in wording of items. The final items of the Divorce Events Schedule for Children (DES-C) are provided in Table 1.

Response Format

As discussed previously, most life events schedules include items tapping both occurrence of events and changes in the frequencies of events. In order to discriminate the occurrence of events from changes in the frequency of events, we developed a response format that included both kinds of information about events. First, we asked children if the event occurred within the past three months and second, whether this event happened more than, less than, or the same as usual during the past three months. That is, an event could occur, but this could be either an increase, decrease, or no change from the usual. Similarly, an event might not occur, and this could be either a decrease or no change from the usual. To obtain a measure of event desirability, we asked children to indicate whether the event was good or bad for them and to rate the degree of goodness or badness using a 7-point scale. This format will allow us to derive scores to examine the relation between adjustment and several different measures of events such as total positive change (e.g., increases in positive events and decreases in negative events), total negative change, total change, as well as total positive events, total negative events, and total events. In this chapter, however, we restrict our attention to the more traditional measure of events, the occurrence of positive and negative events within the past three months (whether or not the occurrence represents a change).

THE RELATION BETWEEN DIVORCE EVENTS, CHILD CHARACTERISTICS, AND ENVIRONMENTAL FACTORS

In this section are presented the results of a large-scale project that has focused on describing the postseparation experiences of children of divorce using the DES–C. Three major issues are addressed. The first concerns assessment of the stability of scores on the DES–C. More specifically, test-retest reliabilities were computed at the individual item level and for summary scores (occurrence of positive events, occurrence of negative events). Although reliability of life-events schedules has rarely been examined, recently researchers have argued convincingly that more attention needs to be given to basic measurement properties of these checklists (e.g., Neugebauer, 1981).

The second issue involves the relation between child characteristics and the events experienced during the process of divorce. Several previous investigators have demonstrated that age of the child is significantly related to divorce adjustment (Kelly & Wallerstein, 1976; Kurdek & Berg, 1983; Kurdek, Blisk, & Siesky, 1981; Wallerstein & Kelly, 1974, 1975, 1980), with older children exhibiting better adjustment. Possible explanations for this developmental effect include: the influence of age-related variables such as internal locus of control and interpersonal reasoning (Kurdek et al., 1981; Kurdek & Berg, 1983), differences in the quality or amount of supportive extrafamilial relationships which may buffer the negative effects of divorce (Felner et al., 1980), and differences in the divorce experiences of older and younger children. We focus on this last factor and examine whether preadolescents (ages 8–11) experience different types of and amounts of events than adolescents (ages 12–15). Another child characteristic that is related to divorce adjustment is gender. Several researchers have shown that boys experience greater social, behavioral, and academic difficulties following parental divorce than girls (Guidubaldi, Cleminshaw, Perry, & Kehle, 1983; Hetherington et al., 1978; Kurdek & Berg, 1983; Wallerstein & Kelly, 1975). Such differential adjustment may be due to boys experiencing more stress during the divorce process (Hetherington, 1979), boys having smaller social support networks, or a combination of these factors. In the present chapter we examine whether the events that occur during the process of divorce differ for boys and girls.

Finally, the relation between two environmental factors and the occurrence of divorce events was examined. Because several studies have demonstrated that children's adjustment is related to decreased financial resources after divorce (e.g., Desimone-Luis, O'Mahoney, & Hunt, 1979; Hodges, Weschler, & Ballantine, 1979) and to time since separation (e.g., Hetherington et al., 1978), the relation between these two factors and divorce events was assessed.

Subjects

Subjects were 131 children from families where parental separation had occurred within the past 30 months. The sample included 53 percent girls and 47 percent boys. These children ranged in age from 8 to 15, and the average age was 11.6 years. Seventy-five percent of the sample were in maternal custody, 8.5 percent were in paternal custody, and the remainder were in joint custody arrangements. The incomes of the custodial or residential parents (reported income included child support) are distributed as follows: under $10,000: 18 percent; $10,000–$15,000: 26 percent, $15,000–$20,000: 18 percent; $20,000–$25,000: 17 percent; $25,000–over $50,000: 21 percent. Eighteen percent of the sample had experienced separation within the last 6 months, 21 percent within the last 12 months, 19 percent within the past 18 months, 26 percent within the last 24 months, and 16 percent within the last 30 months.

Procedure

Subjects were obtained from two sources, court records of requests for marital separation and responses to newspaper articles. Letters describing the study were mailed to several thousand people who had requested a marital separation within the prior two years. Follow-up contact phone calls were made in which an interview was requested with the custodial parent and a child between the ages of eight and fifteen. The child interview lasted 1½ hours and included measures of divorce-related stressful life events (DES-C), perceptions of divorce, psychological symptomatology and competence, and social support. The DES-C consisted of 62 items. For each item children reported whether the event occurred during the past three months, and whether the event was positive, negative, or neutral for them. Finally, if they reported that it was either positive or negative, they rated how good or bad the event was using a 7-point scale. As described previously they were also asked whether or not each event represented a change in their environment. The measures derived for this study were the reported frequency of occurrence of each event and summary scores of the total number of positive and negative events. The parents completed a questionnaire battery about their own divorce adjustment as well as their children's adjustment. A workshop about children's adjustment to divorce was provided for the parents as compensation for participating in the study.

74

Table 1 Frequency, Ratings, Reliability, and Distribution of Divorce Events for Children ($N = 131$)

Event	Frequency (%)	Percentage "good"	Nomothetic category[a]	Reliability	Gender[b]	Age[c]	Income[d]	Length of separation[e]
1. Mom and Dad differ in how they want you to be.	37	47	A	.26				
2. People in your neighborhood say bad things to you about your parents.	18	04	U	.83				
3. You have to do chores around the house.	95	73	A	.63				
4. Dad is unhappy.	52	07	U	.63				
5. Your friends tease you or are mean to you.	30	05	U	.85		Y > O		L > S
6. Dad does extra nice things for you, that you like.	71	97	D	.61			R > P	
7. Mom tells you that she doesn't like you spending time with Dad.	11	20	U	.71				
8. Mom is strict.	42	46	A	.23		Y > O	P > R	
9. You do fun things with Dad.	76	97	D	.91		Y > O	R > P	
10. You have to watch out for, or take care of, your brothers and sisters.	47	79	A	.78				L > S
11. Dad takes care of the things that need to get done for you.	65	95	D	.61				
12. Mom asks you questions about Dad's private life.	33	25	A	.67	F > M		R > P	
13. Dad says bad things about Mom.	26	03	U	.75				
14. Dad is strict.	34	47	A	.50			R > P	
15. Mom says bad things about Dad.	32	05	U	.43	F > M	O > Y		
16. You have free time to do things you like.	93	97	D	-.02				

17. Mom gets mad at you or tells you that you are bad.	64	40	A	.64			S > L
18. Mom and Dad argue in front of you.	34	02	U	.61			
19. Your relatives say bad things to you about your parents.	15	00	U	.64			
20. Dad asks you questions about Mom's private life.	22	03	U	.77	F > M		
21. You spend time with your Father's family.	60	89	D	.64		Y > O	R > P
22. Your NCP misses scheduled visits.	42	13	U	.40			
23. Mom does extra nice things for you, that you like.	77	99	D	.49			S > L
24. Household routines get done smoothly.	71	93	D	.30			
25. You do fun things with Mom.	89	98	D	-.07			
26. You get toys, clothes, and other things you like.	84	98	D				
27. Dad tells you not to tell some things to your Mom.	39	25	A	.51			
28. Dad tells you that he doesn't like you spending time with Mom.	04	00	U	.36			
29. Dad gets mad at you or tells you that you are bad.	40	28	A	.47		Y > O	
30. Mom takes care of the things that need to get done for you.	93	99	D	-.07			P > R
31. Mom tells you not to tell some things to your Dad.	43	39	A	.44			
32. You spend time with Mom.	95	98	D	-f			
33. You spend time with your Mother's family.	74	93	D	.82	F > M		
34. You get to see your old friends.	68	96	D	.61			

(See footnotes on Page 77)

Table 1 Frequency Ratings, Reliability, and Distribution of Divorce Events for Children (*N* = 131) (*Continued*)

Event	Frequency (%)	Percentage "good"	Nomothetic category[a]	Reliability	Gender[b]	Age[c]	Income[d]	Length of separation[e]
35. Dad tells you about things in his life, like problems or his feelings.	53	77	A				R > P	
36. Mom is unhappy.	66	07	U					
37. You are making new friends.	75	99	D					L > S
38. You spend time with Dad.	84	89	D				R > P	
39. You spend time alone, by yourself.	80	80	D	.36		O > Y		
40. You have to give up pets or other things that you like.	29	08	U	.25				
41. Mom tells you about things in her life, like problems or her feelings.	77	74	A	.37				
42. Mom or Dad talk to you about why they got divorced.	54	52	A	.34				S > L
43. Mom or Dad talk to you about which parent you want to live with.	38	38	A	.58				
44. Mom and Dad make you follow different rules while you are at their house.	48	61	A	.72				L > S
45. Your custodial parent works.	89	78	A	.53				
46. Your mother's boyfriend or husband tells you to do things.	28	68	A	.43				
47. Your parents hit each other or physically hurt each other.	04	00	U	.69				
48. Your father's girlfriend or wife tells you to do things.	29	47	A	.61				
49. Dad starts to go out on dates.	41	75	A	.64		Y > O		L > S
50. Dad remarries or has a girlfriend come live with him.	29	47	A	.76			P > R	
51. Dad or Mom told you the divorce was because of you.	03	00	U	-.02		O > Y		

				Reliability[f]	Age[c]	Income[d]	Separation[e]	Sex[b]
52. You change schools.	21	50	A	.87				
53. Mom remarries or has a boyfriend come live with her.	13	65	A	.61				
54. Dad gets a steady girlfriend.	39	63	A	.76	Y > O		L > S	
55. Mom gets a steady boyfriend.	28	80	D	.63			L > S	
56. Mom starts to go out on dates.	42	81	D	.56				
57. Your NCP moves out of town.	09	18	U	.85	Y > O	P > R		
58. Your brothers and sisters live in a different house than you.	19	24	A	.89				
59. You move to a new house.	18	65	A	.83			S > L	
60. You change which parent you live with.	03	40	A	–f				
61. You have to talk to a lawyer or judge.	01	1.00	A	–f				
62. New kids move into your house.	05	71	A	1.00				M > F

[a]A = Ambiguous events, D = Desirable events, U = Undesirable events.
[b]F = Female, M = Male.
[c]Y = Younger (8–11), O = Older (12–15).
[d]R = Richer (over $50,000), P = Poorer (under $10,000).
[e]L = Longer parental separation (25–30 months), S = Shorter parental separation (less than 6 months).
[f]Reliability could not be computed where there was no variance on one of the measures.

77

RESULTS

Table 1 presents the percentage of children endorsing the events as occurring during the past 3 months. As can be seen, these are generally not rare or unusual events, with the median frequency of occurrence in the past 3 months being 45 percent.

Of those children who had experienced the event the percent who said that it was a good event is reported. The results here are generally unsurprising, with children reporting that they do not like family conflict events or bad mouthing of their parents and that they do like doing things with their parents and being taken care of. One area where the children's reports are more positive than might be expected from the prior literature is events that involve the new romantic relationships of the parents. For the eight events in this area, the median percent to whom it occurred who rated it as a good event was 67 percent (range of 47% to 81%).

Events were categorized as being nomothetically positive or negative based on the ratings of children who reported that the event occurred to them. After the suggestion of Dohrenwend and Dohrenwend (1980), it was felt that the ratings of people who had actually experienced the event formed the most appropriate basis for event categorization. The criteria used to make this categorization were as follows. If 80 percent or more of the children reported that the event was either positive or negative, it was so categorized. In order to take into account the magnitude of positive or negative rating, the children's 7-point rating scale of positive or negative was used. The ratings were converted to a 15-point scale (7 points in both the positive and negative directions and zero as the neutral rating). If the mean magnitude rating was greater than one standard deviation away from the neutral point, the event was categorized in that direction. Finally, for one event that occurred to only two children (#61), the consensus judgment of the investigators was used to categorize the event as ambiguous in terms of valence. Using this approach, 16 of the 62 items were categorized as undesirable and 18 as desirable.

Test-retest reliability of the reports of each event was calculated as the correlation of event reports using the phi coefficient. An average of two weeks separated the two administrations of the interview. It should be noted that, since an average of two weeks elapsed between the reports and the period for which they reported was the past three months, one sixth of the reporting period was different. Thus, the correlations obtained are an underestimate of the stability of the children's reports. Nonetheless, the item reliabilities are seen as quite encouraging; median item phi coefficient = .61, range of 1.00 to −.07. The four items with near-zero reliability need to be rewritten. Our impression is that for several of these items children were reporting their current feelings about either their relationship with the mother (e.g., items 25 and 30) or their free time (item 16). Test-retest reliabilities were also computed for four summary scores that were calculated in accord with the traditional life event categories of positive and negative events. Nomothetic positive and negative event scores were calculated using the sums of the items so categorized that occurred to each child. Idiographic positive and negative event scores were calculated using the sums of events that occurred to the children and the children's own valence ratings. Test-retest reliability of these four scores was found to be quite satisfactory: idiographic negative $r(34) = .87$, idiographic positive $r(34) = .77$, nomothetic negative $r(34) = .85$, and nomothetic positive $r(34) = .65$.

Differences in the total number of positive and negative events across age and gender were examined using one-way analysis of variance. More negative events were reported by girls ($\overline{X} = 8.88$) than boys ($\overline{X} = 6.90$), $F(1, 129) = 5.13, p < .05$. The frequency of positive events did not differ across gender. Age effects did not occur for the frequency of positive or negative events.

The effects of length of parental separation and parental income on the summary scores for positive and negative events were assessed as the significance of the linear trend. The analysis for length of separation revealed no significant effects. The analysis of positive events revealed a significant linear trend, indicating that positive events increased with income level, F linear $(1,121) = 6.20, p < .05$. Negative events did not differ significantly across income level. All analyses were computed using both idiographically and nomothetically derived summary scores. Because the results of these anlayses were nearly identical, only those using the nomothetic scores are reported.

An item-by-item analysis of the differential occurrence of events was calculated using χ^2 for gender and age, and Kendall's Tau for income and length of separation. The results of the item analyses are presented in Table 1. Examining those variables where significant effects were obtained for the summary scores reveals an interesting finding for the income variable. Differences were obtained on 11 items for this variable, with the higher-income children reporting more frequent occurrence on seven of these. These seven items all involve contact with dad, usually of a positive nature. No clear pattern of differences emerged for the gender variable.

Although the summary scores for positive and negative events did not differ for time or age, differences were obtained for 11 items for each of these variables. It may be that child age and length of separation are associated with different types of events. For example, with longer separation more events involving a parent's romantic involvement seem to occur. Since these dimensions have not been clearly identified as of yet and because the large number of significance test results in considerable alpha inflation these results should be treated very cautiously.

Discussion and Future Directions

The data will be discussed in terms of (1) the psychometric adequacy of the life event measure, (2) the way in which the results contribute to our understanding of the effects of divorce on children, and (3) the theoretical context of the research and future research directions. Finally, we will return to the theme of which these data are simply a first-step illustration, and indicate how this type of study might be a part of a larger research program to understand the effects of high-risk situations.

From a psychometric point of view, the results are quite encouraging for the use of the scale. Life event measures have been criticized recently (Paykel, 1983) for their poor reliability and validity. It appears that these criticisms may be overly harsh. If items refer to a relatively recent time period (e.g., past three months), and are clearly worded and pretested, adequate reliability (even on a single-item basis) can be obtained. However, the current analyses are just a beginning. As mentioned above, our scoring system includes a rating of whether these events represent a change from the usual frequency of occurrence. Whether these change ratings can be made reliably is a question that needs to be addressed. Life event measures have also been criticized on the grounds that subject reports about events do not correspond to those of a knowledgeable informant (Stone & Neale, 1982). This question also needs to be addressed for the present scale.

The results shed light on children's experience of divorce from a descriptive point of view and raise some interesting questions about previous findings concerning mediators of the effects of divorce on children. Descriptively, it can be useful to observe the frequency of occurrence of events that are of special interest to the investigator. For example, one might select a subclass of events that previous evidence has highlighted as having quite a great deal of impact. For children of divorce, parent conflict has been found to negatively affect child adjustment (Hetherington, Cox, & Cox, 1981; Jacobson, 1978). Children's reports of the frequency of these type of items indicates that approximately 25 to 30 percent of the sample has recently experienced this type of stressor.

The finding that girls experience more negative divorce events than boys is intriguing in light of prior evidence that boys manifest more adjustment problems than girls do after divorce (Guidubaldi et al., 1983; Hetherington et al., 1981). One explanation of this apparent discrepancy is that girls may be more resistant to the effects of stress than are boys. Rutter (1979) proposes that this is the case, although there is little understanding of why this sex difference occurs. A second potential explanation of why boys show greater maladjustment despite girls experiencing greater stress is that girls manifest their distress differently than boys (Eme, 1979) and are not really less affected by the divorce. Hetherington (1972), for example, reports disturbance in relationships with males for female adolescents from divorced families. Boys, on the other hand, appear to express their distress through behaviors such as aggression and noncompliance (Hetherington et al., 1981). Another possible explanation is that girls may have larger and/or more supportive relationships, which may buffer the negative effects of divorce.

A second interesting finding is that household income (including child support) was related to those events that indicate greater involvement with father. Prior literature has reported that both higher income (Wallerstein & Kelly, 1980) and greater contact with father (Hess & Camara, 1979) are related to better child adjustment after divorce. The present finding that the two factors are interrelated leads to the observation that it may be very difficult to assess the effects of one independent of another. If we assume that the higher custodial parent income assessed here reflects the payment of child support, it is not surprising that such payment is associated with greater contact and positive experiences with the child. In that case, these results reaffirm the multiple benefits to the child of a well-functioning child support agreement between the divorced parents.

The life event methodology has been used most often within the context of a stress theoretical model of disorder (Dohrenwend, 1978). Within this model, stress events result in a transient state of distress, and the individual's coping with this distress is a function of his/her personal characteristics (e.g., abilities, beliefs, etc.) and the assistance he/she receives from others (i.e., social support). Investigations of the effects of life event stress on adjustment to risk situations needs to include assessment of each of these kinds of variables.

We, along with others (e.g., Felner et al., 1983), propose that stressful situations are often composed of multiple experiences. Rather than thinking of adjustment to a single stressor (e.g., divorce) therefore, it is more appropriate to think about the series of stressors that may occur as part of the divorce process. The occurrence of disturbance in such situations and the length of time it takes to adjust should reflect the cumulative impact of the multiple stress experiences. Thus, for example, the finding that the level of disturbance peaks one year after divorce and is reduced by two years (Hetherington et al., 1981) is probably in large part due to the kinds of experiences (positive and negative) that occur at those times.

SUMMARY

The central point of this paper is that there is a need for in-depth research on the life situations that epidemiological research has identified as putting children at risk for psychological disorder, and that life event methodology can be a useful tool in such research. Similar to Price (1982), we believe that the development of effective preventive interventions will require the following components: precisely defining the population at risk, specifying what the risk group is at risk for, and developing theories about both the processes through which the risk condition leads to psychological and physical disorders and about how the proposed interventions will modify these processes or the risky situation itself. A thorough understanding of the specific events occurring in a particular risky situation will provide an important part of the data base for theorizing about such mechanisms of action. The current chapter has illustrated a methodology for describing the multiple stressors of risky situations. Furthermore, as part of a larger research program one might identify those aspects of the situation that tend most to lead to disorder. This would be followed by experimental interventions that modify these aspects of the situation. These interventions will provide both an experimental test of the causal relationship and an assessment of the efficacy of preventive interventions.

REFERENCES

Brown, G. W., & Harris, T. (1978). *Social origins of depression.* New York: Free Press.

Cohen, S., & Hoberman, H. M. (1983). Positive events and social supports as buffers of life change stress. *Journal of Applied Psychology, 13,* 99–125.

Desimone-Luis, J., O'Mahoney, K., & Hunt, D. (1979). Children of separation and divorce: Factors influencing adjustment. *Journal of Divorce, 3,* 37–42.

Dohrenwend, B. S. (1978). Social stress and community psychology. *American Journal of Community Psychology, 6,* 1–15.

Dohrenwend, B. S., & Dohrenwend, B. P. (1980). What is a stressful life event? In L. H. Selye (Ed.), *Selye's guide to stress research* (Vol. 1). New York: Van Nostrand Reinhold.

Dohrenwend, B. S., Krasnoff, L., Askenasy, A. R., & Dohrenwend, B. P. (1978). Exemplification of a method for scaling life events: The PERI life events scale. *Journal of Health and Social Behavior, 19,* 205–229.

Douglas, J. W. B., Ross, J. M., & Simpson, H. R. (1968). *All our future.* London: Davies.

Eme, R. (1979). Sex differences in psychopathology: A review. *Psychological Bulletin, 86,* 574–595.

Felner, R. D., Farber, S. S., & Primavera, J. (1980). Children of divorce, stressful life events, and life transitions: A framework for preventative efforts. In R. H. Price, R. F. Ketterer, B. C. Bader & J. Monahan (Eds.), *Prevention in mental health: Research, policy and practice.* Beverly Hills, CA: Sage Publications.

Felner, R. D., Farber, S. S., & Primavera, T. (1983). Transitions and stressful life events: A model for primary prevention. In R. D. Felner, L. A. Tason, T. N. Moritsugu, & S. S. Farber (Eds.) *Preventive psychology: Theory, research and practice.* New York: Pergamon.

Gersten, J. C., Langner, T. S., Eisenberg, J. G., & Orzek, L. (1974). Child behavior and life events: Undesirable change or change per se. In B. S. Dohrenwend and B. P. Dohrenwend (Eds.), *Stressful life events: Their nature and effects*. New York: Wiley.

Gersten, J. C., Langner, T. S., Eisenberg, J. G., & Simcha-Fagan, O. (1977). An evaluation of the etiological role of stressful life-change events in psychological disorders. *Journal of Health and Social Behavior, 18,* 228–244.

Guidubaldi, J., Cleminshaw, H. K., Perry, J. D., & Kehle, T. J. (1983). *Factors affecting the adjustment of children from divorced families*. Paper presented at the annual conference of the American Psychological Association, Anaheim, CA.

Harter, S. (1982). A developmental perspective on some parameters of self-regulation in children. In P. Karoly & F. H. Kanfer (Eds.), *Self-management and behavior change: From theory to practice*. New York: Pergamon.

Hess, R. D., & Camara, K. A. (1979). Post-divorce family relationships as mediating factors in the consequences of divorce for children. *Journal of Social Issues, 35,* 79–96.

Hetherington, E. M. (1979). Divorce: A child's perspective. *American Psychologist, 34,* 851–858.

Hetherington, E. M., Cox, M., & Cox, R. (1978). The aftermath of divorce. In J. H. Steven, Jr., & M. Matthews (Eds.), *Mother-child, father-child relations*. Washington, DC: NAEYLC, 149–176.

Hetherington, E. M., Cox, M., & Cox, R. (1981). Effects of divorce on parents and children. In M. Lamb (Ed.), *Nontraditional families*. Hillsdale, NJ: Erlbaum

Hodges, W. F., Weschler, R. C. & Ballantine, C. (1979). Divorce and the preschool child: Cumulative stress. *Journal of Divorce, 3,* 55–68.

Holmes, T. H., & Rahe, R. H. (1967). The social readjustment rating scale. *Journal of Psychosomatic Research, 11,* 213–218.

Jacobson, D. S. (1978). The impact of marital separation/divorce on children. II: Interparent hostility and child adjustment. *Journal of Divorce, 2,* 3–19.

Johnson, J. H., & McCutcheon, S. M. (1980). Assessing life stress in older children and adolescents: Preliminary findings with the Life Events Checklist. In I. G. Sarason & C. D. Spielbeger (Eds.), *Stress and anxiety* (Vol. 7). Washington, DC: Hemisphere.

Kelly, J. B., & Wallterstein, J. S. (1976). The effects of parental divorce: Experiences of the child in early latency. *American Journal of Orthopsychiatry, 46,* 20–32.

Kurdek, L. A. (1981). An integrative perspective on children's divorce adjustment. *American Psychologist, 36,* 856–866.

Kurdek, L. A., & Berg, B. (1983). Correlates of children's adjustment to their parents' divorce. In L. A. Kurdek (Ed.), *Children and divorce*. San Francisco: Jossey-Bass.

Kurdek, L. A., Blisk, D., & Siesky, A. E. (1981). Correlates of children's long-term adjustment to their parents' divorce. *Developmental Psychology, 17,* 565–579.

Kurdek, L. A., & Blisk, D. (1983). Dimensions and correlates of mothers' divorce experiences. *Journal of Divorce, 6,* 1–24.

Lazarus, R. S., & Launier, R. (1978). Stress related transactions between person and environment. In L. A. Pervin & M. Lewis (Eds.), *Perspectives in interactional psychology*. New York: Plenum.

Links, P. S. (1983). Community surveys of the prevalence of childhood psychiatric disorder: A review. *Child Development, 54,* 531–548.

Neugebauer, R. (1981). The reliability of life-event reports. In B. S. Dohrenwend & B. P. Dohrenwend (Eds.). *Stressful life events and their contexts*. New York: Prodist.

Paykel, E. (1983). *Life events, social support and clinical psychiatric disorder*. Paper presented at the NATO Advanced Research Workshop on Social Support, Chateau de Buras, France.

Price, R. H. (1982). *Priorities for prevention research: Linking risk factor and intervention research*. Paper presented for the Center for Studies of Prevention, National Institute of Mental Health, Washington, DC.

Reich, J. W., & Zautra, A. (1981). Life events and personal causation: Some relationships with satisfaction and distress. *Journal of Personality and Social Psychology, 41,* 1002–1012.

Ross, C. E., & Mirowsky, J. II. (1979). A comparison of life-event-weighting schemes: Change, undesirability, and effect-proportional indices. *Journal of Health and Social Behavior, 20,* 166–177.

Rutter, M. (1979). Protective factors in children's responses to stress and disadvantage. In M. W. Kent & J. E. Rolf (Eds.), *Primary prevention of psychopathology: Vol. III. Social competence in children*. Hanover, NH: University Press of New England.

Rutter, M., Yule, B., Quinton, D., Rowlands, O., Yule, W., & Berger, M. (1978). Attainment and adjustment in two geographic areas. III. Some factors accounting for area differences. *British Journal of Psychiatry, 126,* 520-533.

Sameroff, A. J., & Seifer, R. (1983). Familial risk and child competence. *Child Development, 54,* 1254-1268.

Sandler, I. N., & Block, M. (1979). Life stress and maladaptation of children. *American Journal of Community Psychology, 7,* 425-440.

Sarason, I. G., Johnson, J. H., & Siegel, J. M. (1978). Assessing the impact of life changes: Development of the Life Experience Survey. *Journal of Consulting and Clinical Psychology, 46,* 932-946.

Shepherd, M., Oppenheim, A. N., & Mitchell, S. (1971). *Child Behavior and mental health.* New York: Grune & Stratton.

Stolberg, A. L., & Anker, J. M. (1984). Cognitive and behavioral changes in children resulting from parental divorce and consequent environmental changes. *Journal of Divorce, 7,* 23-41.

Stone, A. A., & Neale, J. M. (1982). Development of a methodology for assessing daily experiences. In A. Baum & J. Singer (Eds.), *Advances in environmental psychology: Vol. III. Environment and health.* Hillsdale, NJ: Erlbaum.

Vinokur, A., & Selzer, M. L. (1975). Desirable versus undesirable life events: Their relationship to stress and mental distress. *Journal of Consulting and Clinical Psychology, 32,* 329-337.

Wallerstein, J. S., & Kelly, J. B. (1974). The effects of parental divorce: The adolescent experience. In E. J. Anthony & C. Koupernik (Eds.), *The child in his family* (Vol. 3) New York: Wiley.

Wallerstein, J. S., & Kelly, J. B. (1975). The effects of parental divorce: Experiences of the preschool child. *Journal of the American Academy of Child Psychiatry, 14,* 600-616.

Wallerstein, J. S., & Kelly, J. B. (1980). *Surviving the breakup: How children and parents cope with divorce.* New York: Basic Books.

Zautra, A., & Sandler, I. (1983). Life event needs assessments: Two models for measuring preventable mental health problems. *Journal of Prevention in Human Sciences, 2,* 35-58.

Zimmerman, M. (1983). Methodological issues in the assessment of life events: A review of issues and research. *Clinical Psychology Review, 3,* 339-370.

II

RELATIVELY HIGH
FREQUENCY CRISIS EVENTS

Parts two and three of this volume deal with crisis intervention as it applies to specific stressors directly impacting children and/or families. Rather than attempting to cover all stressors in this category, we have selected areas that are of great current interest and are being actively researched. In the first of three chapters dealing with relatively high frequency events, Cowen and Hightower (Chapter 4) extend the life events measurement perspective developed by Sandler et al. (Chapter 2) and demonstrate that children experiencing crisis events are more likely to have serious school adjustment problems, and that specific types of stressful events predispose particular patterns of maladjustment. Further, taking a preventive intervention approach, they describe and evaluate a program designed to minimize adjustment problems in children of divorce.

In the next chapter, Stolberg, Kiluk, and Garrison, consistent with the temporal model presented in Chapter 1, provide a temporally based conceptual framework for viewing divorce adjustment, specifying salient stressors for both children and parents and intervention needs at each of four stages. In addition, they describe and evaluate a preventive intervention program for children of divorce and their custodial mothers (the Divorce Adjustment Project), which derives from the general Primary Mental Health Project model developed by Cowen over the last 10 years, and which also served as the stimulus for the development of the intervention program described by Cowen and Hightower in Chapter 4.

In Chapter 6, Melamed and Bush address how illness in a child may produce a crisis for the child and his family. They review the literature on psychological preparation of children for hospitalization, emphasizing the important role parents play as stress mediators. They also describe a study in which patterns of parent-child interaction in a medical setting are measured using a newly developed observational rating scale (Dyadic Prestressor Interaction Scale) and discuss the implications of their findings for teaching parenting strategies.

4

Stressful Life Events and Young Children's School Adjustment

Emory L. Cowen and A. Dirk Hightower
University of Rochester

INTRODUCTION

For nearly three decades we have been involved in the development, implementation, evaluation, and dissemination of the Primary Mental Health Project (PMHP), an innovative array of programs for systematic early detection and prevention of young children's school adjustment problems (Cowen et al., 1975; Cowen, Gesten, & Weissberg, 1980; Cowen, 1980a). PMHP today is very different from the original project; change, nourished both by the clinical experience of line program personnel and consultants and careful research study, has been slow and evolutionary rather than revolutionary.

Studies within PMHP of the effects of stressful life events on young children well illustrate the preceding process. Slowly accreting answers to two broad families of questions, (1) "What relationships are there between experiencing stressful events and school adjustment?" and (2) "What interventions can be developed to forestall the adverse psychological consequences of such events?", have contributed importantly to change in PMHP practice.

The chapter is divided into four sections: (1) an overview of PMHP's rationale, purposes, and operating procedures; (2) a summary of PMHP research relating stressful life events to young children's school adjustment; (3) a review of PMHP-based interventions designed to short-circuit predictable negative sequelae of early stressful events; and (4) implications and future directions, based on work thus far done.

PMHP: RATIONALE AND OPERATING PROCEDURES

PMHP began in 1957 as a pilot-demonstration project in a single school. It was prompted by two sets of clinical observations. First, many classroom teachers reported that about 40 to 60 percent of their time was preempted by the problems of a very few (3 or 4) children, to the detriment of those youngsters, the learning and development of the other children, as well as their own sense of well-being and accomplishment. Equally vexing was the observation of a sharp rise in mental

The interventions and research studies reported in this chapter were supported by a series of grants from the National Institute of Mental Health (MH 14547) and the New York State Department of Education, for which the authors express their sincere appreciation.

health referrals during the transition period between elementary and high school to the point where demand for such services far outstripped available resources. A review of the sometimes thick, cumulative school records of referred youngsters often revealed histories of school adjustment problems that went back as far as the primary grades. Either resources to help them had not been available, or people had hoped that if they waited long enough troubles would go away. Far from vanishing, many early problems became more rooted and spread to new areas.

These clinical observations suggested the need for alternative programming emphasizing the yoked processes of early identification of school adjustment problems and prompt preventive intervention to cut down the flow of later more serious difficulties. They were the wellsprings from which PMHP flowed.

One decade later a Task Force of the Joint Commission on the Mental Health of Children (Glidewell & Swallow, 1969) provided a better documented and codified rationale for PMHP's approach. In a review of 27 incidence studies, the Task Force concluded that roughly 1 in 3 American school children experienced moderate to serious school adjustment problems, and that for 1 in 10 those problems were sufficiently serious to warrant immediate professional help. To the extent that early educational success is a key stepping-stone to other important life adaptations, failing to "cut it" in school increases a child's risk for later adjustive difficulties.

PMHP thus arose in a context of concern about insufficiencies of the then (and still) dominant mental health service-delivery model—a system that provides re-active, repair services to a relatively few people with significant psychological problems. The appealing alternative was to identify problems early on, before they exacted a heavy toll, and to provide effective preventively oriented services to many young school children both to help their immediate adjustment and to cut down the flow of later (individually and socially) costly problems.

PMHP is best seen as a structural model with four main emphases.

1. It focuses on young, modifiable children before problems become rooted and entrenched. The primary school grades are ideal sites for such efforts.

2. It emphasizes active early screening of young children to identify systematically those experiencing significant early school adjustment problems.

3. It expands significantly the reach of early effective helping services to identified children through the use of carefully selected, trained, supervised nonprofessional help-agents—"child-aides."

4. It changes professional roles to emphasize "quarterbacking" activities such as the selection, training, and supervision of nonprofessionals, and consultative and resource functions with school personnel in ways that increase geometrically the reach of early effective helping services.

Those structural components translate into the following step-by-step summary of how PMHP actually works.

1. The project has developed techniques for rapid, accurate early identification of young children's school functioning, which pool data from teachers, mental health professionals, and parents, a group screening battery assessing early intellective and adjustive factors, classroom observations, and teachers' adjustment ratings of young children's behavior problems and competencies (Cowen et al., 1973;

Gesten, 1976; Hightower et al., in press; Lorion, Cowen, & Caldwell, 1975; Weissberg, et al., 1985).

2. Most program referrals are initiated when the teacher perceives ineffective functioning in the child: aggressive, acting-out, and disruptive behaviors; shy, anxious, withdrawn reactions; learning difficulties; and combinations of the preceding. Other school personnel and sometimes parents also make referrals.

3. Screening data are reviewed at an initial assignment conference involving school mental health professionals, teachers, child-aides, and other relevant school personnel. The purposes of that conference are to understand the child's current situation and, on that basis, to set up appropriate intervention goals and strategies. After that aides begin to see referred children regularly, under professional supervision.

4. PMHP schools, depending on pupil enrollment, have anywhere from 2 to 6 half-time child-aides who serve as prime direct help-agents with referred children. Although aides receive focused, time-limited training to help them to function effectively in that role, basically PMHP depends more on *selection* variables than on training variables. Aides are supervised regularly by professionals. They get on-the-job training through case conferences and consultation and are provided additional specialty training options over time. Aides, who are paid at the prevailing hourly rates established by school districts, carry half-time (15–18 hours per week) caseloads of about 10 to 14 children.

5. Teachers and aides typically exchange information and coordinate goals. Substitute teacher time is provided in order to free teachers to participate in PMHP planning and evaluation conferences—a mechanism that increases teachers' sensitivity to the complex relationships between psychological factors and a child's ability to learn. Some teachers have translated such learnings into more effective classroom handling, an important step toward primary prevention.

6. Midyear conferences are held for each child, to take stock and, if necessary, realign goals and procedures. End-of-year termination conferences evaluate children's progress in the program, and formulate recommendations for the next school year.

7. PMHP consultants visit schools regularly to support professionals, provide enrichment and upgrading of skills for program participants, and consider interesting, challenging cases.

8. The PMHP school mental health professional's role differs sharply from the traditional one. Much less time is devoted to direct one-to-one services and much more goes into training, consultative, and resource activities for school personnel and aides. That mode allows PMHP to get at many more problems early, when they are still manageable; to do something about them; and to prevent difficulties, rather than counterpunching when it is too late. Many more children in need are seen, thus augmenting geometrically the reach and clout of the educational and mental health enterprises. The approach, far from implying professional obsolescence, points to new more socially utilitarian professional roles.

Currently the local PMHP is situated in 23 urban and suburban schools. Last year more than 1000 youngsters were seen intensively, with an average of 22 helping contacts per child, for a total of some 22,000 child-serving contacts. Cost-benefit analysis of PMHP's operations (Dorr, 1972) suggests that an increase in project costs of approximately 40 percent expands the reach of services by about 1000 percent.

Both structurally and substantively PMHP has been an evolving rather than a stand-pat project. Thus, over the years, the local program has grown from a pilot-demonstration project in a single school to a program now based in more than a score of urban and suburban schools. Continuous review and change in PMHP program practices has been informed by a productive marriage, since Day 1, between service and research. Thus, research studies are fueled by, and addressed to, live program issues identified by line program personnel and consultants, and research findings in turn are fed back into the program to improve the scope and quality of services to children.

Program evaluation research has been another defining PMHP hallmark from the start. To date, upwards of 20 separate program outcome studies have been done. Collectively those studies provide extensive empirical data testifying to the effectiveness of the approach (Cowen et al., 1975). A recent, comprehensive study (Weissberg, Cowen, Lotyczewski, & Gesten, 1983) evaluating program effectiveness for seven consecutive, independent, annual cohorts of referred children (1974–1981), offers strong evidence that PMHP does indeed enhance the adjustment of many young school children.

As more program experience was logged and effectiveness data was cumulated, PMHP began a systematic three-pronged dissemination effort. Step I consisted of a series of intensive live-in national and regional workshops to bring the approach to the attention of interested school districts. Two additional options were provided for districts interested in implementing (1) follow-up consultation and on-site visits by PMHP staff members to help get new programs off the ground, and (2) short-term internships for program personnel from implementing districts in PMHP CORE (i.e., laboratory-training-demonstration) schools. Later, four Regional PMHP Dissemination Centers were established in different geographic regions around the country—each based on its own viable PMHP offshoot program and each involved in the same three dissemination activities as the parent project.

We have tracked the progress of the dissemination program several times (Cowen, Davidson, & Gesten, 1980; Cowen, Spinell, Wright, & Weissberg, 1983). Currently we estimate that some 150 school districts around the world have established kindred programs in highly varied settings: large and small; urban, suburban, and rural; and socioculturally, racially, and ethnically diverse districts. Collectively, those programs bring effective services to many thousands of children annually. It thus appears that the PMHP's model can be effectively adapted to a broad spectrum of situations.

From the diverse array of new program implementations have come numerous independent evaluations of the effectiveness of the basic approach (e.g., Cowen, Weissberg, et al., 1983). The new programs as a group are diverse and imaginative. Although they all adhere to PMHP's basic structural tenets (cf. above) they vary considerably in terms of depth and types of their professional staffing patterns, types of help-agents used (e.g., full vs. part time, paid nonprofessionals vs. diverse volunteer groups, etc.), formats for recruiting, training, and supervising aides, specific screening procedures used, and funding sources. Such diversity is as it should be, indeed *must* be. Each new program must, in other words, adapt to the realities of its own "pond ecology" (its own needs, resources, belief systems, prevailing practices, etc.).

Currently work is under way with appropriate state offices aiming toward within-state dissemination of the PMHP model. That effort has led to the passage of specific PMHP-enabling legislation, with supporting budget in several states and a sharp increase in the number of new programs. Thus, in small but visible ways, the PMHP approach has had measurable impact on how school mental health services are conceptualized and delivered, and has begun to crack the tough nut of bringing about constructive social change.

Within that historico-developmental context, two points have special relevance for this chapter: (1) PMHP's continuing strong emphasis on objective documentation of its early detection and screening, and program evaluation-procedures, has produced a large data bank of information about young children, and (2) the project's continuing commitment to self-evaluation and to data-based program change designed to improve services to children.

The convergent operation of those two emphases is reflected in our work over the past decade: (1) documenting relationships between stressful life-events and children's school behavior and adjustment, and (2) developing and assessing the efficacy of interventions designed to short-circuit the negative psychological sequelae of such events. The next sections review those two developments.

RELATIONSHIPS BETWEEN STRESSFUL EVENTS AND SCHOOL ADJUSTMENT

Over time, it became increasingly clear clinically that children who experienced stressful life events were susceptible to school adjustment problems. Concurrent changes in cultural standards and values operated to increase the frequency of certain stressful events such as parental divorce and/or single-parent child-rearing (Report of the Select Committee on Children, Youth, and Families, 1983). Those observations gave rise to a series of studies, spanning a decade, of relationships betweeen children's exposure to stressful events and their school adjustment.

In that tradition, Felner, Stolberg, and Cowen (1975) compared the adjustment of young, referred school children who had, as opposed to had not, experienced either of two stressful events (1) parental separation or divorce ($n = 300$) and (2) death or life-threatening illness in the family ($n = 70$), in two consecutive-year samples. Two teacher-rated measures of children's classroom behavior were used as adjustment criteria: the AML Behavioral Rating Scale (Cowen et al., 1973), a brief 11-item screening device; and the Teacher Rating Form (TRF; Clarfield, 1974), a 37-item measure of children's school adjustment problems. Factor analysis of both scales identified the same three problem-clusters: Acting Out, Shy-Anxious, and Learning. In both years groups of children who had experienced those two events were judged to be more maladjusted than *referred* noncrisis controls. Moreover, specific patterns of school problem behaviors were associated with each event. Whereas children of divorce had heightened acting-out problems (e.g., aggression to peers, being disruptive in class, seeking attention) youngsters who had experienced death or life-threatening illness in the family showed elevated shy-anxious behaviors (e.g., shyness, withdrawal; not making friends; tension). Direct comparison of two smaller, demographically matched event-subgroups showed that children of divorce had significantly higher acting-out ratings than children from families in which life-threatening illness or death had occurred—a finding consistent with other literature reviews (Emery, 1982;

Rutter, 1983), whereas the latter group had significantly higher shy-anxious scores.

Another report (Felner, Ginter, Boike, & Cowen, 1981a), also based on two separate studies, extended the earlier findings. The first study compared the school adjustment of three demographically matched PMHP referred groups: (1) parental separation or divorce, (2) death or life-threatening illness in the family, and (3) non-crisis controls. Teachers rated children's (1) problem behaviors on the Classroom Adjustment Rating Scale (CARS; Lorion, Cowen, & Caldwell, 1975), a 41-item adaptation of Clarfield's (1974) TRF, measuring the same three factors, and (2) school competencies using Gesten's (1976) Health Resources Inventory (HRI) which assesses five factors: Good Student, Peer Sociability, Follows Rules, Adaptive Assertiveness, and Frustration Tolerance. Children of divorce had higher Acting-Out scores and lower HRI-rules scores than the other two groups, and were significantly more maladjusted overall than the controls. Children who experienced life-threatening illness or death in the family had significantly higher CARS Shy-Anxious scores than controls.

The second study compared the problem behaviors and competencies of three demographically matched groups of 6- to 9-year-old nonreferred, rural children: (1) 37 children of divorce, (2) 14 children with familial histories of death or life-threatening illness, and (3) 51 noncrisis controls. Both crisis groups were judged to be more maladjusted than the controls. Divorce children again showed elevated Acting-Out profiles compared to the other groups, and had fewer Peer Sociability, Rules, Frustration Tolerance, and overall competencies than controls.

Another related study (Felner, Ginter, Boike, & Cowen, 1981b) assessed the adjustment of the same two crisis groups (i.e., divorce and death/illness), from the perspective of PMHP child-aides instead of teachers. Although the study's design was similar to those used in the prior investigations, the criterion measures changed. Problem behaviors were assessed using the Aide Status Evaluation Form (ASEF; Clarfield, 1974), a measure completed by aides, with a factor structure similar to the TRF and CARS. As in the earlier studies, aides judged children of divorce to have more serious Acting-Out problems and children who experienced death or life-threatening illness to have more serious Shy-Anxious problems. Intervention goals set for these children at referral were also compared using the Aide Goal Form (AGF), a list of 44 goals in working with children, each rated on a 5-point "importance" scale. Goals of reducing Acting-Out behavior were rated as significantly more important for divorce children and those designed to reduce Shy-Anxious behaviors as significantly more important for children from families in which death or life-threatening illness had occurred.

Felner, Farber, Ginter, Boike, and Cowen (1980) examined co-occurrences between parent divorce and death or life-threatening illness in the family and other indicants of family disruption for both urban and suburban PMHP-referred and rural nonreferred, children. In the referred sample, family backgrounds of children of divorce, vs. those from intact families, more often evidenced lack of educational stimulation, economic problems, parental rejections, and difficulty in adjustment to foster placement. In the rural nonreferred sample, children of divorce compared to those from intact families more often had backgrounds associated with lack of educational stimulation, economic difficulties, and more serious family problems overall.

Several recent investigations further round out the picture thus far developed.

In one fairly narrow study, Wyman, Cowen, Hightower, and Pedro-Carroll (1985) demonstrated that latency-aged children of divorce, compared to demographically matched peers from intact families, had heightened anxiety, lower perceived cognitive competence scores, and fewer potential sources of peer support. On a broader scale, Sterling, Cowen, Weissberg, Lotyczewski, and Boike (1985) assessed the frequency of teacher-reported occurrences, with a sample of nearly 1000 1st, 2nd, 3rd, and 4th graders, of 11 recent (i.e., in the past 6 months) stressful life-events: death of a parent, sibling, or close relative; serious illness of a parent, sibling, or close relative; lengthy illness or hospitalization of child; school transfer; parental separation or divorce; parent remarrying; parent losing job; family experiencing severe economic difficulties; change in residence; new child born into family; new adult or child moving into the home.

Overall, teachers reported that 211 children had experienced one or more stressful events during the prior 6 months. Those youngsters, compared to a demographically matched noncrisis group, had significantly more serious school adjustment problems on the CARS and significantly fewer competencies on the HRI. Comparisons among children who had experienced only one event, vs. two, vs. three or more recent stressful events, showed that the three-or-more group had the most serious problems and fewest competencies. In other words, the psychological toll exacted by multiple recent stressful events seemed to cumulate much as lead poisoning. That finding offers support for Rutter's (1983) recent conjecture that the negative effects of stressful events on children may be more nearly multiplicative than additive.

A structurally related study (Lotyczewski, Cowen, & Weissberg, 1986) based on the same large sample identified a cluster of six stressful events associated with physical health and illness: frequent illness, allergies, current medical problems, lengthy illness or hospitalization, frequent visits to school nurse, and physical handicap. The 179 youngsters with one or more such indicators (only nine of whom overlapped with the preceding stressful-events sample) were found to have significantly more serious school adjustment problems and fewer competencies than a demographically matched sample of children with no health problems. Moreover, the 44 children who had two or more health problems had more serious adjustment problems and fewer competencies than the 135 who had experienced only one such problem. Thus, this study's findings parallel structurally those reported by Sterling et al. (1985) for children who had experienced stressful events.

A study by Perez et al. (1982) suggests that the preceding findings generalize to dependent variables other than teacher ratings of children's school adjustment. It compared the social problem-solving skills of demographically matched groups of children who had, vs. had not, experienced certain types of family background problems and/or circumstances. Children whose parents had separated or divorced, compared to those from intact families, were found to be deficient in means-end thinking and role-taking skills.

Cowen, Weissberg, and Guare (1984) approached the same question from a somewhat different perspective. They compared 275 primary graders referred to PMHP for school adjustment problems to a demographically matched sample of 509 nonreferred classmates, with respect to the frequency of occurrence of 39 background descriptive variables reflecting these domains: (1) physical and health characteristics, (2) recent stressful life-events, (3) concurrent school activities and special services, and (4) current family status. For purposes of the present discussion, the most important finding was that recent stressful events (e.g., parental separation or divorce, death or serious illness in the family, parental remarriage, a new adult moving into the home, etc.) occurred on the average about 2½ to 3 times more often in the referred sample. Referred children were also judged to be less attractive physically, have more serious health problems, have less well developed fine and gross motor coordination, require more special services (e.g., speech therapy, remedial education, school nurse visits), participate in fewer extracurricular activities (e.g., after-school sports or recreation programs) and have more serious family problems (e.g., natural father absent from home, father unemployed, adult nonrelatives living in the home).

From the above findings Cowen, Lotyczewski, and Weissberg (1984) developed two composite indices, one for risk factors and one for resources, consisting of items shown to differentiate referred and nonreferred children. In a sample of nearly 1000 urban and suburban primary graders, the correlation between the two indices was −.57. Both indices correlated significantly and in the expected directions with teacher ratings of children's school problem behaviors and competencies (CARS and HRI). Demographically matched subgroups of youngsters with (1) low risk and high resources, (2) high risk and high resources, and (3) high risk and low resources were next compared on the teacher-rated measures of adjustment. Low risk/high resource children were judged consistently to be the best-adjusted group and high risk/low resources children the least well adjusted. Of special interest was the finding that high-risk children with some resources were rated as better adjusted than equally high-risk children who lacked resources. Thus, the presence of resources moderated the adjustive decrement predisposed by exposure to stressful events—a conclusion with implications for conceptualizing and engineering preventive interventions for young children at risk.

One limitation of our own and others' reasearch in this area is that event stressfulness for children has characteristically been assessed from the perspective of adults. As several observers (Anthony, 1974; Segal, 1983) have noted, children and adults may perceive the stressful impact of events differently. Indeed, evidence to support that view is available for older children (Yamamoto, 1979). With that issue in mind, Brown (1985) carried out a study establishing the perceived stressfulness of 22 events from the perspective of 4th, 5th, and 6th graders (i.e., 9- to 12-year-old children). Her questions included the following: (1) How stressful do those youngsters judge various events to be? (2) How do those judgments relate to adult judgments of the stressfulness of the same events? (3) Do children who have actually experienced stressful events judge those events to be more upsetting than those who have not? (4) Are there parametric (e.g., age, sex) differences in the judged stressfulness of events as well as in the frequency of occurrence and sense of upset about events experienced personally? (5) What are the relationships between experiencing stressful events and adjustment in children? (6) To what extent are such relationships moderated by sources of support available to the child? By bringing the child's perspective of event stressfulness into the research arena, Brown, study paved the way for additional research on the effects of stress and its moderation, which can well serve future intervention programs.

In sum, findings from this series of studies in our laboratory add up to a reasonably clear picture internally and are consistent with other literature findings. From several perspectives, it appears that young children who experience stressful life events, particularly parental separation or divorce and life-threatening illness or death in the family, have more serious school adjustment problems and fewer competencies than noncrisis peers. That conclusion holds for referred and non-referred children, and children from urban, suburban, and rural backgrounds. The occurrence of those stressful life events is significantly associated with other signs of familial disruption. Specific types of stressful events predispose specific patterns of maladjustment, with divorce favoring acting-out problems and death or life-threatening illness favoring shy-anxious problems. Additionally, the data suggest that the presence of resources moderates adjustive decrement following risk-enhancing stressful events. Finally, the important perspective of the young child's view of event stressfulness is presently being added to the research framework.

PREVENTIVE INTERVENTIONS FOR YOUNG CHILDREN WHO HAVE EXPERIENCED STRESSFUL LIFE EVENTS

The single most powerful conclusion from the work thus far reported is that stressful events adversely affect young school children's behavior, performance, and adjustment. The very occurrence of a stressful event can be taken as a warning sign that adjustment difficulties, indeed sometimes serious ones, may follow. Although this finding is of interest sui generis, it also poses the intriguing challenge of how to intervene to forestall the otherwise likely negative psychological consequences of stressful events.

In the past, the mental health fields have taken a passive-receptive stance in such matters, that is, they have sought to provide (the best available) repair services for the psychological casualties of stressful events, when and if those people find their way into the formal delivery system. Since problems tend by then to be serious, deeply rooted, and spread out to new areas, therapeutic intervention is difficult and time-consuming, and has a guarded prognosis. A conceptually attractive alternative is to develop before-the-fact preventive interventions for child victims of stressful events, designed to cut down the flow of psychological dysfunction known on base rate to follow their occurrence. The next section reports on the development and evaluation of several such intervention models in our laboratory.

A first effort, within PMHP's broader context, was fueled by our early research findings and by everyday clinical observations of the negative effects of stressful events on children. An initial pilot intervention was targeted to children who had experienced one of four stressful events (i.e., parental separation or divorce, death or life-threatening threatening illness in the family, hospitalization or surgery, and birth of a new sibling) within the preceding two months. Veteran PMHP child-aides were used as interventionists in this program. To prepare them for that work, they received additional training to consider the meaning of crisis for children, the problems it posed for them, and effective methods for working with such youngsters.

Aides worked with referred children for 12 sessions (twice per week for 6 weeks). They helped children to identify and express crisis-related feelings, provided support, and explored adaptive alternatives. Felner, Norton, Cowen, and Farber (1981) reported an evaluation study based on 57 primary graders seen through the program. Thirty-one (54%) were children whose parents had recently separated. The program's goal was to prevent the school adjustment problems that often follow stressful events. Pre-post program evaluations showed significant decreases in children's trait-anxiety levels and teacher-rated shy-anxious scores as well as a significant increase in teacher-rated adaptive assertiveness competence scores.

Both parents and school personnel responded favorably to the program; understandably so, since it dealt with real, vexing, everyday problems they face. Over time the program was modified and expanded and a detailed training manual was written. Each year, new aides are trained for the program, which is now fully integrated into PMHP's mainstream.

In seeking to broaden the pilot intervention our attention turned, on both epidemiological and substantive grounds, to children of divorce. It is now estimated that 40 percent of today's marriages in the US will end in divorce (Glick & Norton, 1979; Hetherington, 1979). Since 60 percent of all divorces involve children, it is further estimated that in any given year at least one million American children will go through the experience of their parents' separating, and that one of two American children born today will spend significant time periods in a single parent family, resulting from parental divorce. Those figures reflect dramatic social change (Report of the Select Committee of Children, Youth, & Families, 1983).

Coupling those powerful epidemiological data with our own group's consistent research findings (cf. above) and those of many other investigators documenting the damaging psychological effects of divorce on children (Felner, Farber, & Primavera, 1980; Emery, 1982? Guidubaldi, Cleminshaw, Perry, & McLoughlin, 1983; Hetherington, 1979; Hetherington, Cox, & Cox, 1978, 1982; Kelly & Wallerstein, 1976; Kurdek, 1981, 1983; Wallerstein, 1983; Wallerstein & Kelly, 1975, 1976, 1980), provides a compelling rationale for preventive intervention. Given the stark nature of those divorce-associated realities it is suprising that there has been so little systematic empirical study of preventive interventions for children of divorce.

Several recent studies have sought to fill that void. Two (Cantor, 1977; Guerney & Jordon, 1979) were small pilot interventions for young children of divorce, resting heavily on principles of support. Each study involved only nine children and was evaluated impressionistically. Cantor (1977) found little evidence of positive change in program children, based on feedback from their parents and teachers. Guerney and Jordon, however, had enough positive feedback from parents and children to be encouraged to start additional groups.

Very recently Stolberg and his associates (Stolberg & Cullen, 1981; Stolberg, Cullen, & Garrison, 1982; Stolberg, Kiluk, & Garrison, this volume) developed a considerably more ambitious intervention for children of divorce, called the Divorce Adjustment Project (DAP). DAP consisted of two main components: (1) The Children's Support Group (CSG), a 12-session intervention for 7- to 13-year-old children, with strong emphases on support and building communication, anger control and relaxation skills, and (2) a parallel 12-session, Single-Parent Support Group (SPSG), also based on mutual support as well as topical discussions oriented to participants as individuals and parents.

Eighty-two mother-child pairs were randomly assigned to one of four conditions: (1) child intervention only, (2) parent intervention only, (3) both parent and child intervention, (4) no intervention (controls). The effects of the intervention were assessed by pre-, post-, and 5-month follow-up evaluations of participants in multiple areas of functioning. Children in the CSG-alone condition improved more than those in other groups on a self-concept measure, whereas parents in the SPSG-alone condition improved more than those in other groups. The combined CSG–SPSG condition did not yield parallel improvement. Gains shown afterward tended to hold up at follow-up; at that time CSG-alone children were found to have improved significantly more than CSG–SPSG youngsters in social skills (Stolberg & Garrison, 1985).

The work done by Stolberg and his associates stimulated the development in our laboratory of a related program for 3rd- to 6th-grade suburban children of divorce (Pedro-Carroll & Cowen, 1985). The new Children of Divorce Intervention Project (CODIP) maintained CSG's emphasis on support and skill-building, though it differed somewhat from DAP both in structure and substance. The two main structural changes were: (1) given the limited effectiveness of DAP's combined parent-child approach, only a child component was used in CODIP, and (2) CODIP focused on a more restricted age band (9-12) than the DAP intervention. With respect to content, CODIP (1) added an early focal affective component to provide children opportunities to discuss and better understand divorce-related feelings and experiences; (2) made extensive use of group discussions, filmstrips, and role-playings of emotionally laden, divorce-related experiences to supplement CSG's cognitive skill building components; (3) reduced the number of anger-control sessions from five to three; and (4) emphasized Wallerstein's (1983) first four divorce-related mastery challenges in leader training, as a framework for establishing intervention goals.

The 10-week CODIP intervention includes three major substantive blocks. The first three sessions comprise the program's focal affective component. They build a climate of support by providing opportunities for children to get to know each other, share common experiences, and talk about divorce-related feelings. The exercises help to reduce the isolation and sense of stigma that some youngsters feel. Later, role-playings, skits, and a vividly realistic filmstrip on divorce are used to demonstrate and generate discussion on (1) relationships between events, including divorce, and feelings; (2) how strong feelings (e.g., fear and anxiety) affect behavior; and (3) issues of attribution and blame, and concerns about the future that the divorce precipitates. The intent of these sessions, other than to build support, is to put children in touch with feelings about the divorce and to reduce their sense of isolation and being different.

Sessions four through six comprise the program's cognitive skill-building component. Children first learn about self-statements, which are sequential statements to oneself that can be used to deal effectively with problems, and then are taught a 6-step sequence for resolving interpersonal problems. Empathic, supportive discussion of problem resolutions by group members fosters further group cohesion. Important distinctions are made between problems beyond children's control (e.g., parent reconciliation) vs. those within their control (e.g., ways of communicating their feelings about the divorce). Being able to deal effectively with the latter increases children's sense of mastery and comfort with others, and helps to realize one of Wallerstein's (1983) key mastery tasks, that is, disengaging from parental conflict and resuming the child's agenda.

Sessions seven through nine emphasize appropriate expression and control of anger. Circumstances precipitating anger and its various forms of expression are considered first. Children then describe personal anger experiences and begin to

discuss appropriate and inappropriate ways of dealing with anger and their consequences. The strong emotion of anger thus enters the group's shared experience,
and opportunities are provided for catharsis and mutual support around divorce-
related, anger-eliciting experiences. Next, alternatives for dealing with anger,
another of Wallerstein's (1983) key mastery tasks, are considered, including
approaches that reflect good (i.e., "makes things better") and poor ("makes things
worse") control. The process is catalyzed by role-playing divorce-related, anger-
provoking situations, with feedback on their handling by peers. The ultimate
goal of these sessions is for the children to develop adaptive ways of dealing with
anger. The 10th (final) session is both to wind down and to evaluate the group
experience, including feelings about its ending.

The 10-week CODIP intervention was targeted to 72, 3rd- to 6th-grade children
of divorce in 4 suburban schools. Two subgroups, matched for sex, age, school,
and adjustment level, were randomly assigned as immediate- ($n = 40$) and delayed-
($n = 32$) intervention (control) groups. Within the E-condition, 5 mixed-sex
subgroups were formed, each with 8 or 9 children from the same school and at
the same, or adjacent, grade levels. Those groups met for weekly 1-hour sessions
in their respective home schools. After the intervention ended, and a second,
posttesting round was completed, children who had served as delayed controls
during the initial intervention period were seen in groups for a condensed 5-week
intervention, but were not evaluated again.

Groups were co-led by school mental health professionals assisted in one case
by a graduate student and in another by an experienced PMHP child-aide. Leaders
received extensive training before the program started dealing both with the effects
of divorce on latency-aged children and with specific skills (e.g., group dynamics)
needed to conduct the program. Weekly supervisory and discussion meetings
were held for group leaders, while the program was under way.

A comprehensive, objective, pre-post evaluation of CODIP, tapping multiple
perspectives, was conducted. Teachers reported significant decreases in participants'
school problem behaviors (i.e., aggressive, shy-anxious, and learning problems)
and significant increases in such school competencies as peer sociability, following
rules, frustration tolerance, and adaptive assertiveness. Parents reported improved
communication with their children specifically in divorce-related matters and more
generally about children's feelings, problems, experiences, and accomplishments.
Program children had significantly lower scores on an anxiety measure. They also
reported that being in the program improved their understanding both of their
parents' divorce and their own feelings about that event, and helped them to learn
to solve problems better and to feel less alone and/or different from others. Group
leaders judged similarly positive program outcomes to have occurred in the participants. Beyond the preceding objective outcome data, all four respondent groups
offered strongly positive comments about the program and its effects. A recent
replication with a new sample of 4th- through 6th-grade children of divorce
provided confirming data (Pedro-Carroll, Cowen, Hightower, & Guare, in press).

OVERVIEW AND FUTURE DIRECTIONS

Studies in our laboratory, over a 10-year period, document important relationships between stressful events that young children experience and school adjustment problems. Consistent with data reported by other investigators, the findings

apply to normal and referred children from various sociodemographic strata in urban, suburban, and rural settings. We have also found that specific stressful events are associated with specific types of school adjustment problems and that the presence of resources moderates the psychologically damaging effects of those events.

Although those findings have been informative, other goals remain. One, emphasized by Rutter (1983), is to chart further and more specifically the adverse consequences associated with particular stressful events. Others are to understand better the different forms such reactions take in diverse age and sociodemographic groups, and the in vivo factors that moderate the stressfulness of life events for children. These are essential building blocks for fashioning informed preventive interventions for affected groups.

A noteworthy development of the past decade is the perceptible shift in focus from a psychology of illness to a psychology of health. An important porthole to that development comes from the study of invulnerable, or resilient, children (Garmezy, 1975, 1976, 1981, 1983; Garmezy, Masten, Nordstrom, & Ferrarese, 1979). The concept is based on this observation: Given the most profound adversities imaginable, (i.e., experiencing the ravages of war or concentration camp, death of a loved one, victimization by chronic brutality, extreme poverty, separation or abandonment, or combinations of such factors) described by Garmezy (1983) as "stressors of marked gravity," some children not only surmount the adversity, but are competent and well adjusted in spite of it. What factors make them "invincible" despite overpowering odds against them?

Werner and Smith's (1982) recent book *Vulnerable But Invincible: A Study of Resilient Children*, the 3rd volume based on their 20-year longitudinal study of 700 children of Kauai, is a monumental step toward answering that question. About 200 of the 700 youngsters in that cohort, exposed to profound insults of biology, poverty, and family disequilibrium, developed serious learning and/or behavior problems in the first two decades of life. But 1 in 10 exposed to exactly the same profound stressors "remained invincible and developed into competent autonomous young adults." The book summarizes a careful empirical search for the wellsprings of invincibility. Although those ingredients varied somewhat for different age and sex groups, three influential clusters were found to favor invincibility: (1) being active, socially engaging and relatively autonomous in infancy and early childhood; (2) having a source of genuine closeness and support within the family; and (3) having significant peer and nonfamilial support sources (e.g., teachers, neighbors, clergymen). Certainly such knowledge has important implications for developing more effective preventive interventions for children who experience situation and/or event adversities.

If stressful events do indeed predispose maladjustment in children, as is strongly suggested by our own findings and those of others, effective before-the-fact interventions are needed to short-circuit predictably negative psychological problems and to bolster psychological wellness (Cowen, 1977, 1980b, 1982). CODIP's importance, for example lies in its demonstration that child maladjustment is not an inevitable consequence of parental divorce. That is an encouraging, but still limited and fallible, finding. Noting some of those limitations explicitly helps to structure a future agenda in program development and research.

For one thing, generalization of the CODIP's findings is restricted by the relatively small sample of suburban, white, middle-class children that the program served. The model must be extended to older and younger children with diverse sociodemographic attributes to probe the full range of its potential applicability. That process will necessarily require significant changes in program content and format, to be developmentally and socioculturally appropriate to new and different groups. Pinpointing CODIP's active and inert components is also a precondition for strengthening future programs. Similarly, CODIP findings reflect only the short term. To assess the durability and robustness of those encouraging proximal outcomes, follow-up over a longer period of time is essential. Finally, of course, the stressful life event of parental divorce is but one of a myriad of stressors, each with its own special profile of consequences, that impinge significantly on children's psychological well-being. A fine articulation of even-consequence taxonomies, in a context that respects developmental and sociodemographic variables, is needed to frame a needed, much broader array of meaningful preventive interventions for affected groups.

The conceptual roots of the preventive approach we are advocating differ qualitatively from mental health's previous unswerving emphasis on repairing things that have already gone wrong. The new paradigm (Bloom, 1979) begins by identifying stressful events with damaging psychological effects, then charts specific consequences associated with those events and finally develops preventive interventions based on such knowledge designed to short-circuit otherwise predictable, negative psychological sequelae.

The work reported in this chapter falls squarely within the framework of that new paradigm. Important psychological consequences of stressful events in young schoolchildren have been identified and effective preventive interventions to short-circuit such consequences have been modeled. Extensions of the latter work, in the directions proposed, offer an intriguing primary prevention pathway for forestalling the debilitating problems that many children in modern society experience following stressful events.

REFERENCES

Anthony, E. J. (1974). A risk-vulnerability intervention model for children of psychotic patients. In E. J. Anthony & C. Koupernik (Eds.), *The child in his family: Children at psychiatric risk.* New York: Wiley.

Bloom, B. L. (1979). Prevention of mental disorders: Recent advances in theory and practice. *Community Mental Health Journal, 15,* 179–191.

Brown, L. P. (1985). Stressful life-events as perceived by children. Unpublished doctoral dissertation, University of Rochester.

Cantor, D. W. (1977). School-based groups for children of divorce. *Journal of Divorce, 1,* 183–187.

Clarfield, S. P. (1974). The development of a teacher referral form for identifying early school maladaptation. *American Journal of Community Psychology, 2,* 199–210.

Cowen, E. L. (1977). Baby-steps toward primary prevention. *American Journal of Community Psychology, 5,* 1–22.

Cowen, E. L. (1980a). The Primary Mental Health Project: Yesterday, today, and tomorrow. *Journal of Special Education, 14,* 133–154.

Cowen, E. L. (1980b). The wooing of primary prevention. *American Journal of Community Psychology, 8,* 258–284.

Cowen, E. L. (1982). The special number: A compleat roadmap. In E. L. Cowen (Ed.), "Research in primary prevention in mental health," special issue. *American Journal of Community Psychology, 10,* 239–250.

Cowen, E. L., Davidson, E., & Gesten, E. L. (1980). Program dissemination and the modification of delivery practices in school mental health. *Professional Psychology, 11,* 36–47.

Cowen, E. L., Dorr, D., Clarfield, S. P., Kreling, B., McWilliams, S. A., Pokracki, F., Pratt, D. M., Terrell, D. L., & Wilson, A. B. (1973). The AML: A quick screening device for early detection of school maladaptation. *American Journal of Community Psychology, 1*, 12-35.

Cowen, E. L., Gesten, E. L., & Weissberg, R. P. (1980). An interrelated network of preventively oriented school based mental health approaches. In R. H. Price & P. Politzer (Eds.), *Evaluation and action in the community context.* New York: Academic Press.

Cowen, E. L., Lotyczewski, B. S., & Weissberg, R. P. (1984). Risk and resource indicators and their relationship to young children's school adjustment. *American Journal of Community Psychology, 12*, 353-367.

Cowen, E. L., Spinell, A., Wright, S., & Weissberg, R. P. (1983). Continuing dissemination of a school-based early detection and prevention model. *Professional Psychology, 14*, 118-127.

Cowen, E. L., Trost, M. A., Lorion, R. P., Dorr, D., Izzo, L. D., & Isaacson, R. V. (1975). *New ways in school mental health: Early detection and prevention of school maladaptation.* New York: Human Sciences Press.

Cowen, E. L., Weissberg, R. P., & Guare, J. (1984). Differential attributes of children referred to a school mental health project. *Journal of Abnormal Child Psychology, 12*, 397-409.

Cowen, E. L., Weissberg, R. P., Lotyczewski, B. S., et al. (1983). Validity generalization of school-based preventive mental health program. *Professional Psychology, 14*, 613-623.

Dorr, D. (1972). An ounce of prevention, *Mental Hygiene, 56*, 25-27.

Emery, R. E. (1982). Interparental conflict and the children of discord and divorce. *Psychological Bulletin, 92*, 310-330.

Felner, R. D., Farber, S. S., Ginter, M. A. , Boike, M. F., & Cowen, E. L. (1980). Family stress and organization following parental divorce or death. *Journal of Divorce, 4*, 67-76.

Felner, R. D., Farber, S. S., & Primavera, J. (1980). Children of divorce, stressful life events, and transitions: A framework for preventive efforts. In R. H. Price, R. F. Ketterer, B. C. Bader, & J. Monahan (Eds.), *Prevention in mental health: Research, policy and practice.* Beverly Hills, CA: Sage Publications.

Felner, R. D., Ginter, M. A., Boike, M. F., & Cowen, E. L. (1981a). Parental death or divorce and the school adjustment of young children. *American Journal of Community Psychology, 9*, 181-191.

Felner, R. D., Ginter, M. A., Boike, M. F., & Cowen, E. L. (1981b). Parental death or divorce in childhood: Problems, interventions and outcomes in a school based project. *Journal of Prevention, 1*, 240-246.

Felner, R. D., Norton, P. L., Cowen, E. L., & Farber, S. S. (1981). A prevention program for children experiencing life crisis. *Professional Psychology, 12*, 446-452.

Felner, R. D., Stolberg, A. L., & Cowen, E. L. (1975). Crisis events and school mental health referral patterns of young children. *Journal of Consulting and Clinical Psychology, 43*, 305-310.

Garmezy, N. (1975). The experimental study of children vulnerable to psychopathology. In A. Davids (Ed.), *Child personality and psychopathology: Current topics (Vol. 2).* New York: Wiley-Interscience.

Garmezy, N. (1976). *Vulnerable and invulnerable children: Theory, research and intervention.* Washington, DC: American Psychological Association.

Garmezy, N. (1981). Children under stress: Perspectives on antecedents and correlates of vulnerability and resistance to psychopathology. In A. I. Rabin, J. Aronoff, A. M. Barclay, & R. A. Zucker (Eds.), *Further explorations in personality.* New York: Wiley Interscience.

Garmezy, N. (1983). Stressors of childhood. In N. Garmezy & M. Rutter (Eds.). *Stress, coping and development in children.* New York: McGraw-Hill.

Garmezy, N., Masten, A., Nordstrom, L., & Ferrarese, M. (1979). The nature of competence in normal and deviant children. In M. W. Kent & J. E. Rolf (Eds.), *The primary prevention of psychopathology, (Vol. 3): Social Competence in children.* Hanover, NH: University Press of New England.

Gesten, E. (1976). A Health Resources Inventory: The development of a measure of the personal and social competence of primary grade children. *Journal of Consulting and Clinical Psychology, 44*, 775-786.

Glick, P. C., & Norton, A. J. (1979). *Marrying, divorcing and living together in the U. S. today.* Washington, DC: Population Reference Bureau, Inc.

Glidewell, J. C., & Swallow, C. S. (1969). *The prevalence of maladjustment in elementary schools: A report prepared for the Joint Commission on the Mental Health of Children.* Chicago: University of Chicago Press.

Guerney, L., & Jordon, L. (1979). Children of divorce: A community support group. *Journal of Divorce, 2,* 283–294.

Guidubaldi, J., Cleminshaw, H. K., Perry, S. D., & McLoughlin, C. S. (1983). The impact of parental divorce on children: Report of the nationwide NASP study. *School Psychology Review, 12,* 300–323.

Hetherington, E. M. (1979). Divorce: A child's perspective. *American Psychologist, 34,* 841–858.

Hetherington, E. M., Cox, M., & Cox, R. (1978). The aftermath of divorce. In J. H. Stevens & M. Mathews (Eds.), *Mother/child relationships.* Washington, DC: National Association for the Education of Young Children.

Hetherington, E. M., Cox, M., & Cox, R. (1982). Effects of divorce on parents and children. In M. E. Lamb (Ed.), *Nontraditional families: Parenting and child development.* Hillsdale, NJ: Erlbaum.

Hightower, A. D., Work, W. C., Cowen, E. L., Spinell, A. P., Lotyczewski, B. S., Guare, J., Rohrbeck, C. A., & Brown, L. P. (in press). The Teacher-Child Rating Scale: A brief objective measure of young school children's problem behaviors and competencies. *School Psychology Review.*

Kelly, J. B., & Wallerstein, J. S. (1976). The effects of parental divorce: Experiences of the child in early latency. *American Journal of Orthopsychiatry, 46,* 20–23.

Kurdek, L. A. (1981). An integrative perspective on children's divorce adjustment. *American Psychologist, 36,* 856–866.

Kurdek, L. A. (Ed.). (1983). *Children and divorce.* San Francisco: Jossey-Bass.

Lorion, R. P., Cowen, E. L., & Caldwell, R. A. (1975). Normative and parametric analyses of school maladjustment. *American Journal of Community Psychology, 3,* 293–301.

Lotyczewski, B. S., Cowen, E. L., & Weissberg, R. P. (1986). Adjustment correlates of physical and health problems in young children. *Journal of Special Education, 20.*

Pedro-Carroll, J. L., & Cowen, E. L. (1985). The Children of Divorce Intervention Project: An investigation of the efficacy of a school-based prevention program. *Journal of Consulting and Clinical Psychology, 53,* 603–611.

Pedro-Carroll, J. L., Cowen, E. L., Hightower, A. D., & Guare, J. C. (in press). Preventive intervention with latency-aged children of divorce: A replication study. *American Journal of Community Psychology, 14.*

Perez, V., Gesten, E. L., Cowen, E. L., Weissberg, R. P., Rapkin, B., & Boike, M. (1982). Relationships between family background problems and social problem-solving skills of young normal children. *Journal of Primary Prevention, 2,* 80–90.

Report of the Select Committee on Children, Youth, and Families, 98th Congress (1983). *U. S. children and their families: Current conditions and recent trends.* Washington, DC: Foundation for Child Development.

Rutter, M. (1983). Stress, coping, and development: Some issues and questions. In N. Garmezy & M. Rutter (Eds.), *Stress, coping and development in children.* New York: McGraw-Hill.

Segal, J. (1983). Utilization of stress and coping research: Issues of public education and public policy. In N. Garmezy & M. Rutter (Eds.), *Stress, coping and development in children.* New York: McGraw-Hill.

Sterling, S., Cowen, E. L., Weissberg, R. P., Lotyczewski, B. S., & Boike, M. (1985). Recent stressful life events and young children's school adjustment. *American Journal of Community Psychology, 13,* 31–48.

Stolberg, A. L., & Cullen, P. M. (1981). *Divorce Adjustment Project, Children's Support Group: A procedures manual.* Richmond, VA: Virginia Commonwealth University.

Stolberg, A. L., Cullen, P. M., & Garrison, K. M. (1982). Divorce Adjustment Project: Preventive programming for children of divorce. *Journal of Preventive Psychiatry, 1,* 365–368.

Stolberg, A. L., & Garrison, K. M. (1985). Evaluating a primary prevention program for children of divorce: The Divorce Adjustment Project. *American Journal of Community Psychology, 13,* 111–124.

Wallerstein, J. S. (1983). Children of divorce: Stress and developmental tasks. In N. Garmezy & M. Rutter (Eds.), *Stress, coping and development in children.* New York: McGraw-Hill.

Wallerstein, J. S., & Kelly, J. B. (1975). The effects of parental divorce: Experiences of the preschool child. *Journal of the American Academy of Child Psychiatry, 14,* 600–616.

Wallerstein, J. S., & Kelly, J. B. (1976). The effects of parental divorce: Experiences of the child in later latency. *American Journal of Orthopsychiatry, 46,* 256–269.

Wallerstein, J. S., & Kelly, J. B. (1980). *Surviving the breakup: How children and parents cope with divorce.* New York: Basic Books.

Weissberg, R. P., Cowen, E. L., Lotyczewski, B. S., & Gesten, E. L. (1983). The Primary Mental Health Project: Seven consecutive years of program outcome research. *Journal of Consulting and Clinical Psychology, 51,* 100–107.

Weissberg, R. P., Cowen, E. L., Lotyczewski, B. S., Boike, M., Orara, N. A., Stalonas, P., Sterling, S., & Gesten, E. L. (1985). Normative and parametric aspects of school problem behaviors and competencies. (Manuscript in Preparation).

Werner, E. E., & Smith, R. S. (1982). *Vulnerable but invincible: A study of resilient children.* New York: McGraw-Hill.

Wyman, P. A., Cowen, E. L., Hightower, A. D., & Pedro-Carroll, J. L. (1985). Perceived competence, self-esteem and anxiety in latency-aged children of divorce. *Journal of Child Clinical Psychology, 14,* 20–26.

Yamamoto, K. (1979). Children's ratings of experiences. *Developmental Psychology, 15,* 581–582.

5

A Temporal Model of Divorce Adjustment with Implications for Primary Prevention

Arnold L. Stolberg, Diane J. Kiluk, and Katherine M. Garrison
Virginia Commonwealth University

INTRODUCTION

This chapter describes the divorce adjustment process based on the temporal model of adjustment to life crises from Chapter 1 in this volume. A comprehensive primary prevention program for divorcing families is, then, based on this temporally sequenced stage model. Finally, the procedures and program evaluation of one component of this prevention strategy, the Divorce Adjustment Project, are presented.

A TEMPORAL MODEL OF THE DIVORCE ADJUSTMENT PROCESS

Cognitive, affective, behavioral, and psychophysiological problems have been reported in many children of divorce (Coddington & Troxell, 1980; Hetherington, 1979; Kurdek, 1981). Cognitive experiences inlcude self-blame, feeling different than one's peers, and heightened sensitivity to interpersonal incompatibility (Kelly & Berg, 1978; Kurdek & Siesky, 1980a, 1980b). Deficits in prosocial behavior and high frequencies of acting-out and aggressive behaviors have also been found among children of divorce (Stolberg, Camplair, Currier, & Wells, in press). Their academic performance is often hampered by classroom behaviors that interfere with performance and require special handling (Guidubaldi, Perry & Cleminshaw, 1983) and they are more often diagnosed as having serious illnesses than peers from intact families (Coddington & Troxell, 1980; Jacobs & Charles, 1980).

Divorced adults also tend to experience a range of problems greater than normal. They use inpatient and outpatient mental health services at a higher rate than married adults (Bloom, 1975). Anxiety, depression, anger, rejection, incompetence, poor self-concept, and psychophysiological disease are among presenting problems (Bloom, Asher, & White, 1978; Hetherington, Cox, & Cox, 1977).

A model of divorce adjustment may clarify processes that lead to these problem patterns and to more adaptive functioning. The components included in this model should be:

This research was supported in part by a grant from the National Institute of Mental Health (RO1 MH 34462). The authors wish to thank the staff of the Chesterfield County (Virginia) school and mental health systems.

1. Objective event of physical separation,
2. Temporal proximity to the separation,
3. Environmental, familial, and individual factors that mediate the impact of the separation,
4. Subjective evaluation of the separation, and
5. Individual's psychological response to the event.

The divorce adjustment process, thus, involves temporally sequenced stages, each with its own set of demands. The stressfulness of each stage is moderated or intensified by the presence of environmental, familial, and individual conditions. The psychological functioning of the family member is, thus, influenced by the specific stage-linked demands facing the family members as moderated by external and internal influences.

The four periods or stages of the divorce adjustment process are predecision, final separation, adjustment to the separation, and recovery/redefinition. External/ environmental stress mediators include social supports and divorce-related environmental change. Perceptions of the self and of the separation, adaptability to change, parenting skills, and economic stability are internal/familial stress mediators. Optimal divorce adjustment results from economic and social supports, minimal environmental change, positive self-perceptions, and mastery-oriented coping and parenting skills (Fig. 1).

TEMPORAL STAGES OF DIVORCE ADJUSTMENT

Temporal proximity to life-crisis events has been hypothesized to mediate an individual's reaction to that event and to moderate the needs associated with adaptive responding to that event (Auerbach, Chapter 1, this volume). Operationalizing divorce as a series of time-linked stages explains the relationship between divorce-related events, the demands on the individual resulting from these circumstances, and the psychological adaptation of the individual (Hetherington, Cox, and Cox, 1981; Wallerstein & Kelly, 1980).

A model for stages of divorce can be extrapolated from a general model of stages of stress responses (Auerbach, this volume; Chiriboga & Cutler, 1977; Lazarus, 1966). An anticipation or "predecision" period occurs before the separation. Marital discord is the most extreme at this time. A decision to divorce has yet to be reached. An impact or "final separation" period follows the physical separation and may last for several months. Longterm adaptation during the period of "adjustment to the separation" overlaps the final separation period and begins immediately after the physical separation. It may last for several years (Hetherington et al., 1981). Divorce, unlike some other stressors, may be assumed to involve a fourth stage, the recovery/redefinition period, in which the individual redefines relationships with family members and others.

Predecision Period

Significant conflict and consideration of marital separation are primary elements of the predecision period. It has been called the marital point of no return, when an individual's emotional investment in the marriage begins to be withdrawn (Federico, 1979). Denial of emotional withdrawal and unconscious use of marriage

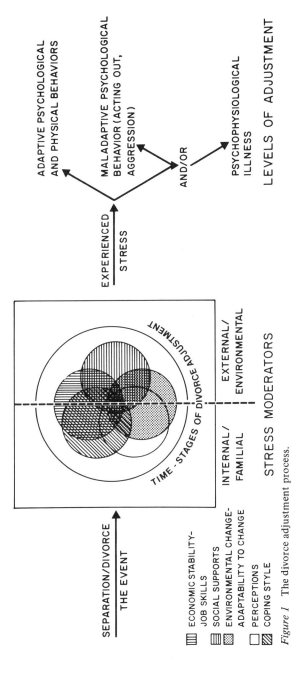

SEPARATION/DIVORCE
THE EVENT

ECONOMIC STABILITY-
JOB SKILLS
SOCIAL SUPPORTS
ENVIRONMENTAL CHANGE-
ADAPTABILITY TO CHANGE
PERCEPTIONS
COPING STYLE

TIME - STAGES OF DIVORCE ADJUSTMENT

INTERNAL/
FAMILIAL

EXTERNAL/
ENVIRONMENTAL

STRESS MODERATORS

EXPERIENCED
STRESS

ADAPTIVE PSYCHOLOGICAL
AND PHYSICAL BEHAVIORS

MALADAPTIVE PSYCHOLOGICAL
BEHAVIOR (ACTING OUT,
AGGRESSION)

AND/OR

PSYCHOPHYSIOLOGICAL
ILLNESS

LEVELS OF ADJUSTMENT

Figure 1   The divorce adjustment process.

termination strategies are common adult behaviors and may result in substantial stress. The amount of time required to reach a final decision to separate is variable. Further, entry into and retreat from this stage may occur several times as the partners attempt to resolve their conflicts and to avoid separation and divorce.

Problematic responses to predecision-period stressors are severe for women and children (Chiriboga & Cutler, 1977). Women frequently report trouble sleeping, loneliness, depression, pessimism, and a lack of self-concern. This period has been reported to be the most stressful for children (Luepnitz, 1979). Children have been reported to be acutely aware of their parents' marital problems despite efforts to keep this knowledge from the children (Cantor, 1979). Children view the reasons for parental hostility as stressful, trivial, and incomprehensible. Longer predecision periods have been associated with lower self-esteem in children (Berg & Kelly, 1979).

Competing demands and marital discord are primary stressors in this period (Emery, 1982). Partners compare the potential success of the separation and the marriage. Marital success is based on the couple's ability to resolve current conflicts or to accept the current circumstances as permanent. A successful separation is determined by the anticipated ability of the family member to master postdivorce demands and is dependent upon social supports, life, job and parenting skills, and economic stability. Current, problematic circumstances are compared to frequently exaggerated or underestimated postdivorce circumstances. Thus, reaching an objective decision is quite difficult.

Final Separation Period

The decision to divorce marks the beginning of the final separation period, which generally lasts several months. The emotional impact of this period is thought to be equal to the stressfulness of the predecision period and greater than that of later stages (Chiriboga & Cutler, 1977; Goode, 1956; Weiss, 1979). The stressfulness of the final separation period is attributed in part to the fact that separation is an inconclusive marital status and is, therefore, more stressful than divorce.

This is a time of considerable trauma for children. The anger of latency-aged children reportedly results from evaluations of divorce as unjustified (Wallerstein & Kelly, 1980). Children who had thought of their homes as happy found this period substantially more traumatic than did children who had recognized the family conflict (Landis, 1960).

A study of parental separation indicated that parental adjustment involved four major areas: resolving legal conflicts, caring for children, rebuilding social networks, and working to achieve emotional adjustment (Spanier & Casto, 1979). The legal system presented major problems for one-fifth of the subjects. Child care concerns involved worries about custody arrangements and the effect of the divorce on the children. Difficulty in adjusting to the separation was related to the availability of a stable social support network and was problematic for more than 84 percent of this sample. Emotional adjustment was further mediated by the anticipated consequences of the separation and attachment remaining for the spouse.

The separating adult's emotional needs compete with parenting demands. Many parents cite "making it through to tomorrow" as their major goal (Stolberg, 1982). The feeling of being emotionally overwhelmed may result in a lack of attention to the child's needs. Projecting child care responsibilities to sources outside the family may be inferred from data of admission to a prevention program for separating families (Stolberg & Cullen, 1983). Custodial mothers progressing through the final separation period sought enrollment only in intervention components that focused on child and parenting matters. Mothers in other stages did not show this selective interest.

The negative impact of this stage on children results primarily from alterations in the parent-child relationship. Parents' reduced physical and emotional availability is frequently interpreted by children as parental rejection (Stolberg & Anker, 1983). Changes in living conditions may significantly alter the child's developmental experience and demand the acquisition of new skills (Stolberg & Anker, 1983; Wallerstein, 1983). The development of internal controls is hampered by the loss of external controls (e.g., parental rules and limits). Greater environmental demands facing adults tend to reduce parental availability and are associated with impulse control problems in their children (Stolberg & Anker, 1983; Stolberg, Camplair, et al., in press). Defining one's place in the interpersonal world is made more difficult by changes in parent-child and peer relationships. Moving to a new neighborhood and changing schools requires special social and academic skills.

Period of Adjustment to the Separation

The separated adult directs attention to matters of renewed stability (e.g., job, education, child care and parenting, home maintenance, financial planning, etc.) and to regaining emotional equilibrium during the period of adjustment to the separation. A new stability is reportedly reached in many families two years after the separation (Hetherington et al., 1977), marking the end of the third adjustment period.

A new lifestyle evolves and many expected and unanticipated problems are confronted. Spanier and Casto (1979) found the periods of final separation and of adjustment to the separation to be interrelated and bidirectional, noting:

> Those who successfully launch a new lifestyle have less difficulty dealing with problems related to dissolution of the marriage than do those who have problems adopting a new lifestyle. Other problems with the marital dissolution, such as feelings of regret, attachment and bitterness toward the spouse actually may increase over time if failures in creating a new lifestyle become apparent.

Economics, children, and social and emotional adjustment are primary concerns of this adjustment stage. Emotional stability reportedly increases and economic instability continues for women, often affecting emotional adjustment (Spanier & Casto, 1979). Custodial parents feel more parenting pressures, while noncustodians feel deprived of their children. Growing apart from old friends and changing lifestyles make social adjustment more difficult. A longitudinal study of divorcing families showed that economic and social problems were greatest one year after the separation, with adults reporting that "things got worse before they got better" (Hetherington et al., 1977).

The children's experience during this period is influenced by the parents' success at meeting their life demands. Increased parental stability often means greater physical and emotional availability and improved parenting. A new predictability in life circumstances is identified within a few months of the separation (Stolberg,

1982). A general visitation schedule is set up with the noncustodian, and his/her whereabouts are frequently known. If the family moves to a new neighborhood and school, the setting becomes somewhat familiar and experience in meeting related demands is gained.

Recovery/Redefinition Period

Many of the stresses of separation are diminished and roles in the family redefined during the fourth and last period of adjustment, recovery and redefinition. Children who were preschoolers at the separation often display marked improvement in functioning two to five years after the divorce (Hetherington et al., 1981). Differences in adjustment and experienced stress in divorced and married women reportedly disappear three years after filing for divorce (Spivey, 1979).

For most individuals, divorce culminates in a recognition of family redefinition rather than a termination of family relationships (Pais & White, 1979). Nuclear families become binuclear systems (Ahrons, 1980). Referring to the previous stages as "emotional separation," Fitzgerald (1980) characterized this period as psychic divorce, an attitudinal and emotional state marking a relatively complete recovery from the divorce trauma.

Reaching a permanent stability within the family (Fitzgerald, 1980) and redefining relationships among family members are the major demands of the recovery/ redefinition period (Hetherington et al., 1977). The stability of the family results from the parents' recovery from divorce-related affective distress and from their ability to successfully master divorce-related demands. A redefinition of the self and an acceptance of the divorce state results from this newly established stability.

Stable interactional patterns between each parent and the children are structured (Pais & White, 1979). Remarriage for the former spouses requires a meshing of the new families and the old. Family members seek (1) both real and perceived successful outcomes to coping and skills mastery efforts, (2) awareness and acceptance of family members' new roles, (3) reduced anger toward the former spouse and increased cooperation around parenting matters, and (4) the reestablishment of an independent and satisfying social life.

While this final stage of the divorce adjustment process holds the promise of recovery for many children, chronic maladjustment resulting from parental divorce is common in some, especially boys. Anger continues for some children several years after the marital dissolution (Wallerstein & Kelly, 1980). Almost half of the children in this study seemed to be in a state of chronic maladjustment. Boys who were preschool-aged at the divorce were found to experience more enduring problems than girls two and five years after separation (Hetherington et al., 1977; 1981).

NEED STATES MEDIATING ADAPTATION TO DIVORCE

Psychological and physical adjustment to marital separation is mediated by three categories of determinants: individual-cognitive, individual-behavioral, and environmental-familial (Stolberg et al., in press). The individual-cognitive factor is comprised of perceptions and expectancies of the divorce as a desirable or undesirable event (Chiriboga, Coho, Stein, & Roberts, 1979), adaptability of the individual to change (Stolberg & Anker, 1983; Stolberg et al., in press), and the individual's coping style. Behavioral skills, including job, parenting, and home and family maintenance skills, make up the individual-behavioral factor. The presence or absence of a stable social support system (Everly, 1978; Goldstein, 1981; Heller & Schneider, 1978; Spanier & Casto, 1979), economic stability (Colletta, 1978), and the extent of positively and negatively evaluated environmental change (Stolberg and Anker, 1983; Stolberg et al., in press) comprise the environmental-familial factor.

The presence of elements of each of these three factors in the postdivorce environment facilitate the adaptive functioning of the family member. The extent to which negatively evaluated environmental change is minimized, positively evaluated change is maximized, and all change is responded to with optimism and the acquisition of necessary skills substantially influences the family members' postseparation and divorce adjustment. The presence of stable social and economic supports further facilitates this adjustment process.

The importance of these need factors varies over time, following a general pattern of crisis adjustment articulated in Chapter 1 in this volume. The closer the temporal proximity to the crisis event of marital separation, the more affectively mediated will be the family members' needs. Temporal distance, both before and after the event, is associated with needs for education and skills acquisition. Positive perceptions of and response flexibility to separation-related environmental changes, coping patterns, and stable social supports take priority in the stages surrounding the separation. Skill acquisition, behavioral adaptability, and concrete economic resources become more important as temporal distance is gained (Fig. 2).

APPLICATION OF THE TEMPORAL ADJUSTMENT MODEL TO PRIMARY PREVENTION PROGRAMMING

The priority and perceived viability of prevention programs for families of divorce is demonstrated by the financial support provided by the National Institute of Mental Health. Preliminary results of these efforts are encouraging. Improved

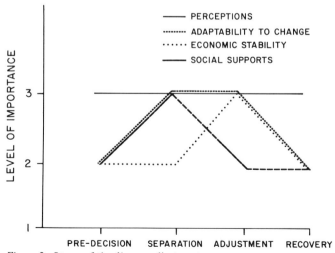

Figure 2 Stages of the divorce adjustment process

self-concept (Stolberg and Garrison, 1985), reductions in behavior problems and anxiety in children (Warren, Grew, Konanc, Ilgen, & Amara, 1982), and improved social skills (Stolberg & Garrison, 1985) have been reported outcomes in child participants in these programs. Improved adult adjustment and greater control over environmental events have been observed in adult participants (Stolberg and Garrison, 1985).

Essential components of primary prevention programs are those procedures which relate to person and environmental factors mediating crisis-related adjustment (Dohrenwend & Dohrenwend, 1974). Factors identified in this review fit that requirement exactly and translate into content areas for a comprehensive prevention strategy for divorcing families. Economic stability, perceptions of the stressful event/separation and cognitive adaptability are mediating factors in the individual. Parenting effectiveness, social supports, and divorce-related environmental changes are external/environmental mediators of adjustment, as shown in Fig. 1. Time since separation moderates the importance of each of the adjustment determinants.

The use of the distinction between first-order (individual-oriented) and second-order (environment-focused) change programs (Watzlawick, Weakland, & Fische, 1974) may provide a structure for incorporating temporal aspects of the adjustment process into the prevention strategy. Interventions can be aimed both at preventing processes that interfere with adjustment (e.g., increasing environmental change, disintegrating support systems) and at assisting family members in mastering separation-related demands.

Early shapers of the adjustment process are professionals, family members, and friends who assist in making important separation decisions (Coogler, 1978; Kappleman & Black, 1978; Deredyn, 1977). Important psychological adjustment processes are frequently ignored. Custodial, financial, and residential arrangements may be based on anger at the spouse and on the adversarial requirements of the legal system, not on important developmental considerations. As a consequence, environmental change and intraparent hostility may be maximized and social supports, financial flexibility, and parent availability may be minimized. Second-order change programs that shape the attitudes, values, and directives of "primary decision influencers" (e.g., extended family, clergy, physicians, attorneys) through educational programming may yield a tangible appreciation of psychological factors and may have an important effect very early in the adjustment process.

First-order change programs are directed at the individual and are intended to assist the family member in mastering life demands brought about by the separation. The content of such programs can be designed to meet the demands of each adjustment stage. Adults' predecision-period needs include emotional support and objective information. Resolving self-perception conflicts, family castigations, and emotional distress is assisted by a stable support system (Wilcox, 1981). Evaluating the potential for success of the marriage and separation requires an objective perspective on current circumstances and an experienced awareness of future problems. Educational and supportive programs may assist in evaluating current and future circumstances, in building support systems, and in developing future career, economic, and family goals.

The predecision period brings children a different set of problems. Parents' marital hostility is most extreme during this period and may have the most deleterious long-term psychological consequences (Emery, 1982; Stolberg et al., in press). Thus, the child needs to be distanced or buffered from prolonged and direct exposure to intraparental hostility. Further, only particularly strong parent-child relationships have been observed to mitigate the effects of marital turmoil and discord (Hetherington, Cox & Cox, 1979). Thus, interventions must focus on maintaining or developing the quality of the parent-child relationship.

The emotional state of the now-separated adult dictates the content of final-separation-period interventions. Stable emotional support systems must be established and new family and household demands must be reduced. It follows, then, that the establishment of a social support system, including external assistance in attending to legal matters and child care responsibilities must be the foundation of parents' interventions offered during this period.

Parents are less physically and emotionally available to children, yet their presence is required for children to successfully master developmental tasks (Wallerstein, 1983). Intervention strategies for children may have to take a temporary *in loco parentis* role and might assist the child in meeting normal developmental tasks (Stolberg & Cullen, 1983). Clarification of the child's role in the divorce, identifying and developing sources of stability and consistency in his/her life and the acquisition of impulse control skills may achieve such goals.

The period of adjustment to the separation is characterized by adults' reduced affective distress and increased attention to life demands. Home and family responsibilities that were shared by marriage partners must now be mastered alone. The separated adults may not possess important and specific skills and therefore must learn to perform crucial functions previously carried out by their former partner, such as cooking, financial planning, home maintenance, and child discipline and/or rearing (Stolberg & Anker, 1983). Thus, the separated adults in this adjustment stage primarily need to acquire skills. Emotional and social supports that assist in coping with the new demands and changed social circumstances are secondary needs.

Of greatest significance to the child is the parents' active participation in their child's developmental experience. Thus, the child's external assistance needs remain essentially as they were in the final separation period, with the amount of extra-familial assistance being determined by the parents' ability to accept their normal role in the family and in the child's development.

Redefining family relationships and establishing permanent stability in the family are demands of the recovery/redefinition period. Enhancing family members' adjustment during this stage is substantially dependent on the successful resolution of earlier stage demands. Thus, the most effective preventive interventions may be those initiated earliest in the divorce adjustment process.

DIVORCE ADJUSTMENT PROJECT: A FIRST–ORDER CHANGE PREVENTION PROGRAM

The following is a description of the Divorce Adjustment Project, a first-order change, primary prevention program for children of divorce and their custodial mothers. The major goals of this project are to increase adaptive psychological skills and to reduce the intensity and duration of the cognitive and behavioral difficulties often experienced by these children. Targeted skill areas include academic, social, and group and individual activities. Typical problems include acting out, poor self-concept, and academic failure.

METHOD

Subjects

Subjects were 82 mothers and their 7- to 13-year-old children (median = 10.7 years), made up of 43 boys and 39 girls. Maximum separation time was 33 months (median = 16.73 months). The mean education of the mothers, all of whom had been married only once, was 13.7 years. Parents and children had no prior histories of using mental health services either within or outside of the school.

Subjects were recruited from the local public school system, the local chapter of Parents Without Partners (PWP), and newspaper advertisements. Letters describing the project and its admission criteria were sent both to all parents of 4th-through 6th-grade children in 3 schools and to active members of PWP. Out of 180 divorce families in the school groups contacted, 44 agreed to participate in the program. Eighteen others came from responses to the PWP letters and the remaining 20 were mothers who responded to the newspaper advertisements.

Instruments

Parent adjustment and skills were assessed by the Fisher Divorce Adjustment Scale (Fisher, 1978), the Life Experiences Survey (Sarason, Johnson, & Siegel, 1978) and the Single Parenting Questionnaire (Stolberg & Ullman, 1985). Children's adjustment was assessed by the Child Behavior Checklist (Achenbach, 1981) and the Piers-Harris Self-Concept Scale (Piers & Harris, 1969).

Intervention Program

Children's Support Group (CSG)

The Children's Support Group (Stolberg, Cullen, Garrison & Brophy, 1981) is a 12-session psychoeducational program designed to help 7- to 13-year-old children meet behavioral and affective demands on them associated with parental divorce. Each one-hour session was divided into two sections. Part I was for discussing a specific session-linked topic (e.g., Whose fault is it? What do I do on vacations? Do I worry about my dad? I wish my parents would get back together.) Part II focused on the teaching, modeling, and rehearsal of specific cognitive-behavioral skills, e.g., problem-solving skills (Finch & Kendall, 1979), anger control skills (Novaco, 1975), and communication skills and relaxation skills (Koeppen, 1974).

Groups, with a maximum size of 8 children, were led by two school-based education and mental health professionals. Group activities were specified in a program procedures manual (Stolberg, et al., 1981). The sequence began with basic, concrete applications (e.g., problem-solving skills applied to mathematics problems), and ended with more complex skills, based on earlier ones, now applied to complex family problems (e.g., communication, anger, and relaxation skills applied to solving the problem of what to say when your father doesn't make his Saturday date).

Single Parents' Support Group (SPSG)

The Single Parents' Support Group (Garrison, Stolberg, Mallonee, Carpenter, & Antrim, 1983) is a 12-week support and skill building program for divorced, custodial mothers. The group focused on the development of participants both as individuals and as parents. Individual-focused sessions include topics such as "The Social Me," "The Working Me," "The Sexual Me," and "Controlling My Feelings." Parent-focused sessions include topics such as "Communicating with My Child," "Disciplining My Child," and "Communicating with My Former Spouse about Childrearing Matters."

Participants determined the sequence of topics for SPSGs based on a list of 20 topical options provided by group leaders. Procedures associated with each topic were described in a program procedures manual (Garrison et al., 1983).

Procedures

Subjects were assigned to one of three intervention groups or to a no-treatment control group ($n = 24$). Group 1 ($n = 25$) involved children's participation in the school-based Children's Support Group, with no adult participation. Group 2 ($n = 22$) involved children's participation in the Children's Support Group concurrent with parents' involvement in the Single Parents' Support Groups. Group 3 ($n = 11$) involved parents' participation in the SPSG, with no child participation.

Data for the three intervention groups were collected before, immediately after, and five months after participation in the respective intervention group. The initial data for no-treatment controls were collected after they agreed to participate, and post-data for that group were collected five months later.

RESULTS

Program outcome data were analyzed in three steps. Eleven analyses of covariance were run using preintervention scores for each criterion measure as covariates and pre-post change scores for the same measures as the dependent variables. Next, 11 analyses of covariance were calculated on postfollow-up change scores for the 3 intervention groups. Again, prescores were used as covariates. T-tests were used as subsequent tests to identify the specific group differences. Analyses of covariance with prescores as covariates were used to partial out the effect of preintervention group differences, thus providing some correction for the lack of randomization to groups.

Analyses of covariance on pre-post change scores yielded significant treatment effects on the Piers-Harris Self Concept Scale $[F(3,78) = 3.51, p < .01]$, the Fisher Divorce Adjustment Scale $[F(3,78) = 2.69, p < .05]$, and the 3 Life Experiences Survey scales: Total Events $[F(3,78) = 5.85, p < .001]$, Positive Evaluations $[F(3,78) = 3.94, p < .01]$, and Negative Evaluations $[F(3,78) = 5.25, p < .01]$. Piers-Harris Self Concept Scores (Fig. 3) increased significantly more in children in the Children's Support Group alone than those of children in the combined intervention group $[t(37) = 2.24, p < .05]$. and in the no-treatment control group $[t(32) = 2.08, p < 05]$. Parents' improvement on Fisher Divorce Adjustment Scale was significantly greater for Single Parents' Support Group members than that for parents in the combined intervention group $[t(28) = 2.14, p < .05]$ and directionally greater than that for the no-treatment controls $[t(16) = 1.84, p < .08]$. The Life Experiences Survey total score decreased

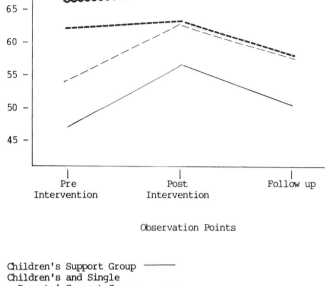

Observation Points

Children's Support Group ————
Children's and Single
  Parents' Support Groups ------·
Single Parents' Support   — — —
  Groups
No Treatment Controls   ∿∿∿

Figure 3 Piers-Harris Self-Concept Scale score by treatment groups

more for no-treatment control group members than for the Children's Support Group alone members [$t(41) = 2.69, p < .01$]. Changes in Life Experiences Survey Positive Evaluation scores were greater for the combined intervention group members than for Children's Support Group alone [$t(45) = 3.25, p < .01$] and no-treatment parents [$t(43) = -2.17, p < .05$]. Positively evaluated events decreased after intervention. Single Parents' Support Group alone [$t(14) = -21.8, p < .05$] and no-treatment [$t(43) = -3.02, p < .01$] group members reported significantly greater increases in the Life Experiences Survey Negative Evaluation score than the combined intervention group.

Analyses of covariance using mean postfollow-up change scores for the 3 intervention groups and all variables reflected only additional change since posttesting. Significant pre-post gains were either maintained or did not change differentially across groups. A significant intervention effect was found for the Child Behavior Checklist Social Skills change score [$F(2,53) = 4.19, p < .01$] (Fig. 4). Prosocial social skills of Children's Support Group alone children ($M = 6.56$) improved more than those of the combined intervention children ($M = 2.23$) at follow up [$t(34) = 2.51, p < .01$].

DISCUSSION

Two of the three Divorce Adjustment Project interventions effectively achieved important prevention and enhancement goals. The Children's Support Group alone condition resulted in substantial increases in children's self-concept at the end of intervention and yielded increases in adaptive social skills at follow up. The Single Parents' Group alone prevented deterioration in parents' adjustment, which was found in the other groups at posttesting, and in fact strengthened adjustment for its participants. The improved adjustment found after intervention in participants of these two groups was either maintained or did not change differentially across groups at follow up.

The success of the CSG can be attributed to its skill and support components. Support components may have helped children to understand their parents' divorce, to accurately define their roles in the process and to improve their self-concepts. Enhanced social adjustment may be linked to skills taught and an improved ability to solve social problems.

Improved social skills in children from the CSG alone groups was not observed until follow up. Apparently, time was needed to practice learned skills before differences in behavior appeared. The enhanced functioning of these youngsters however appears to reflect program effects.

The combined Children's Support Group and Single Parents' Support Group

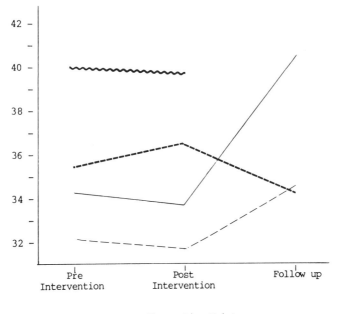

Children's Support Group —————
Children's and Single
  Parents' Support Groups ------.
Single Parents' Support — — —
  Groups
No Treatment Controls ~~~~~

Figure 4 Child Behavior Checklist Social Skills score by treatment groups

intervention did not yield anticipated outcomes. Indeed group members differed in only two respects from controls. Parents reported fewer increases in negatively evaluated change events and greater reductions in positively evaluated events, reflecting a decrease in emotional responses to environmental events.

The goals of this program were to prevent psychological problems in children of divorce. Children's self-concept and prosocial social skills improved only for members of the CSG alone intervention. While parents' participation in the SPSG intervention facilitated adult adjustment, it did not affect their children's adjustment. Single parenting skills were not differentially influenced by this intervention. It appears that intervention programs must emphasize important child development processes to significantly influence child adjustment.

Prevention strategies are meaningful to the extent that they can be exported to other settings and can achieve similar results. The work of Pedro-Carroll and Cowen (1984) demonstrates the replicability of DAP findings. She introduced several modifications in the original CSG program placing more weight on emotional support and expression, and less on concrete applications of the skills taught. The time since divorce had been as much as six years.

Pedro-Carroll and Cowen reported significant reductions in problem behaviors (e.g., acting out) and increases in competencies (e.g., effective learning and interpersonal functioning, adaptive assertiveness, appropriate school behavior, coping with failure and social pressures) in children who participated in her modified CSG, compared to those who did not. Adjustive gains in program children were judged to have taken place by teachers, parents, group leaders, and child self-ratings.

The prospective utility of the current primary prevention program is enhanced by her findings. Children's prosocial skills were enhanced and their adjustment improved. Program procedures manuals assisted in the implementation of the CSG in another setting. We might expect similar results in other groups, at least in populations who have not yet experienced psychological problems.

Future interventions may well profit, as Pedro-Carroll and Cowen's findings suggest, from a stronger emphasis on emotional support and expression. In addition, increased attention to child development concerns (e.g., effective single parenting, continued contact with the noncustodian, etc.) and decreased concentration on adult adjustment may further improve the effectiveness of the program. Concurrent children's and parents' groups did not yield desired psychological outcomes. They can be omitted. Future program evaluations can also identify a wider range of intervention effects if assessment measures are used that tap both prosocial and maladaptive behaviors, in multiple settings, as rated by several observers.

Prevention programming efforts in general might benefit from some of the procedures used in this project. The intervention strategy was firmly based on a model of divorce adjustment and individual-developmental, familial, and environmental processes normally facilitating and interfering with postdivorce adjustment. Program effectiveness may be attributed to the goodness of fit between these real needs and the procedures utilized. Several intervention strategies were used and evaluated comparatively; each had its own well defined methodologies. Moreover, the detailed program procedures manual facilitated Pedro-Carroll and Cowen's replication project and thus stands as a useful program implementation tool for other service settings. That document also allows for refinement of the intervention design, as in Pedro-Carroll and Cowen's work, with a clear linkage of procedural changes and outcome improvements. The failure of the SPSG to influence child adjustment suggests that prevention efforts, in general must focus directly on child development processes and less on parent adjustment if promotion goals are to be achieved.

REFERENCES

Achenbach, T. M. (1981). Behavioral problems and competencies reported by parents of normal and disturbed children aged 4 through 16. *Monographs of the Society for Research in Child Development*, Serial No. 188.

Ahrons, C. B. (1980). Divorce: A crisis of family transition and change. *Family Relations, 4*, 533–540.

Berg, B., & Kelly, R. (1979). The measured self-esteem of children from broken, rejected, and accepted families. *Journal of Divorce, 2*, 363–369.

Bloom, B. L. (1975). *Changing patterns in psychiatric care.* New York: Human Sciences Press.

Bloom, B. L., Asher, S. G., & White, S. W. (1978). Marital disruption as stressor: A review and analysis. *Psychological Bulletin, 85*, 867–894.

Cantor, D. (1979). Divorce: A view from the children. *Journal of Divorce, 2*, 357–362.

Chiriboga, D. A., Coho, A., Stein, J. A., & Roberts, J. (1979). Divorce, stress and social supports: A study in help-seeking behavior. *Journal of Divorce, 2*, 121–135.

Chiriboga, D. A., & Cutler, L. (1977). Stress responses among divorcing men and women. *Journal of Divorce, 2*, 95–106.

Coddington, R. D., & Troxell, J. R. (1980). The effect of emotional factors on football injury rates–A pilot study. *Journal of Human Stress, 14*, 3–5.

Colletta, N. D. (1978). Divorced mothers at two income levels: Stress, support and child-rearing. Unpublished master's thesis, Cornell University, Ithaca, NY.

Coogler, O. J. (1978). *Structured mediation in divorce settlement: A handbook for marital mediations.* Lexington, MA: Lexington Books.

Deredyn, A. P. (1977). Children in divorce: Interventions in the phase of separation. *Pediatrics, 60*, 20–27.

Dohrenwend, B. P., & Dohrenwend, B. S. (1974). Social and cultural influences on psychopathology. *Annual Review of Psychology, 25*, 417–452.

Emery, R. E. (1982). Interpersonal conflict and the children of discord and divorce. *Psychological Bulletin, 92*, 310–330.

Everly, K. G. (1978). Leisure networks and role strain: A study of divorced women with custody. *Dissertation Abstracts International, 6*, 3865A.

Federico, J. (1979). The marital termination period of the divorce adjustment process. *Journal of Divorce, 2*, 93–106.

Finch, A.J., & Kendall, P. S. (1979). Impulsive behaviors: From research to treatment. In A. J. Finch & P. S. Kendall (Eds.), *Clinical treatment and research in child psychopathology.* New York: Spectrum Publications.

Fisher, B. (1978). *When your relationship ends.* Boulder, CO: Family Relations Learning Center.

Fitzgerald, R. V. (1980). What patients should expect after divorce. *Medical Aspects of Human Sexuality, 11*, 73–92.

Garrison, K. M., Stolberg, A. L., Mallonnee, D., Carpenter, J., & Antrim, Z. (1983). The Single Parents' Support Group: A procedures manual. Unpublished manual, Divorce Adjustment Project, Virginia Commonwealth University, Richmond.

Goldstein, M. (1981). Major factors acting on the early adolescent. In C. D. Moore (Ed.), *Adolescence and stress.* Rockville, MD: National Institute of Mental Health.

Goode, W. J. (1956). *Women in divorce.* New York: Free Press.

Guidubaldi, J., Perry, J. D., & Cleminshaw, H. K. (1983). The legacy of parental divorce: A nationwide study of family status and selected mediating variables on children's academic and social competencies. *School Psychology Review, 12*, 300–323.

Heller, D. B., & Schneider, C. D. (1978). Interpersonal methods for coping with stress: Helping families of dying children. *Omega, 8*, 319–331.

Hetherington, E. M. (1979). Divorce: A child's perspective. *American Psychologist, 34,* 851–858.

Hetherington, E. M., Cox, M., & Cox, R. (1977). The aftermath of divorce. In J. H. Stevens, Jr. & M. Matthews (Eds.), *Mother-child, father-child relations.* Washington, DC: National Association for the Education of Young Children.

Hetherington, E. M., Cox, M. & Cox, R. (1979). Family interactions and the social, emotional and cognitive development of children following divorce. In V. Vaughan & T. Brazelton (Eds.), *The family setting priorities.* New York: Science and Medicine.

Hetherington, E. M., Cox, M., & Cox, R. (1981). Effects of divorce on parents and children. In M. Lamb (Ed.), *Nontraditional families.* Hillsdale, NJ: Erlbaum.

Jacobs, T. J., & Charles, E. (1980). Life events and the occurrence of cancer in children. *Psychosomatic Medicine, 1,* 11–24.

Kappelman, M. M., & Black, J. (1980). Children and divorce: The pediatrician's responsibility. *Pediatric Annals, 9,* 342–351.

Kelly, R., & Berg, S. (1978). Measuring children's relations to divorce. *Journal of Clinical Psychology, 34,* 215–221.

Koeppen, A. S. (1974). Relaxation training for children. *Elementary School Guidance Counseling, 9,* 14–21.

Kurdek, L. A. (1981). An integrative perspective on children's divorce adjustment. *American Psychologist, 35,* 856–866.

Kurdek, L. A., & Siesky, A. E. (1980a). Children's perceptions of their parents' divorce. *Journal of Divorce, 3,* 339–378.

Kurdek, L. A., & Siesky, A. E. (1980b). The effects of divorce on children: The relationship between parent and child perspectives. *Journal of Divorce, 4,* 85–99.

Landis, J. (1960). The trauma of children when parents divorce. *Marriage and Family Living, 22,* 7–13.

Lazarus, R. S. (1966). *Psychological stress and the coping process.* New York: McGraw-Hill.

Luepnitz, D. A. (1979). Which aspects of divorce affect children? *Family Coordinator, 1,* 79–85.

Novaco, R. W. (1975). *Anger control: The development and evaluation of an experimental treatment.* Lexington, MA: Lexington Books.

Pais, J., & White, P. (1979). Family redefinition: A review of the literature toward a model of divorce adjustment. *Journal of Divorce, 3,* 271–281.

Pedro-Carroll, J. A. L., & Cowen, E. L. (1985). The Divorce Intervention Project: An investigation of the efficacy of a school-based prevention program. *Journal of Consulting Clinical Psychology, 53,* 603–611.

Piers, E. V., & Harris, D. B. (1969). *The Piers-Harris children's self-concept scale.* Nashville, TN: Counselor Recordings and Tests.

Sarason, I., Johnson, J., & Siegel, J. (1978). Assessing the impact of life changes: Development of the Life Experiences Survey. *Journal of Consulting and Clinical Psychology, 46,* 932–946.

Spanier, G., & Casto, R. (1979). Adjustment to separation and divorce: An analysis of fifty case studies. *Journal of Divorce, 2,* 241–253.

Spivey, P. B. (1979). Maladjustment, personality characteristics and stress in divorced women. *Dissertation Abstracts International, 10,* 5090B.

Stolberg, A.L. (1982). A stage-linked model of divorce adjustment and primary prevention (NIMH Research Grant Application No. RO1 MH 34462). Rockville, MD: National Institute of Mental Health.

Stolberg, A. L., & Anker, J. M. (1983). Cognitive and behavioral changes in children resulting from parental divorce and consequent environmental changes. *Journal of Divorce, 7,* 23–41.

Stolberg, A. L., Camplair, C., Currier, K., & Wells, M. (in press). Individual, familial and environmental determinants of children's post-divorce adjustment and maladjustment. *Journal of Divorce.*

Stolberg, A. L., & Cullen, P. M. (1983). Preventive interventions for families of divorce: The Divorce Adjustment Project. In L. Kurdek (Ed.), *New directions in child development: Children and divorce.* San Francisco: Jossey-Bass.

Stolberg, A. L., Cullen, P. M., Garrison, K. M., & Brophy, C. J. (1981). The Children's Support Group: A procedures manual. Unpublished manual. Divorce Adjustment Project, Virginia Commonwealth University, Richmond.

Stolberg, A. L., & Garrison, K. M. (1985). Evaluating a primary prevention program for children of divorce: The Divorce Adjustment Project. *American Journal of Community Psychology, 13,* 111–124.

Stolberg, A. L., & Ullman, A. J. (1985). Assessing dimensions of single parenting: The Single Parenting Questionnaire. *Journal of Divorce, 8,* 31–45.

Wallerstein, J. S. (1983). Children of divorce: The psychological tasks of the child. *American Journal of Orthopsychiatry, 53,* 230–243.

Wallerstein, J. S., & Kelly, J. B. (1980). *Surviving the breakup: How children and parents cope with divorce.* New York: Basic Books.

Warren, N. J., Grew, R. S., Konanc, J. T., Ilgen, E. R., & Amara, I. (1982). Parenting after divorce: Evaluation of prevention programs for divorcing families. American Psychological Association Conference, Washington, DC.

Watzlawick, P., Weakland, J. H., & Fische, R. (1974). *Change: Principles of problem formation and problem resolution.* New York: Norton.

Wilcox, B. L. (1981). Social support, life stress and psychological adjustment: A test of the buffering hypothesis. *American Journal of Community Psychology, 4,* 371–386.

6

Parent–Child Influences
during Medical Procedures

Barbara G. Melamed
University of Florida

Joseph P. Bush
Virginia Commonwealth University

MEDICAL INTERVENTION AS A CRISIS
FOR THE FAMILY

The process of becoming a medical patient has many aspects of a "life crisis" for the sick child as well as the entire family (Auerbach, 1980). This problem is large, as each year over 5 million children are admitted to hospitals for diagnostic or treatment procedures. A 1979 American Hospital Association survey reported that there are over 16 million pediatric patient bed days per year (Traughber & Cataldo, 1982). An estimated 45 percent of all children have been admitted to the hospital by the time they reach age 7 (Davies, Butler, & Goldstein, 1972).

The magnitude of this "crisis" is even more significant because we are not certain which families are most vulnerable to this kind of stress-evoking situation. These situations typically involve individuals who ordinarily function adequately but who may become anxious to the point where emotional equilibrium is disrupted and normal coping behaviors are rendered ineffective.

The current chapter attempts to identify a taxonomy of stressors facing a family entering the health care system because of an acute illness in one of their children. The adaptive and nonadaptive strategies employed by the family to deal with these stressful events have rarely been studied. Intervention procedures seem to be applied in an indiscriminate fashion with little regard for developmental differences or coping abilities. The chapter attempts to reorganize the data into areas that will lead to systematic research emphasizing the individualizing of medical preparation.

A survey of hospitals providing pediatric care for nonchronic conditions reported that over 70 percent of these hospitals routinely use psychological preparation for children undergoing diagnostic or surgical procedures (Peterson & Ridley-Johnson, 1980). It is too often assumed that all children can benefit to some extent by receiving support and information about what to expect. In fact, children's prehospital adjustment and personality may make them more or less prone to psychological consequences from the hosptial experience. Some children

Support for this chapter was provided by grants DE05305 and T32DE07133 from the National Institute of Dental Research.

may become sensitized by hospital preparation if they are too young to understand or if they distort the information being presented (Melamed, Dearborn, & Hermecz, 1983).

Although estimates of behavioral disturbances resulting from the hospital experience range from 10 to 92 percent of all children hospitalized, only a small percentage acutally suffer severe transient or long-term disturbance (Melamed, Robbins, & Fernandez, 1982). In fact, a rarely cited finding demonstrates that 25 percent of the children were rated as improved in behavior after a hospital stay (Vernon, Foley, & Schulman, 1967). Thus, the emotional climate offered by the hospital and its personnel can be constructive for many children by (1) serving as a refuge from emotional strains, (2) promoting emotional education, (3) encouraging normal patterns of growth and development, (4) enhancing the parent-child relationship, (5) teaching and providing good nutrition, and (6) providing a sense of mastery and shaping adaptive behavior (Shore, Geiser, & Wolman, 1965).

Thus, the task of the pediatric psychologist is to identify the factors that exacerbate emotional distress accompanying hospitalization, to pinpoint which families are at risk for developing disturbances without intervention, and to determine the most appropriate intervention for the particular child and parents in a specific hospital environment.

Sources of Stress

The child's encounter with health care settings, whether as a hospital patient or as an outpatient, often involves various kinds of stress such as separation from familiar persons, painful experiences such as injections, and the need to cooperate with various unfamiliar and sometimes frightening medical procedures. Although the severity of the illness or physical dysfunction can exacerbate the stress with its concomitant pain, at least some portion of children's reactions can be attributed to the aversive properties of the setting itself (Traughber & Cataldo, 1982). The children are often restricted in movement, isolated from their peer group, and lack the information or ability to control their situation.

For the parent, there is another array of concerns that have to do with the seriousness of the problem—physical burdens of illness, special diets or regimens, and the financial strain. The parent must often cope with his or her uncertainty about outcome, try to mitigate the child's fears, pain, and discomforts, juggle his or her own expectations and past experiences, as well as maintain continuing familial, occupational, marital, and personal role behaviors (Melamed, Robbins, & Fernandez, 1982).

The psychological effect upon siblings of a serious illness of one child has been shown to depend on when, how long, and how much they are deprived of the things they want. They experience guilt about not being sick. Some siblings develop a protective attitude toward the sick child. However, the deprivations of parental affection and attention and deprivation of material wants because of the sick child's needs creates resentment that in some cases becomes very deep and destructive. Although there are few empirical studies of siblings of acutely ill children, studies of siblings of chronically ill children show them to be at risk for adjustment problems (Breslau, Weitzman, & Messenger, 1981).

Factors that Mediate the Impact of the Hospital Experience

The effects of hospital experiences are far from uniform and depend upon a multitude of factors including psychosocial characteristics of the family and factors specific to the illness. Some of the factors that mediate the relationship between severity of illness and the child's response to it include the age of the child, the child's cognitive style and coping skills repertoire, his or her interpretation of the meaning of the illness, and the supportive nature of the family relationships.

The younger the child, the more vulnerable he/she is to separation from familiar adults. In younger children, the meaning of the illness may be misinterpreted as punishment for breaking rules (Perrin & Gerrity, 1981). Children under seven years of age are usually less able to profit from preparation programs that focus on providing information about how to cope with medical procedures. They require a more concrete preparation close in time to the events that they must handle. There is some recent evidence (Melamed et al., 1983) that children who are under the age of eight and have had previous surgery are most vulnerable and may even be sensitized by receiving information about impending events.

The parent of the younger child is most likely to assist in the care of the ill child if his/her own anxiety is lessened by adequate preparation. In families with close relationships, children showed more withdrawal and upset when the parent was absent (Brown, 1979). Mothers who are themselves anxious and highly accepting of hospital authority tend to have children who are distressed and withdrawn. Thus, the task of the clinician is also to assess the parents' needs and abilities in order to decide how involved they should become in their children's medical treatment.

Thus, in examining the effects of psychological preparation of families for medical treatment, one must evaluate the individual needs of the family members, their abilities to cope with the stressors, and their intellectual and emotional states over the course of the illness. Vernon and his colleagues (1967) have identified three variables that are the focus of many programs that prepare children for surgery or hospitalization: providing information, encouraging emotional expression, and establishing a trusting relationship.

LITERATURE REVIEW ON PREPARATION OF CHILDREN

Child-Focused Interventions

The majority of currently utilized preparatory programs, employ direct intervention with the child. While a considerable variety of preparatory techniques have been described and evaluated, they may be classified according to three salient dimensions. The first dimension references the modality of intervention, such as information provision, desensitization, or training in and rehearsal of relaxation techniques. The second dimension is concerned with situational parameters, such as time and physical setting, in the context of which intervention occurs. The third important dimension of preparatory techniques is that of specificity. This references the population of children for whom the intervention has been empirically determined to be effective, defined in terms of individual child characteristics.

It will be seen that these dimensions must be considered together in order to optimize the impact of preparatory efforts.

Intervention Modalities

Research on techniques for preparing children to undergo medical procedures has primarily utilized pedodontic and pediatric surgery situations. Specific intervention modalities have included direct provision of information and coping skills training, information provision, and coping skills training presented by means of exposure to various types of models, relaxation and systematic desensitization, and preparatory play. These modalities do not represent distinct categories. An intervention intended to present hospital information via modeling, for instance, may also function as desensitization by providing the opportunity for controlled exposure to medically related stimuli. There appear to be three variables in any preparatory intervention procedure, which that technique may or may not explicitly specify, impacting significantly on outcome. These variables are: information communicated to the child; emotional impact of the interaction between the child and the individual(s) delivering the intervention; and parental participation in the child's preparation.

Information has been found by several researchers to benefit patients undergoing a variety of medical procedures (Kendall & Watson, 1981). In a study of 4- to 17-year-old children hospitalized for elective surgery, Melamed et al. (1983) found that subjects who scored higher on a hospital information test, regardless of whether or not they had previously been shown a hospital information film, were rated by their mothers four weeks after surgery as having adjusted better to the hospital experience and as manifesting fewer posthospitalization behavioral problems than lower-scoring subjects.

Information has been described as improving adjustment to medical procedures by correcting the child's negative fantasies about medical experiences (Becker, 1972) and by reducing the child's uncertainty about what is in store, thereby diminishing fear of the unknown and abetting anticipatory cognitive coping (Duffy, 1972). In addition, information provision necessary occurs in an interpersonal context. The child may receive emotional support, either directly or in more subtle ways, from the behavior of a care-giving adult or danger-control authority (Parcel & Meyer, 1978) endeavoring to help them cope and, at least by implication, recognizing their anxiety.

The use of models to present preparatory information to children involves factors that blur the distinction between information provision and coping skills training, as the model is depicted in some way interacting with the medical stimuli in question. Even if the "model" is an age-peer on a videotape who simply describes, for example, the procedures involved in undergoing dental prophylaxis, his or her affective tone and syntactic presentation implicitly model cognitive coping strategies.

In general, models have been found effective. Melamed and Siegel (1975) reported more favorable postoperative indices in children exposed to an age-peer model than in children viewing unrelated material. Studies have suggested that children benefit more if the model explicitly demonstrates use of coping procedures to overcome initial fearfulness than if she or he demonstrates only successful coping, beginning at a mastery level (Arata, Klorman, Chandler, & Sveen, 1977). Furthermore, having children actually practice the modeled coping skills has been shown to increase their usage of the skills and to decrease anxiety and disruptiveness during dental treatment relative to children observing the same model without structured practice (Klingman, Melamed, Cuthbert, & Hermecz, 1984).

Systematic desensitization in employing relaxation has also been effectively used to reduce children's disruptiveness in a dental setting (Machen & Johnson, 1979). Preparatory play with medically related toys is one of the more traditional approaches to helping children cope with these experiences. The effectiveness of this approach, which has not fared as favorably in the research literature as modeling procedures, may be attributable to the desensitizing of medical stimuli through association with pleasurable play activity. Alternatively, children may use medical toys to accomplish "the work of worry" (Burstein & Meichenbaum, 1979; Janis, 1958) in a relatively nonthreatening context. Both interpretations suggest that the child, in order to be prepared to adapt to the fear-arousing stimuli, must become aroused and then experience a reduction of anxious arousal.

Situational Parameters

The mediating effects of situational variables on preparatory intervention have been largely neglected in empirical research. A great many studies do not even specify the physical setting in which intervention occurs, leaving the reader to speculate about possible confounding. Likewise, few researchers have attempted to systematically evaluate the interpersonal context in which preparatory intervention is delivered. Fernald and Corry (1981) compared responses to arm venipuncture or finger stick between children receiving "empathic" and "directive" informational preparation. While not a methodologically rigorous investigation, results did show concordance between negative interpersonal impacts as reported by children and negative behavioral responses in the latter group. Auerbach, Martelli, and Mercuri (1983) demonstrated that information provided by an impersonal agent was not as satisfying as that provided by an empathic person. Another important situational parameter, which will be considered in some detail, involves timing of preparatory intervention.

Individual Characteristics

Several research studies have shown that the effects of preparatory intervention vary with the age of the child (Ferguson, 1979; Melamed, Meyer, Gee, & Soule, 1976). More generally, differing outcomes may be associated with various matches among intervention modality, situational parameters, and individual child characteristics. Findings supporting the specificity of intervention effects, reviewed in Melamed, Robbins, and Fernandez (1982), belie the widely held "intuitive psychology" belief that all children can benefit from preparation. Many children get through intensive medical procedures without the benefit of any preparation and show no adverse effects (Vernon, Schulman, & Foley, 1966). It is important that we optimize our therapeutic efficiency and efficacy and minimize iatrogenic effects (Melamed et al., 1982) by developing and utilizing an empirical data base defining the predicted outcome of which intervention with which child in which situation.

A detailed review of research documenting the importance of each of a number of individual child characteristics would be too lengthy to include in this chapter. However, some of the dimensions found to be of importance have included the developmental level of the child's concepts of physical illness (Simeonsson, Buckley, & Monson, 1979), coping style (Burstein & Meichenbaum, 1979; Knight et al., 1979), age (Brain & Maclay, 1968; Prugh, Staub, Sands, Kirschenbaum, & Lenihan, 1953), and prior medical experiences (Arata et al., 1977; Melamed, 1981).

Family Factors

Relatively little empirical research has addressed the role of family (as distinct from parental) factors in preparing children for potentially stressful medical procedures. In contrast, family coping and intrafamilial support have been considered with respect to severe chronic disease in childhood. For example, Kaplan and his colleagues (Kaplan, Smith, Grobstein, & Fischman, 1973) have proposed a sequential model of phase-specific coping tasks associated with the characteristic stages of chronic illness: diagnosis, remission, exacerbation, and terminal state. Their recommendations are primarily concerned with preservation of family functioning, important for the continued well-being of all family members as well as providing support for the sick child. While different coping strategies may be appropriate for different individuals, the method chosen by each family member influences the adjustment of all others, and particularly difficult problems may be caused by highly discrepant coping among family members.

Prugh and his colleagues (1953) called attention over 30 years ago to the potential emotional disequilibrium in families resulting from behavioral disturbances often associated with hospitalization of young children. Preparatory intervention programs have focused almost exclusively on improving the adjustment and minimizing adverse psychosocial sequelae of the hospitalized child. Few if any interventions have been reported that focus either on familial facilitation of this goal or on mitigating the effects of adverse child reactions to acute disease or brief hospitalization on other family members or on the family system as a whole.

Parents as Therapeutic Agents

A question of great concern to health care professionals is whether or not to encourage parental participation during pediatric and pedodontic procedures. Current trends in hospital practice (Roskies, Mongeon, & Gagnon-Lefebvre, 1978) as well as in psychological preparation for elective surgery (Wolfer & Visintainer, 1975) place increased emphasis on the role of parents. In the case of the child requiring hospitalization, the parent might have varying degress of involvement ranging from merely being the agent who delivers and retrieves the child from the hospital to being an intricately involved member of the child care team. In the outpatient care of children in most clinics, the parent is expected to provide information about the child's medical condition as well as providing support in order to enhance cooperation.

Parental Anxiety

The emotional contagion hypothesis (Escalona, 1953; Visintainer & Wolfer, 1975) states that parental anxiety is communicated to the child by nonverbal as well as verbal means, which in turn increases the child's anxiety level. This hypothesis is broadly supported by empirical studies correlating parental and child state anxiety in medical situations (Bailey, Talbot, & Taylor, 1973; Sides, 1977). However, data from studies employing interventions to reduce parental anxiety have suggested that decreased parental anxiety by itself is insufficient to improve children's reactions to medical procedures (Pinkham & Fields, 1976; Wright, Alpern, & Leake, 1973).

A second model accounting for parents' effects on children's handling of stressful medical procedures is the crisis-parenting hypothesis (Bush, 1983). This model emphasizes the increased importance of parenting when children face stressors (Kaplan et al., 1973). Support for this model was demonstrated by Vernon et al. (1966) in their study of 2- to 6-year-old children hospitalized for elective surgery. They compared the effect of maternal presence on children's behavior during a relatively nonstressful hospital procedure (admission) with a more highly stressful procedure (anesthesia induction). During the less stressful procedure, children evidenced little upset, and maternal presence or absence had no significant effect. During the highly stressful procedure, however, maternal presence was negatively related to children's distress levels.

Studies have shown that parents often become highly anxious when accompanying their children in medical situations. Gofman, Buckman, and Schade (1957) interviewed 100 parents at the time of their children's admission to the hospital. They reported that all of these parents described themselves as anxious, 57 of them calling it "overwhelming." They described over half of the parents as having been plainly unable to provide adequate support to the child. Similar results were obtained by Skipper, Leonard, and Rhymes (1968).

The crisis-parenting hypothesis thus states that high parental anxiety during or just prior to crises may lead to disorganized parental functioning (Duffy, 1972; Robinson, 1968), and consequently to less adequate parental support for the child's coping efforts at a time when such support is likely to be crucial. On the other hand, the hypothesis also states that effective parenting in crisis situations may help children cope successfully and even benefit from the experience.

Parental Presence

To the extent that parental anxiety is not perfectly correlated with child fear and noncooperativeness during medical procedures, the crisis-parenting hypothesis may account for much of this variance in terms of competent parenting behavior in the setting. It is not surprising, according to either model, that studies of the effect of parental absence or presence that do not take into account parental anxiety or parenting behaviors have at times failed to show main effects (Allen & Evans, 1968; Venham, Murray, & Gaulin-Kremer, 1979).

Shaw and Routh (1982) randomly assigned parents of children in two age groups (18 months and 5 years) to be present or absent during well-child examinations. More crying was observed in the younger children whose mothers were excluded. However, during the actual injections, children in the mother-present group received the most negative ratings. It was concluded that while protest may occur with separation, presence of mother may serve as a discriminative cue for or to reinforce overt expression of anxiety. Similar findings were reported in another study, comparing 4- to 6-year-old with 7- to 10-year-old children receiving venipunctures (Gross, Stern, Levin, Dale, & Wojnilower, 1983).

Venham and his colleagues (1979) published one of the only studies in which actual parenting behaviors during children's dental appointments were studied. Parents were given a choice as to whether or not they wished to accompany their children in the operatory. No differences were found in how well children adjusted during the procedures between groups whose parents were or were not present. It was found that the quality of the interaction between child and mother varied with the intensity of the child's response during treatment, and that parents demonstrated a variety of behaviors including ignoring, coercing, reassuring and instructing their children.

On the other hand, Hanallah and Rosales (1983) demonstrated that when parents of preschoolers having surgery elected to stay with their children during anesthesia induction, there was a significant decrease in the number of very upset children relative to children unaccompanied by a parent. It may be the case that the decision of parents to stay or not indicates something about the current status of their relationship with their children.

Prugh et al. (1953) pointed out that this possibility may significantly confound studies of the effects of parental presence. They found that parents who visited their hospitalized children less frequently were more likely than frequently visiting parents to have nonsatisfactory relationships with these children. Several authors (Dimock, 1960; Gofman et al., 1957; Brown, 1979) have contended that the quality of this relationship is a crucial variable influencing the child's hospital adjustment.

Couture (1976) attempted to control for this variable by randomly assigning parents of 3- to 6-year-old hospitalized children to a limited visiting, unlimited visiting, or rooming-in condition. Significantly less problematic behavior was observed in children of parents who roomed in. This replicated the earlier finding, not incorporating random assignment of parents to visiting conditions, of Brain and Maclay (1968), who found better in-hospital and posthospitalization adjustment in young children whose mothers roomed in.

These results, then, indicate that parental presence may or may not help children in medical situations. The overall unclarity of the results of studies of parent presence, particularly in conjunction with previously reported findings regarding the correlates of parental anxiety levels, suggests the need for further investigation into differential effects associated with differences in how the parent interacts with the ill child, in addition to the age of the child.

Child-Rearing Variables

The task facing parents in helping their children cope with stressful medical procedures is more complex than simply being present or telling the child what to expect. In addition to coping with his or her own anxiety, the parent must respond appropriately to the individual child's changing needs. Researchers have looked at child-rearing variables in order to explore the relationship between parenting in a variety of stressful situations and the child's responses in the medical situation. Levy (1959) found a significant relationship between observer ratings of hospitalized children's behavior at several stresspoints and parents' prior provision of stress-response training specific to hospitalization. A low but significant positive correlation was obtained between parents' provision of general and of hospital-specific stress-response training.

Venham et al. (1979) found significant associations between observational and physiological measures of 3- to 5-year-old children's anxiety during dental treatment and observational and self-report measures of the child rearing practiced at home by parents. Children who were more anxious during treatment had parents who tended to avoid the use of reward and punishment, while low child anxiety was related to maternal responsivity and the organization of the home environment. Zabin and Melamed (1980) mailed a self-report measure of parenting behavior in response to children's fearful avoidance in a variety of common stressful situations, to parents of 4- to 12-year-old children within one year after hospitalization for elective surgery. Paternal use of punishment was found to be associated with high self-reported state anxiety in the child. High preoperative anxiety was observed in children whose parents reported reinforcing the child's dependency and/or avoidance behaviors. On the other hand, lower pre- and postoperative anxiety was found in children whose parents used more modeling and reassurance.

Heffernan and Azarnoff (1971) found a significant interaction between children's previous anxiety during outpatient medical examinations (rated retrospectively by mother) and mother's suppressiveness of the child's crying when frightened. Among children rated by mother as previously nonfearful, those with suppressive mothers reported high anxiety, while those with nonsuppressive mothers reported low anxiety about the impending examination. Children of suppressive mothers reported greater anticipatory anxiety regardless of maternally reported child anxiety on previous visits.

Parent-Focused Preparatory Interventions

Research has also been conducted on the impact of parent-focused preparatory intervention for children about to undergo medical procedures. Seidl and Pilliteri (1967) indicate that interest in such programs has been increasing, and Roskies and her colleagues (1978) have described emerging trends in nursing as involving parents more fully in the hospital care of young children.

Wright et al. (1973) sent mothers of 3- to 6-year-olds scheduled for dental treatment a preappointment letter intended to provide information and give advice. Mothers receiving the letter had lower Taylor Manifest Anxiety at time of appointment than control group mothers. This effect was not accompanied, however, by any significant differences in observer ratings of children's cooperativeness during treatment. Similar results were subsequently obtained by Pinkham and Fields (1976).

Wolfer and Visintainer (1975) identified five "stresspoints" in hospitalization, just prior to each of which nurses provided child–parent units with information and reassurance. Children receiving stresspoint preparation were rated as more cooperative and less upset during stresspoint procedures, as well as showing more favorable postoperative indices than control group children. Parents in the stresspoint nursing group self-reported less anxiety than control group parents.

These findings support the efficacy of preprocedural support and information as ways of reducing mothers' anxiety, as well as providing evidence that preparing parents and children together is helpful to both. They do not, however, establish that reductions in maternal anxiety cause or even facilitate reduction of child anxiety or contribute in any other way to improving the child's adjustment to the medical experience.

Somewhat stronger evidence that parent-focused preparation may help children was provided by Skipper et al. (1968). Mothers of children hospitalized for tonsillectomy were given preparatory information by nurses who avoided paying any more attention to the children than was received by control group children. Mothers receiving "supportive information" reported less stress, and their children received more favorable ratings on several postoperative indices than controls. The authors interpreted their results as indicating that the intervention enabled mothers to more effectively assist their children in coping with the stress of hospitalization. While their interpretation is consistent with the crisis-parenting hypothesis, their results may also be accounted for by the emotional contagion hypothesis, as they did not document any differences between parenting behaviors of experimental and control group mothers. Similar conclusions were drawn by Peterson and Shigetomi (1981), looking at 2- to 10-year-olds hospitalized for elective tonsillectomy. Again, however, their study included no measure of parental compliance with training—whether these parents actually did anything different with their children than parents not so prepared.

These results were replicated and extended by Zastowny, Kirschenbaum, and Meng (in press), who manipulated parenting activities more explicitly. Six- to ten-year-old children who had been hospitalized for elective surgery were included in one of three treatment groups. "Control group" parents and children viewed a coping model film two weeks prior to admission, and parents were encouraged to spend extra time with their children during those two weeks. In the "anxiety reduction group" parents were also trained in relaxation. Finally, in the "coping skills group" all the above interventions were delivered and parents viewed a videotape modeling parental use of these techniques to facilitate a child's coping at hospitalization stresspoints and were given a booklet to help them adapt these techniques with their own children. In comparison to "control group" children, children in the "coping skills group" were rated by parents as behaving less problematically at home both during the preadmission week and during the second postdischarge week, and these parents rated themselves as less stressed during the prehospitalization period. "Coping skills" children were also rated by observers as engaging in fewer maladaptive behaviors than "controls" during six hospitalization stresspoints. While providing some of the strongest evidence currently available that preparatory intervention can differentially enhance parental facilitation of children's coping with medical stressors, this study does not specify the facilitative parental behaviors involved, nor does it evaluate whether there were in fact any differences between groups in what parents actually did.

Summary

Research has supported the commonsense proposition that parents influence how their children handle stressful medical experiences. Correlational studies have established that parental anxiety as well as certain self-reported childrearing practices covary with children's adjustment, and parent-focused interventions have been favorably evaluated. Unfortunately, there has been a lack of research on parenting behavior in the medical setting. Until such research has been carried out, we will not know what parents actually do while interacting with a stressed child, nor what the effects of various parenting behaviors are. Clearly, an understanding of parenting in the crisis situation will have to precede identification of targets and prescription of interventions designed to modify crisis parenting behaviors.

Naturalistic Patterns of Parent-Child Interactions under Stress

In an attempt to address this need, our current research involves development of an observational scale that will measure parent-child interaction during stressful medical events. We have thus far been successful in developing a highly reliable instrument and have obtained encouraging data which support some of the hypotheses that exist in the child development literature.

First, from the emotional contagion hypothesis, it was predicted that agitated mothers would have children who showed more signs of distress. It was also anticipated that younger children would show this effect more strongly, that is, with increasing age emotional contagion from mother would become relatively less dominant as a determinant of the child's anxiety level.

Second, from the crisis-parenting hypothesis, it was predicted that agitated mothers would show more disorganization of parenting in terms of helping their children cope with stress, and that this would have a negative effect on the children. Thus, it was expected that parents who showed more agitation and used more ignoring or distracting with their children in the stressful situation would have children who did not use exploration in order to overcome their fears and who were high in distress.

Method

Subjects were 50 dyads, consisting of children between 4 and 10 years of age, seen as outpatients in the Urology, Gastroenterology, Elective Surgery, or Infectious Diseases clinics at Shands Teaching Hospital, J. Hillis Miller Health Center, University of Florida, in 1982, and their mothers. Children with severe chronic disabilities were excluded, as were any children who would be accompanied into the examination room by anyone other than mother alone. Patients were heterogeneous with respect to race, socioeconomic status, and diagnosis, but comparable with respect to their being referred by primary care physicians for specialized medical attention or postsurgical follow-up.

Self-report measures of anxiety were administered to mothers and children (Spielberger, Gorusch, & Lushene, 1970; Melamed & Siegel, 1975) prior to their entry into examination room, and mothers rated their children's reactions to past medical visits and expected reaction to the current visit, as well as completing a questionnaire describing their own coping style (Billings & Moos, 1981). Mothers were also asked to rate the stressfulness for them of their child's current health crisis on a four-point scale.

After the child's clinic visit was completed, the examining physician listed the child's diagnosis and rated its severity on a 10-point scale ranging from "entirely trivial" to "imminently life-threatening." Also at this time, mothers were rated by observers on their anxiety, cooperativeness with the physician during the exam, and helpfulness to the child in coping during the exam. Mothers were asked whether they got to ask the physician all the questions they had.

An observational scale of mother and child behaviors while waiting for the physician in the clinic examination room, the Dyadic Prestressor Interaction Scale (DPIS) was constructed after review of related literature and extensive narrative-descriptive clinic observation (Bush, 1983). Four classes of child behaviors and six of parent behaviors were selected, and four specific behaviors were operationally defined within each class. Behaviors were chosen according to criteria of objective definability, theoretical and empirically established relevance to the purposes of the research, and regularity of occurrence in the outpatient clinic situation.

Child behavior categories were adpated from Bretherton and Ainsworth's (1974) functional systems of behavior in a strange situation. The classes are attachment, distress, exploration, and social-affiliative behaviors. In order to adapt these classes for purposes of this study, four face-valid constituent behaviors were operationally defined for each class. Parent behavior classes were structured in the same way and correspond to dimensions of parent behavior suggested by past research as relating to children's behaviors in stressful medical situations. The classes of parent behaviors are information provision, reassuring, ignoring, distracting, restraining, and agitation.

The DPIS was used to rate videotaped mother–child interactions obtained while the patients were waiting for the physicians in the clinic examination rooms. Observers made instantaneous scan ratings (Altmann, 1974) of each of the 10 DPIS behavior categories every 5 seconds, on all dyads for whom at least 5 minutes of videotaped interaction was obtained, up to a maximum of 10 minutes.

Inter-observer reliability of DPIS ratings was evaluated by comparing ratings made by three independent observers on each of the 50 videotapes. Observers were trained in group sessions in which pilot subjects' videotapes were rated and disagreements discussed, until a criterion of 90 percent agreement for all behavior categories was attained. A repeated-measures ANOVA procedure, described by Winer (1962), was used to assess the inter-observer reliability of ratings made by three independent observers. Obtained reliability coefficiencies were in excess of .90 for eight of the behavior categories, with child distress observations falling at .77 and maternal restraining at .60 (Bush, 1983).

Results and Discussion

The purpose of this study was to investigate the interactive behavior of parents with their children in a stressful medical situation. It was predicted that the behavior of mothers in the clinic examination rooms would be related to distress and coping behaviors observed contemporaneously in their children. More specific predictions were made on the basis of the two theoretical models that have been discussed as accounting for parental influences on children's adjustment in stressful situations.

The four child behavior categories were found to measure four reasonably independent functional systems. Only two significant correlations ($p < .05$) were found among child categories. Children high in distress were likely to be low ($r = -.43, p < .01$) in social-affiliative responses. Children who were high in distress were likely to spend less time ($r = .78, p < .05$) exploring the situation. Parent behaviors were somewhat more interrelated. Significant within-parent correlations largely involved ignoring behavior, which was defined as active nonresponding by a mother occupying herself to the exclusion of the child (e.g., reading, snoozing). Ignoring was negatively correlated with each of the four parent behavior categories with which it could not by definition co-occur simultaneously: reassuring ($r = -.30, p < .05$); distracting ($r = -.59, p < .0001$); informing ($r = -.34, p < .05$); and restraining ($r = -.38, p < .01$). Ignoring and agitation were positively correlated

($r = .31$, $p < .05$), and more agitated mothers provided less information to their children ($r = -.28, p < .05$).

Analysis of correlations between parent and child behaviors revealed three patterns which appeared to represent simultaneous reciprocal interactions. Attachment in children was associated with parental reassuring ($r = .56$, $p < .0001$). Though free to vary independently, behaviors scored as attachment (e.g., reaching for mother) were often observed occurring together with parental reassuring behaviors (e.g., picking the child up). A second reciprocal interaction involved mothers using distraction with children engaging in nonmedical play or affiliation ($r = .77$, $p < .0001$) and mothers providing information with children who were exploring the environment ($r = .57, p < .0001$).

As predicted by the emotional contagion hypothesis, distress of the child was associated with parental agitation ($r = .32$, $p < .05$) as well as with parental reassuring ($r = .39$, $p < .01$). Low child distress was associated with maternal distracting ($r = -.31$, $p < .05$). While it might be suspected that parental agitation elicited children's distress whereas parental reassurance was responsive to children's distress and distraction reduced or inhibited it, these correlational data are inconclusive as to causality or causal direction. Further research employing sequential analysis techniques (Gottman, 1979) by means of which such causal inferences may be evaluated is currently underway.

The remaining parent-child correlations consisted of tendencies for parental ignoring to be associated with less exploration by children of their current situation ($r = .30$, $p < .05$), and with children's engaging in less social-affiliative behavior ($r = -.46, p < .001$).

Patterns of relationship between combinations of parent behaviors and combinations of child behaviors were examined by canonical correlation analysis. In addition, age interactions with maternal behaviors were examined. The first canonical function, R^2 of .67 ($p < .0001$), showed that mothers who used much distracting and little reassuring had children who showed more social-affiliative behavior.

The second canonical function showed that mothers who employed less reassuring and provided more information had children who were high in exploring ($R^2 = .48$, $p < .0001$). This effect was age-related. Even though the overall frequencies of both exploring and informing behaviors were unrelated to the child's age, these variables were more strongly associated among younger than older children. Older children were apparently more able to engage in exploring the stressful situation regardless of mother's acting as a source of information than were younger children.

The third canonical function showed that parents who used a lot of reassuring had children who showed a lot of distress. These children also showed high levels of exploration as well as engaging in frequent social-affiliative and attachment behaviors ($R^2 = .45, p < .0001$).

The last canonical function supported the prediction drawn from the crisis-parenting hypothesis. It showed that parents who were highly agitated and who ignored their children a great deal or tended to make use of distracting had children who showed little attachment and were high in distress ($r^2 = .26, p < .01$). More distracting was used with younger children when they showed distress. Also, maternal ignoring was more likely to be associated with distress in younger children than in older children.

Mothers' self-reported trait anxiety was correlated with their ratings of the child's difficulties with previous medical visits ($r = .48$, $p < .001$) and with their ratings of the stressfulness of their children's current health problems ($r = .35$, $p < .05$). Mothers with higher degrees of medical concerns were rated by observers as less effective in helping their children cope with examination procedures ($r = .25$, $p < .05$). Parents who reported high state anxiety reported that they did not get to ask the doctor all the questions they had ($r = .37$, $p < .001$). Parents rated by observers as less anxious, on the other hand, were rated as more cooperative with the examining physician ($r = .27$, $p < .05$).

Summary

These results supported the prediction that children are responsive to parental anxiety. Highly anxious mothers who tended to show agitation and ignoring had children who engaged in less exploration and remained more attached to their mothers while awaiting the exams. These mothers provided little information, although they often provided reassurance, particularly for the youngest children. On the positive side, mothers who were not highly agitated interacted more with their children and used distraction to keep them from being distressed. The effectiveness of distracting and informing were found to be dependent upon the interactive context in which they occurred, that is, upon what else a mother did while interacting with her child in the examining room. These results suggest that parents can be identified as to their skills in helping their children. The next step, of course, is to attempt to teach the parent more effective parenting strategies. Rather than use standard behavioral packages (e.g., teach relaxation or distraction), it is important to do a functional analysis of individual patterns of interacting.

METHODOLOGICAL ISSUES

Defining the Problem

The first task of the scientist-clinician is to identify the taxonomy of stress. What are the situations, people, events, and transactions that evoke the fear that takes place within the medical context? The second task is to provide depdendent variables that reflect both the emotional responses of the patients and the physical concomitants of their adjustment. The outcomes of our interventions must also have medical relevance if we hope to catch the attention of the medical community. We have many methods based on established psychological principles that have been applied to this task. In this section, the complexity of the measurement problem is described. Then psychological interventions derived from social learning theory in our work with preparation of children for medical procedures will be used to identify the methodological issues that remain unsolved. These include the need to consider the moderator variables: age, sex, cognitive-developmental level, medical diagnosis, length of hospitalization, previous experience with medical procedures and the hospital, nature and timing of preparation for the hospital, and prehospital psychological adjustment. The importance of communication between patient and doctor and involvement of family in preparation of medical patients in reducing anxiety and enhancing adherence to health regimens is demonstrated.

There are many sources for defining the psychological stress associated with medical care. We can ask the patient what he or she experiences. We can observe the patient's adjustment and physiological reaction in anticipation of, during, and after the examination. We can observe the medical outcome, such as time to recovery, need for pain medication, vomiting, nausea, and other postoperative indices. We can also collect information from the staff, obtain physicians' and nurses' ratings, and assess the family's reactions. It is important to obtain reliable and valid indices in each of these areas, as it is likely that our treatment efforts will affect them differentially.

It is important to look at the context in which measurement is obtained. The reactions to hospitalization that the child presents depend upon a number of variables, such as potential separation from parents and home, the child's adaptive and coping capacity, the fantasies that the child elaborates, entering a strange new environment, the parents' attitudes, medical procedures that may be painful and unexpected, observing the fate of other children, forced dependency and restriction of mobility, the developmental stage of the child, and the nature of the illness.

Psychological assessment in pediatric settings must take into account the cognitive, emotional and social dimensions of the involved individuals. The cognitive development of the child can influence the meaning attributed to the medical experience (Simeonsson et al., 1979). Younger children may see the procedures as punishment for bad behavior, whereas older children are able to verbalize the germ theory of disease. The prehospital characteristics of the family can also affect a hospital experience (Brown, 1979). Thus, the age of the child is critical in terms of determining the type of preparation that would be optimal and whether the parents' involvement must be considered.

There are a wide range of measures that have been used to study the outcome of psychological intervention. This may partly explain the lack of convergence of findings when one compares different studies without standardized measures. The use of broad-based therapeutic strategies may have the effect of differentially altering behaviors that are reflected, to varying extents, by subjective, behavioral, or physiological indices. The need for multidimensional assessment at this stage of development is predicated on the fact that some intervention procedures affect certain response modes, whereas other interventions may produce changes on other measures. Also, there are individual differences between patients' emotional responses, resulting in variability as to which measure may tap the most clinically significant response modality.

Coping with the impact of disease on normal developmental tasks and on family life is a complex psychological process. In addition to the typical measures of stress associated with anxiety such as self-report, behavioral, and physiological indices (Melamed & Johnson, 1979), the assessment must tap the array of behavioral and habit disorders that may be related to the hospital experiences. Thus, feeding problems, enuresis, encopresis, and aggression, which have been found to occur in about 32 percent of children who have undergone a hospital experience, must also be included.

Developing a psychological profile of the child directly relates to determining appropriate intervention strategies both in terms of initial decisions and ongoing reevaluations. The use of a developmental approach has been recommended. The child must be viewed within the context of his or her family. The hospitalization allows the staff to observe interactions between mother and child. At-risk parenting, poor mothering, or maladaptive interactions may contribute to adjustment problems both in the hospital and several months later. Therefore, in addition to individual measures of coping and anxiety, interactive behaviors should be assessed.

The current review does not include children with neurological impairments or chronic and terminal illnesses. Children with acute illness or short-term hospitalization concerns need to be evaluated in terms of characteristics that contribute to more adequate coping. Intervention approaches that can enhance emotional and social development by allowing greater control over transient painful or psychological stressors are available. The psychologist's task is to identify children and families at risk if intervention is not employed. Selection of preparatory packages should then be geared to the level of cognitive, social, and emotional development of the child. The parent, who is much more familiar with the child's language system, should be our primary consultant in this task.

Identification of children at risk for maladaptive responses may be assisted by use of information obtained from the parent by means of questionnaires such as the Vineland Social Maurity Scale (Doll, 1965), the Child Development Questionnaire (Zabin & Melamed, 1980), or behavior problem checklists (Achenbach, 1979; Quay, 1977; Walker, 1970). Children with problems in hyperactivity may be particularly at risk for adverse reactions to hospitalization, which often demands isolation and restriction of mobility.

In short, children's reactions to hospitalization may be observed by self-reported concerns, behavioral reactions such as crying, clinging, fearfulness, withdrawal, aggressiveness, and physiological changes such as elevated pulse rate, blood pressure, and temperature. Cost effectiveness of preparation can be documented by such indices as number of days in the hospital, amount of analgesics required, return to school or work. Johnson and Melamed (1978) reviewed the available literature on children's fears concerning hospital or medical stress and concluded that self-report measures are the least reliable in terms of the range of measures evaluated. Although behavioral measures have superior validity, they are not easy to obtain since they require the observation and coding of many instances of behavior. Physiological indices can be obtained through measures often routinely recorded during the examination and hospital stay, including heart rate, blood pressure, and temperature.

Timing of Preparation

There is some disagreement surrounding the selection of an optimal time of preparation. For example, data exist suggesting that some child patients can be sensitized by advance preparation (Shipley, Butt, & Horwitz, 1979; Shipley, Butt, Horwitz, & Farbry, 1978). Melamed and her colleagues (1976) found that a modeling film sensitized children under 7 years old when they were prepared a week in advance of elective surgery. Ferguson (1979) demonstrated a similar effect using a different videotape. A wide range of dependent measures indicated that younger children (3 to 5 years) benefitted more from videotaped modeling at time of admission, whereas older children (6 to 7 years) did equally well with verbal preparation at home one week in advance.

Recently, we compared same-day preparation of children admitted on the day of schedule elective surgery with a similar group of children admitted and prepared the night prior to surgery (Faust & Melamed, 1984). Children admitted the same day as surgery were better off viewing an unrelated film rather than a slide-tape presentation providing information about what would occur. Although children exposed to the hospital-relevant presentation did demonstrate more information than children who watched the control film (regardless of age, IQ, previous hospital experience, and time of preparation), they did not necessarily cope better with impending surgery.

Thus, information will not help a child if it only serves to increase arousal. There were autonomic and self-reported arousal differences between children prepared the same day as surgery and those prepared the night before. Arousal, however, is not necessarily a maladaptive response in the child preparing to cope with a stressful medical procedure. According to Janis (1958), moderate levels of physiological arousal may facilitate a coping response to stress. In-hospital children prepared with the hospital-relevant presentation adapted better to the stressful event as a result of showing sufficient, but not overwhelming, anticipatory anxiety. Although these children showed increases in heart rate while viewing the hospital-relevant presentation, they had decreased palmar sweating. This pattern of physiological activation may indicate active cognitive processing (Lacey, 1967) and physiological habituation of the fear response (i.e., cholinergic palmar sweating reduction). Support for this hypothesis that active engagement of adaptive mechanisms accompanies moderate levels of anticipatory arousal was also evident in the self-reported anxiety among children prepared in-hospital the night before surgery, which tended to decline after viewing of the hospital-relevant presentation. In contrast, children prepared the same day as surgery showed increases both in heart rate and palmar sweating. These children showed almost no decrease in self-reported anxiety after viewing the hospital-relevant presentation. Apparently, showing the hospital-relevant materials to these children created more anticipatory anxiety than the moderate amount optimal for coping. It was too late for these children to make use of the information provided to allay their fears because of the immediacy of the surgery. A distracting film seemed more effective in preparing children admitted on the same day as scheduled surgery. Children in this group who saw the control film showed an increase in heart rate and reduced palmar sweating. Self-report of hospital fears decreased significantly for these children after viewing the distracting film. They went into surgery with less anticipatory anxiety.

These results suggest that optimal time of preparation may vary as a function of child's age and that arousal may be a key mediating variable. Perhaps it is the case that, particularly with younger children, preparation either too far in advance or too immediately prior to the stressful event results in arousal that is less likely to be used in adaptive coping efforts. However, this effect has been demonstrated only for preparatory interventions utilizing audiovisual media. Visintainer and Wolfer (1975) replicated their finding that stresspoint preparation—consisting of information and reassurance provided to parent-child units immediately prior to five stressful experiences during hospitalization for elective surgery—was effective with 3- to 12-year-olds relative to a relationship-supportive care control group. In this replication a second experimental group was prepared in a single initial session. Children receiving immediate stresspoint preparation were less upset on a variety of measures than children receiving single-session preparation. While this study does not report data elucidating the mediating effects of preparation-induced anticipatory arousal, it does suggest that highly specific preparation provided immediately prior to medical stressors, with the parent(s) present, may be more helpful than the same preparation provided further in advance.

The complexity and incompleteness of the research data on optimal time of preparation argues strongly in favor of increased efforts to systematically study the time course of crisis experiences (Auerbach, Chapter 1, this volume). Different stages in the crisis experience impose different stresses and demand different types of coping responses in the optimally adapting individual. Research is needed to define these stages in the pediatric medical setting. Furthermore, analysis of coping tasks and effective crisis preparation/intervention must also take into account the developmental status of the child. For example, preparation emphasizing active ideational anticipation of temporally remote stressful events would probably be inappropriate for very young children. Elicitation of moderate levels of anticipatory arousal might be beneficial in advance of, but not immediately prior to, the stressful procedure, or it might be elicited by different stimuli. Highly specified behavioral instructions, perhaps in conjunction with relaxation induction, might be preferable for younger children and for preparation immediately prior to the event. Speculations such as these need to be derived from the developmental and crisis literatures and subjected to empirical test.

It is also clear that stress does not in all cases devolve from a single discrete "crisis event." Rather, there is more likely to be a series of events or protracted states constituting the crisis experience. For example, hospitalization for elective surgery involves not only anesthesia induction when the patient is about to be operated on, but also postoperative recovery, hospital admission, separation from significant others, a variety of presurgical procedures such as injections and sometimes highly invasive examinations, and the initial learning that surgery needs to be done. While passing through this crisis, the individual is simultaneously at a variety of stages in the time course of each of these smaller constituent crisis events. There will certainly be individual differences in the relative significance of each. Intervention that facilitates adjustment to a particular event may not help or may even exacerbate reaction to another event. Some preparatory interventions even appear to introduce a new stressor (anticipatory arousal) in order to facilitate the patient's coping with a more significant upcoming stressor. Intervention provided immediately prior to a "target event" is also likely to be distally preparatory to another stressful event, to follow in the aftermath of yet another, and so on.

Compliance and Generalization

Few of the studies evaluating preparatory interventions utilizing coping skills training have included any kind of check on whether the child and/or parent actually makes use of the technique in the target sitatuion. Still fewer studies assess generalization of skills to other stressful situations.

Klingman et al. (1984) reported data suggesting not only that children vary in the extent to which they utilize coping skills taught in a modeling film, but that this variability is linked both to intervention parameters and to outcome criteria. Children high in dental fears were shown a videotape with a child model demonstrating coping techniques (deep breathing and relaxation, positive distracting imagery, comforting self-talk). For half the children, the tape included pauses during which they were to practice the coping techniques. Children in the "participant modeling" group reported using these skills during dental treatment more than children who received coping skills training without structured practice, as well as showing more favorable anxiety and cooperativeness ratings.

This study indicates an important direction for future research: What factors help children use coping skills in the crisis situation? Clearly, this question applies both to skills acquired through preparatory training and to skills already in the child's behavioral repertoire.

The role of parenting behaviors might be expected to be critical in this connection. For example, parents might direct the child's attention to similarities between the medical context and other more familiar stressful situations with which the child has coped competently. Parents might also reinforce rehearsal and skill utilization during relatively less stressful events (e.g., blood test) prior to a more highly stressful procedure (e.g., anesthesia induction). Parents might help to cue the child's response or to draw the child's attention to discriminative stimuli indicating its appropriateness, or they might help to shape it. If research indicates that parenting behaviors such as these are facilitative, further studies would be in order evaluating interventions training parents in their use.

Generalization of coping skills acquired in the medical setting is also a desirable outcome of preparatory intervention which might be facilitated by parental participation. Studies of behavioral sequelae following pediatric hospitalization by Vernon et al. (1966) and by Prugh et al. (1953) have identified a minority of children in whom overall psychological benefit was an apparent result of the experience. Anecdotal explanations for findings such as these have included improved self concept owing to mastery of anxiety, correction of pathological conditions that previously interfered with adaptation, and alleviation of guilt by functioning as punishment for violation of superego prohibitions. These findings do not relate directly, however, to the question of generalization of coping skills to future medical crises or to other crisis situations. Peterson and Shigetomi (1982), in a follow-up to their previous intervention study (Peterson & Shigetomi, 1981), found that few parents reported that they had continued to use the facilitative parenting skills taught during the original study. Research is needed on how generalization may be assessed and how parent may be trained to maximize the generality of skills acquired through successful coping with a stressful medical experience.

SUMMARY AND CONCLUSIONS

One of the primary tasks of a psychologist prior to intervening in the preparation of children for medical procedures is to identify factors that may exacerbate the distress accompanying medical intervention. In this task, the existing research literature has provided an abundance of evidence regarding interpersonal, intrapersonal, and situational factors that influence the degree of anxiety evoked.

It is also clear from the literature that not everyone requires assistance for dealing with these situations and that the majority of individuals can cope with acute illness and medical procedures without long-term problems (Melamed, Robbins, & Fernandez, 1982). Thus, a second task is to identify what skills are required for adaptive coping and what factors identify individuals or families at risk for excessive emotional distress. The existing data base in this area is far from satisfactory since the large majority of studies evaluate treatment packages across a broad range of unselected individuals and using a variety of outcome measures of limited comparability.

The next decade of research needs to include a more developmental focus in which the characteristics of the individual can be more clearly identified within the familial and environmental context of treatment. Longitudinal research is necessary to confirm the effects of previous experience and maturational effects on the ability of children to cope with health care procedures.

The role of the family during adjustment to acute illness or surgery depends not only on the nature of the problem but also upon the cohesiveness and flexibility of family functioning. Although the role of family factors influencing chronic illness has been studied (Johnson, 1980), the nature of their interactions in the face of acute distress has been largely neglected. Although it has long been recognized that parental anxiety is communicated to the children by nonverbal as well as verbal cues and that this can have disruptive effects on children's coping, little research has been undertaken regarding the nature of these interactions. Few theories exist that directly predict the pertinent behaviors to be studied. However, there does exist a wealth of theoretical work on the effects of stranger anxiety and maternal deprivation on children which should have implications in this area (Rutter, 1981). Our own research efforts are extending the Bowlby and Ainsworth separation anxiety models by looking developmentally at children's ability to cope with medical procedures, as well as applying social learning theory in which both the individual's characteristics and the situational context are regarded as influencing adaptive functioning.

The taxonomy of stressors facing individuals has been assessed by means of self-report, behavioral observation, and physiological stress indices during medical procedures. Adults' concerns regarding their children's welfare focus largely on the fear of painful events and uncertain outcomes. For children, there is ample evidence that individual factors, including intellectual and developmental factors, previous experiences with medical stressors, as well as the nature of the parent-child interaction, must all be considered in determining that which evokes fear. Children's concerns are often related to age and depend on their cognitive functioning level. For children under five, protest behaviors are exhibited when separation is threatened or even when the parent is present during a noxious procedure such as a blood test. These children most likely view the parent as a source of relief from distress, and the crying may be a discriminative cue to elicit parent response. However, older youngsters who have had other separation experiences can usually cope with an upcoming dental or medical visit when information is provided by an empathic adult. Modeling may facilitate these children's ability to cope. Children closer to five tend to show more instrumental behavior such as information seeking before the examination and more emotionally expressive behavior during the exam. Younger children are more threatened by concrete events (being touched with instruments) and older children by symbolic events in coping with outpatient medical visits (Hyson, 1983). Thus, with increasing age, fear responses and coping behaviors become more realistic, anticipatory, and goal directed. Therefore, it is important to provide developmentally appropriate assistance to children. An individual functional analysis of the child's already existing coping repertoire should precede choice of a preparation technique.

The effects of parental participation depend upon the previous nature of that relationship and the availability of other support individuals such as nurses or physicians during stressful medical events. Studies where parents have been included in preparation have not led to conclusive findings in that the behavior of the parent has not been considered. The advisability of using parents as agents to promote children's adjustment cannot be evaluated without understanding their strategies for coping with stress, their level of anxiety, and the expectations they have for their children's abilities to cope. The previous level of support that the parent has shown the child is likely to affect the probability that the child will look toward the parent for support in the current situation.

Timing of preparation has also been a neglected variable in the evaluation of preparatory intervention. Our previous research found that taking the child's age into account in determining optimal timing of preparation was critical. Younger children prepared too far in advance were more aroused at the actual time of admission. Children with previous surgery who were under 8 years of age can even be sensitized by informational modeling.

Longitudinal research would allow us to understand how previous experience affects children's coping. Yet most studies have focused on a unique experience or on single stress exposures. Thus, defining the taxonomy of situations that arouse medical concerns can allow us to observe the reactions of children and their parents over a series of seemingly different situations that may in fact elicit similar concerns.

A greater integration of theory with measurement may lead to a greater degree of prediction based on areas of research often previously neglected, such as attachment and social learning theory.

REFERENCES

Achenbach, T. M. (1979). The child behavior profile: An empirically-based system for assessing children's behavior problems and competencies. *International Journal of Mental Health, 7,* 24-42.

Allen, B. P., & Evans, R. O. (1968). Videotape recording in social psychological research: An illustrative study in pedodontia. *Psychological Reports, 23,* 1115-1119.

Altmann, J. (1974). Observational study of behavior: Sampling methods. *Behaviour, 49,* 227-267.

Arata, C. L., Klorman, R., Chandler, M. J., & Sveen, O. B. (1977). Decreasing pedontic patients' uncooperativeness with coping and mastery models. *Journal of Dental Research, 56,* B160.

Auerbach, S. M. (1980). Surgery-induced stress. In R. H. Woody (Ed.), *Encyclopedia of clinical assessment* (Vol. II). San Francisco: Jossey-Bass.

Auerbach, S. M., Martelli, M., & Mercuri, L. (1983). Anxiety, information, interpersonal impacts and adjustment to a stressful health care situation. *Journal of Personality and Social Psychology, 44,* 1284-1296.

Bailey, P. M., Talbot, A., & Taylor, P. P. (1973). A comparison of maternal anxiety levels with anxiety levels manifested in the child dental patient. *Journal of Dentistry for Children, 40,* 277-284.

Becker, R. D. (1972). Therapeutic approaches to psychopathological reactions to hospitalization. *International Journal of Child Psychotherapy, 2,* 64-97.

Billings, A. G., & Moos, R. H. (1981). The role of coping responses and social resources in attenuating the stress of life events. *Journal of Behavioral Medicine, 4*(2), 139-157.

Brain, D. J., & Maclay, I. (1968). Controlled study of mothers and children in hospital. *British Medical Journal, 1,* 278-280.

Breslau, N., Weitzman, M., & Messenger, K. (1981). Psychological functioning of siblings of displaced children. *Pediatrics, 67*(3), 344-353.

Bretherton, I., & Ainsworth, M. D. (1974). Responses of one-year-olds to a stranger in a strange situation. In M. Lewis & L. A. Rosenblum (Eds.), *The origins of fear.* New York: Wiley, pp. 131-164.

Brown, B. (1979). Beyond separation. In D. Hall & M. Stacey (Eds.), *Beyond separation.* London: Routledge and Kegan Paul.

Burstein, S., & Meichenbaum, D. (1979). The work of worrying in children undergoing surgery. *Journal of Abnormal Child Psychology, 7*(2), 121-132.

Bush, J. P. (1983). *An observational study of mother-child interactions in a stressful medical situation.* Unpublished doctoral dissertation, University of Virginia.

Couture, C. J. (1976). The psychological responses of young children to brief hospitalization and surgery: The role of parent-child contact and age. *Dissertation Abstracts International, 37,* 1427B.

Davies, R., Butler, N., & Goldstein, H. (1972). *From birth to seven: The second report of the National Child Development Study.* (1958 cohort). London: National Children's Bureau.

Dimock, H. G. (1960). *The child in hospital: A study of his emotional and social well-being.* Philadelphia: Davis.

Doll, E. A. (1965). *Vineland Social Maturity Scale: Manual of directions* (Rev. ed.). Minneapolis, MN: American Guidance Service.

Duffy, J. C. (1972). Emotional reactions of children to hospitalization. *Minnesota Medicine, 55,* 1168-1170.

Escalona, S. (1953). Emotional development in the first year of life. In M. J. Senn (Ed.), *Problems of infancy and childhood.* Mineola, NY: Foundation.

Faust, J., & Melamed, B. G. (1984). The influence of arousal, previous experience, and age on surgery preparation of same-day and in-hospital pediatric patients. *Journal of Consulting and Clinical Psychology, 52*(3).

Ferguson, B. F. (1979). Preparing young children for hospitalization: A comparison of two methods. *Pediatrics, 64,* 656-664.

Fernald, C. D., & Corry, J. J. (1981). Empathetic versus directive preparation of children for needles. *Journal of the Association for the Care of Children's Health, 10,* 44-47.

Gofman, H., Buckman, E., & Schade, G. (1957). Parents' emotional responses to children's hospitalization. *American Journal of Diseases of Children, 93,* 157-164.

Gottman, J. M. (1979). Time-series analysis of continuous data in dyads. In M. E. Lamb, S. J. Suomi, & G. R. Stephenson (Eds.), *Social interaction analysis.* Madison, WI: University of Wisconsin Press, pp. 207-229.

Gross, A. M., Stern, R. M., Levin, R. B., Dale, J., & Wojnilower, D. A. (1983). The effect of mother-child separation on the behavior of children experiencing a diagnostic medical procedure. *Journal of Consulting and Clinical Psychology, 51,* 783-785.

Hanallah, R. S., & Rosales, J. K. (1983). Experience with parents' presence during anesthesia induction in children. *Canadian Anesthesiology Society Journal, 30,* 286-289.

Heffernan, M., & Azarnoff, P. (1971). Factors in reducing children's anxiety about clinic visits. *HSMHA Health Reports, 86*(12), 1131-1135.

Hyson, M. C. (1983). Going to the doctor: A developmental study of stress and coping. *Journal of Child Psychology and Psychiatry, 24,* 247-259.

Janis, I. L. (1958). *Psychological stress.* New York: Wiley.

Johnson, S. B. (1980). Psychosocial factors in juvenile diabetes: A review. *Journal of Behavioral Medicine, 3,* 95-116.

Johnson, S., & Melamed, B. G. (1978). Assessment and treatment of fears in children. In B. Lahey & A. Kazdin (Eds.), *Advances in child clinical psychology.* New York: Plenum.

Kaplan, D. M., Smith, A., Grobstein, R., & Fischman, S. E. (1973). Family mediation of stress. *Social Work, 18,* 60-69.

Kendall, P. C., & Watson, D. (1981). Psychological preparation for stressful medical procedures. In C. A. Prokop & L. A. Bradley (Eds.), *Medical psychology.* New York: Academic Press, pp. 60-69.

Klingman, A., Melamed, B. G., Cuthbert, M., & Hermecz, D. A. (1984). Effects of participant modeling on information acquisition and skill utilization. *Journal of Consulting and Clinical Psychology, 52*(3).

Knight, R. B., Atkins, A., Eagle, C. J., Evans, N., Finkelstein, J. W., Fukushima, D., Katz, J., & Weiner, H. (1979). Psychological stress, ego defenses, and cortisol production in children hospitalized for elective surgery. *Psychosomatic Medicine, 41,* 40-49.

Lacey, J. I. (1967). Somatic response patterning and stress: Some revisions of activation theory. In M. H. Appley & R. Trumball (Eds.), *Psychological stress: Issues in research.* New York: Appleton-Century.

Levy, E. (1959). Children's behavior under stress and its relation to training by parents to respond to stressful situations. *Child Development, 30,* 307-324.

Machen, J., & Johnson, R., (1979). Desensitization, model learning, and the dental behavior of children. *Journal of Dental Research, 53,* 83-89.

Melamed, B. G. (1981). Effects of preparatory intervention on adjustment of children to medical procedures. In M. Rosenbaum, M. Franks, & Y. Jaffee (Eds.), *Perspectives on behavior therapy in the eighties.* New York: Springer.

Melamed, B. G., Dearborn, M., & Hermecz, D. A. (1983). Necessary consideration for surgery preparation: Age and previous experience. *Psychosomatic Medicine, 45,* 517-525.

Melamed, B. G., & Johnson, S. B. (1979). Assessment of chronic illness: Asthma and diabetes. In E. Mash & L. Terdal (Eds.), *Behavioral assessment of childhood disorders.* New York: Guilford.

Melamed, B. G., Meyer, R., Gee, C., & Soule, L. (1976). The influence of time and type of preparation on children's adjustment to hospitalization. *Journal of Pediatric Psychology, 1*(4), 31-37.

Melamed, B. G., Robbins, R. L., & Fernandez, J. (1982). Factors to be considered in psychological preparation for surgery. In D. Routh & M. Wolraich (Eds.), *Advances in behavioral pediatrics.* New York: JAI Press.

Melamed, B. G., & Siegel, L. J. (1975). Reduction of anxiety in children facing hospitalization and surgery by use of filmed modeling. *Journal of Consulting and Clinical Psychology, 43*(4), 511-521.

Parcel, G. S., & Meyer, M. P. (1978). Development of an instrument to measure children's locus of control. *Health Education Monographs,* 149-159.

Perrin, E. C., & Gerrity, P. S. (1981). There's a demon in your belly: Children's understanding of illness. *Pediatrics, 67*(6), 851-859.

Peterson, L., & Ridley-Johnson, R. (1980). Pediatric hospital response to a survey on presurgical preparation for children. *Journal of Pediatric Psychology, 5*(1), 1-7.

Peterson, L., & Shigetomi, C. (1981). Use of coping techniques to reduce anxiety in hospitalized children. *Behavior Therapy, 12,* 1-14.

Peterson, L., & Shigetomi, C. (1982). One-year follow-up of elective surgery child patients receiving preoperative preparation. *Journal of Pediatric Psychology, 7*(1), 43-48.

Pinkham, J., & Fields, H. W. (1976). The effects of preappointment procedures on maternal manifest anxiety. *Journal of Dentistry for Children, 43,* 180-183.

Prugh, D. G., Staub, E. M., Sands, H. H., Kirschenbaum, R. M., & Lenihan, E. A. (1953). A study of the emotional reactions of children and families to hospitalization and illness. *American Journal of Orthopsychiatry, 23,* 70-106.

Quay, H. C. (1977). Psychopathic behavior: Reflections on the nature, origins, and treatment. In F. Weizmann & I. Uzgiris (Eds.), *The structuring of experience.* New York: Plenum.

Robinson, D. (1968). Mothers' fear, their children's well-being in hospital, and the study of illness behavior. *British Journal of Preventive Social Medicine, 22,* 228-233.

Roskies, E., Mongeon, M., & Gagnon-Lefebvre, B. (1978). Increasing maternal participation in the hospitalization of young children. *Medical Care, 16*(9), 765-777.

Rutter, M. (1981). *Maternal deprivation reassessed* (2nd ed.). New York: Penguin Books.

Seidl, F. W., & Pilliteri, A. (1967). Development of an attitude scale on parental participation. *Nursing Research, 16*(1), 71-73.

Shaw, E. G., & Routh, D. K. (1982). Effect of mothers' presence on children's reaction to aversive procedures. *Journal of Pediatric Psychology, 7,* 33-42.

Shipley, R. M., Butt, J. H., & Horwitz, E. A. (1979). Preparation to reexperience a stressful medical examination: Effect of repetitious videotape exposure and coping style. *Journal of Consulting and Clinical Psychology, 46,* 499-507.

Shipley, R. M., Butt, J. H., Horwitz, E., & Farbry, J. E. (1978). Preparation for a stressful medical procedure: Effect of amount of prestimulus exposure and coping style. *Journal of Consulting and Clinical Psychology, 46,* 499-507.

Shore, M. F., Geiser, R. L., & Wolman, H. M. (1965). Constructive uses of hospital experience. *Children, 12,* 3-8.

Sides, J. P. (1977). Emotional responses of children to physical illness and hospitalization. *Dissertation Abstracts International, 38,* 917B.

Simeonsson, R., Buckley, L., & Monson, L. (1979). Conceptions of illness causality in hospitalized children. *Journal of Pediatric Psychology, 4,* 77-84.

Skipper, J. K., Leonard, R. C., & Rhymes, J. (1968). Child hsopitalization and social interaction: An experimental study of mothers' feelings of stress, adaptation, and satisfaction. *Medical Care, 6*(6), 496–506.

Spielberger, C. D., Gorusch, P. L., & Lushene, R. (1970). *State-trait anxiety inventory.* Palo Alto, CA: Consulting Psychologists.

Traughber, B., & Cataldo, M. (1982). Biobehavioral effects of pediatric hospitalization. In J. Tuma (Ed.), *Handbook for the practice of pediatric psychology.* New York: Wiley.

Venham, L. L., Murray, P., & Gaulin-Kremer, E. (1979). Child-rearing variables affecting the preschool child's response to dental stress. *Journal of Dental Research, 58,* 2042–2045.

Vernon, D. T., Foley, F. M., & Schulman, J. J. (1967). Effect of mother-child separation and birth order on young children's responses to two potentially stressful experiences. *Journal of Personality and Social Psychology, 5*(2), 162–174.

Vernon, D. T., Schulman, J. J., & Foley, F. M. (1966). Changes in children's behavior after hospitalization. *American Journal of Diseases of Children, 111,* 581–593.

Visintainer, M. A., & Wolfer, J. A. (1975). Psychological preparation for surgical pediatric patients: The effect on children's and parents' stress responses and adjustment. *Pediatrics, 64*(5), 646–655.

Walker, H. M. (1970). *Walker Behavior Problem Checklist.* Los Angeles: Western Psychological Services.

Winer, B. J. (1962). *Statistical principles in experimental design.* New York: McGraw-Hill.

Wolfer, J. A., & Visintainer, M. A. (1975). Pediatric surgical patients' and parents' stress responses and adjustment. *Nursing Research, 24*(4), 244–255.

Wright, G. Z., Alpern, G. D., & Leake, J. L. (1973). The modifiability of maternal anxiety as it relates to children's cooperative dental behavior. *Journal of Dentistry for Children, 40,* 265–271.

Zabin, M. A., & Melamed, B. G. (1980). Relationship between parental discipline and children's ability to cope with stress. *Journal of Behavioral Assessment, 2*(1), 17–38.

Zastowny, T. R., Kirschenbaum, D. S., & Meng, A. L. (in press). Coping skills training for children: Effects on distress before, during, and after hospitalization for surgery. *Health Psychology.*

III

RELATIVELY LOW FREQUENCY CRISIS EVENTS

The five chapters comprising the third section of this volume deal with crisis events that, although less prevalent than those considered earlier, are generally deemed (with one exception) to be of more pervasive and devastating impact. Swift's chapter (7) on sexual abuse of children deals with a topic of great current concern in this country. She carefully analyzes intervention procedures appropriate at each of the four temporal stages outlined by Auerbach in Chapter 1, but notes that the temporal model (which is oriented around single events) often cannot be applied "cleanly" to child sexual abuse. Because the abuser is often well known to the child and the abuse had thus been concealed, the child "has either been victimized over an extended period of time or has suffered abuse on multiple occasions." In the second part of her chapter, Swift describes and evaluates a Type 3 poststress intervention program geared at professionals charged with identifying and treating sexually abused children.

In Chapter 8, Kupst identifies five temporal stages associated with pediatric leukemia, pinpoints particularly salient stressors at each of these stages, and discusses how intervention needs for siblings of the ill child and the entire family change over the course of the illness. She also presents longitudinal outcome data assessing the effects of a family intervention project oriented around her five-stage model. Auerbach and Spirito (Chapter 9) similarly approach crisis intervention programming in natural disasters from a temporal stage standpoint, and detail a cognitively based stress inoculation program for treating postdisaster fears in children.

Chapters 10 and 11 differ from the preceding presentations in that they deal with stressors that are less transitory and more pervasive in their continuing impact on the victims and their families. In Chapter 10, Kerr reviews the literature indicating that physical handicaps in children are indeed associated with higher stress levels in the children and their families, presents a field theory analysis of crisis and stress as it pertains to physical disability, relates this approach to the temporal model of crisis intervention, and presents specific intervention suggestions for stresses associated with physical disability in children. In Chapter 12 on Holocaust survivors and their families, Goldwasser demonstrates how exposure to an extremely destructive crisis-inducing event may have long-lasting consequences that in effect produce "personality trait" changes in otherwise normally functioning individuals; these pervasive behavior changes disrupt family functioning and saddle the victims' children with a burden that they sometimes perpetuate in their own children. In the latter part of his chapter, Goldwasser reviews the emerging literature on intervention with survivor children and also makes recommendations on helping grandchildren of survivors understand and deal with their grandparents' experiences.

7

Community Intervention in Sexual Child Abuse

Carolyn F. Swift
Wellesley College

Sexual abuse is a major crisis in the lives of the victimized children and their families. This chapter begins by defining the problem and briefly reviewing the methodological issues involved in conducting research in this area. Next, Auerbach's four-type intervention model, which was previously defined in this book, is used as the context for presenting the results of a Type 3 community intervention. A summary of the ecological characteristics of sexual child abuse and its impact on victims is then presented. The chapter ends with suggestions for future programming.

INTRODUCTION: PROBLEM DEFINITION

The sexual abuse of children is becoming an increasingly frequent life crisis. It has been estimated that somewhere between a fourth and a third of the U. S. population experience one or more unwanted sexual interactions with adults while growing up (Finkelhor, 1985; Landis, 1956; Russell, 1984; Walters, 1975). Reports of victimization of female children range as high as 38 percent. While still under-reported, victimization of male children is currently estimated to be between 5 and 30 percent, depending on the source (Finkelhor, 1985; Landis, 1956; Swift, 1978).

The immediate emotional and behavioral sequelae of sexual child abuse include nightmares, phobias, multiple fears, regression (e.g., bedwetting, thumbsucking), disruption of eating and sleeping habits, somatic complaints (particularly chronic abdominal pain), preoccupation with sexual activity, and escape behaviors such as truancy or running away (Burgess & Holmstrom, 1974, 1980; Krasner, Meyer, & Carroll, 1977; Lewis & Sarrel, 1969). Victimized children are usually reluctant to report the abuse out of fear of being punished by the abuser. Therefore, indirect allusions to discomfort with or dislike of an adult in the child's life, in combination with one or more of the above signs, should signal the need for an investigation.

LIMITATIONS OF THE BODY OF EXISTING RESEARCH

Four factors contribute to the difficulty in establishing reliable statistics on incidence:

1. Varying definitions of what constitutes sexual child abuse,
2. Underreporting by both professionals and the public,

3. The disadvantage of the child victim relative to the adult abuser vis-à-vis identifying, labeling, and reporting the incident, and

4. Societal taboos that have effectively masked this problem from public and scientific attention until relatively recently.

There are no incidence data that are not methodologically flawed. Up to one-half of the cases that come to professional attention are not reported to child protective service agencies (James, Womack, & Strauss, 1978; NCCAN, 1981) even though such reporting is mandated by law. The number of cases that never surface to professional or public attention is unknown, but has been estimated to be three to four times the number of reported cases (Finkelhor & Hotaling, 1983).

Until a decade ago there were less than 500 children for whom a usable body of data was available for study of adult-child sexual interactions (Gagnon, 1970). The difficulties inherent in attempting to gather systematic data on sexual abuse of children range from ethical considerations to the technical complexities of observing and measuring private events. Retrospective studies—adult reports of recollections of childhood sexual experiences—are found most commonly in the literature and form the data base for theory construction and projected research. Such studies suffer the obvious flaws of memory deficit and distortion. Compounding the issue of reliability raised by selective and distorted recall is the issue of the representativeness of the responding sample. Many of the surveys are biased in the direction of middle-class college-educated populations. It is the norm in sex research that reporting is done by the articulate and the willing. Caution is required in generalizing the results to the larger population, presumed to include the inarticulate and those unwilling to disclose their sexual histories. The phenomenon of sexual child abuse is being reported with increasing frequency, both in the research literature (Raigrodski, 1983) and the popular press. Whether increased reports reflect increased incidence or more accurate estimates of incidence and prevalence is not clear. What is clear is that a substantial proportion of children—conservatively estimated to be 30 percent—suffers sexual abuse in our culture.

CRISIS INTERVENTION IN SEXUAL CHILD ABUSE

"Virtually every form of crisis intervention involves preparing individuals for a stressor they are about to confront, or helping them recover from the effects of one that has already impacted on them," states Auerbach in Chapter 1 of this volume. The state of development of crisis intervention in sexual child abuse is such that the child victim is usually reacting to both situations simultaneously. Most abusers are well known to the child. They are often family members (Krasner et al., 1977; Swift, 1977). In these situations rarely is an initial abusive incident reported to authorities. A variety of forces combine to conceal the abuse, with the result that in most of the cases coming to official attention the child has either been victimized over an extended period of time or has suffered abuse on multiple occasions. If there is no official intervention the abuse is likely to continue. There is a critical need to identify these cases earlier, before both the severity and duration of abuse effect irreversible adjustment problems in the child victims (Steele & Alexander, 1981). Both pre- and postvictimization intervention, therefore, is usually appropriate. For these reasons all four of Auerbach's intervention categories, as previously described in this volume, are relevant.

Type 1

Distal prestress interventions are directed to prevention, and are targeted to individuals who are unaware that they are at risk. Type 1 interventions for sexual child abuse are appropriate for all children, since a substantial proportion are abused and there is currently no accurate means of predicting which children will be victimized. The most popular interventions of this type, outside the family, are programs designed to educate children about potential sexual abuse and equip them with appropriate coping behaviors (Kleven, 1981; Cooper, Lutter, & Phelps, 1983).

In an exemplary program that has been replicated in 50 communities across Ohio, California, and Massachusetts, elementary school children and their parents and teachers are targeted for educational interventions designed to prevent sexual victimization of children. The Child Assault Prevention (CAP) training is based on a theoretical model that identifies children's vulnerability as the critical condition underlying sexual abuse. According to this model—which parallels a feminist analysis of rape (Sparks & Bar On, 1982)—powerlessness and isolation in abuse situations, together with the general public's ignorance of the prevalence of sexual child abuse, contribute to vulnerability and perpetuate conditions associated with abuse. The CAP procedures for obtaining broad community support prior to implementing the training workshops ensure parental and administrative cooperation. Less than one percent of the children in targeted schools has been denied permission by parents to participate. The children's workshops are previewed in detail in the adult workshops, which are conducted one week prior to the children's training. The school workshops involve role plays and guided discussions focusing on abuse situations. Assertiveness and communication skills stress the rights of children to control their own bodies. Children are also taught how to build networks for peer support to reduce isolation and powerlessness. Community resources are identified so that children, their families and teachers will know "who to tell" and where to turn for help. Specific goals of the children's workshops are "(1) To help children identify potentially threatening situations, (2) to enable children to strategize realistic options, (3) to model alternative behavior, (4) to provide children with an opportunity to practice alternative behavior" (Cooper et al., 1983). In the seven years of operation 40,000 children and 10,000 adults in the original CAP community (Franklin County, Ohio) have received the 1½- to 2-hour workshops. The model has also been adapted for use with other vulnerable populations—the chronically ill, the mentally retarded, the developmentally disabled, and hearing impaired children. A national training conference is planned.

Type 1 interventions are particularly relevant for populations of children considered to be at high risk for sexual abuse. Siblings of incest victims are at high risk, since sexual abuse of more than one child is common in incest cases. Programs that combine legal sanctions with professional counseling and/or self-help groups appear to be most successful in preventing the spread of abuse to siblings. Giarretto (1981) pioneered this model in Santa Clara, California. After discovering, in his early work (Giarretto, 1977) that neither punishment nor therapy alone were effective in stopping incestuous fathers from abuse, he initiated a program that included both. Working with the local court system he developed a program requiring incestuous fathers to participate in professional counseling as a condition of release or probation. As his caseload grew he started self-help groups for family members. These groups—Parents United and Daughters and Sons United—now have chapters across the country. Giarretto has developed training programs for professionals, and has provided treatment for over 4000 children and their families over the last 10 years. He claims a recidivism rate of less than one percent.

Children in families with stepfathers may also be at higher risk than the norm. In the National Incidence Study fathers were the abusers in 30 percent of the cases and stepfathers or mothers' paramours in 40 percent (Finkelhor & Hotaling, 1983). In commenting on the suprisingly high incidence of stepfather abuse these authors note:

> *The percentage of stepfathers in the population of sexual abusers far outstrips the percentage that would be expected based on the number of children living with step-fathers in the population at large. In 1980 approximately ten percent of children lived with a stepfather. If natural fathers committed sexual abuse to the same degree as stepfathers, we would expect the ratio to be more along the order of nine natural fathers for one stepfather. The fact that the ratio is so much lower than that suggests clearly that children are at higher risk for sexual abuse at the hands of stepfathers than natural fathers. (1983, p. 10)*

According to the study reported later in this chapter, father abuse accounted for 26 percent of the cases and abuse by the stepfather, foster father, or mother's/ sister's boyfriend accounted for 28 percent. It is unclear to what extent these data represent the actual incidence of stepfather abuse and to what extent they reflect a differential pattern of reporting. The children may have greater loyalty to natural fathers based on a longer history in the relationship, and mothers may be less conflicted in reporting stepfather abuse. This phenomenon merits additional research.

Type 2

Proximal prestress interventions target individuals who are confronted with an imminent crisis; they are faced with mobilizing resources either to prevent it or to minimize its impact. Type 2 interventions are appropriate for two categories of children: siblings of victims and victims themselves. The victim's siblings in incest situations may have observed or been told of the abuse and may suffer anxiety as a result. Interventions here should both guarantee the siblings' safety and reduce their associated anxiety related to fear of abuse.

Some Type 2 interventions have as their goal the prevention of further abuse of an already sexually victimized child. A common approach in incest cases is to separate the abuser and victim by removing one or the other from the home or by denying custody or visitation rights. If the two are not separated the victim may continue to be sexually victimized, and may be punished for revealing the secret (Herman, 1982). In separations enforced by police and protective service workers the person most often removed from the home is the child. Such action places additional hardships on the victim, who is removed from the traditional supports of family, home, friends, neighborhood and school, and forced to adapt to a new setting—a foster family, group home, or institution. For these reasons professionals choosing separation as an intervention are increasingly choosing to remove the offender, rather than the victim, from the home (Finkelhor, 1984). Another Type 2 approach with victims is to teach the child specific escape or defense behavior. This is particularly appropriate in cases in which the social service and law enforcement systems have failed to either stop the abusive behavior or to separate the victim from the abuser through alternative living arrangements. The CAP program, described earlier, exemplifies theis approach (Cooper et al., 1983). By teaching children assertive defensive behhaviors as well as where to turn for help, such educational programs may prevent additional victimization.

One of the obstacles to mobilizing Type 1 or 2 interventions with risk populations is the persistent tendency for those involved, both professionals and family members, "to interpret warning cues in 'normal' terms" (Auerbach, Chapter 1, this volume). Denial of incest is most commonly attributed to the mother, but in fact pervades the behavioral response of all those associated with the phenomenon. "The reporting process for sexual abuse may not be blocked at the level of 'official reporting' but at the level of recognition. Professionals still are not trained to suspect and diagnose sexual abuse, and we suspect they have emotional and personal blocks to discovering it as well" (Finkelhor & Hotaling, 1983, p. 3). There is no experimentally established profile of the incestuous abuser. Even if there were the risks of labeling false positives would pose problems for information dissemination campaigns. The problem here parallels the potential damage involved in the labeling that would result from screening elementary school children for juvenile delinquency. One of the difficulties in implementing Type 1 and 2 interventions directly with children is in achieving appropriate balance between alerting them about possible abuse from loved ones and avoiding inducing paranoia about demonstrations of affection from parents and other relatives. In attempting to address these issues the CAP Leader's Manual (Cooper et al., 1983) suggests answers to questions commonly asked by parents:

Q: "Will this workshop frighten, rather than educate, children?"
A: "One of the things we have found is that children are already very aware of assault. Watching television and overhearing adults discuss sensitive topics has exposed them to much more violence than they will ever face in their lifetimes. The fear is already there. Unfortunately, the skill to handle the fear is not. Like teaching children to cross the street safely or to get out of a burning building, assault prevention makes children feel safer and more confident." (pp. 106-107)
Q: "I want my children to trust people, especially relatives and close friends. My children are spontaneously affectionate and I'm afraid they will lose that trait if we talk to them about assault."
A: "Children choose who they will be affectionate with, based on their trust of the adult. This does not change because children learn that someone they know may try to touch them in a bad way; it simply gives them the right and the skill to stop that type of touching. Children who have control over how and by whom their bodies can be touched will still be comfortable returning truly affectionate behavior." (pp. 108-109)

Data from adult female victims of sexual assault suggest possible means of avoiding abuse in children. Bart (1981) and McIntyre (1981) have demonstrated the successful avoidance of sexual assault by women who physically and verbally resist their assaulters. Rape avoiders demonstrate more independence, both physically and psychologically, than those women who are raped by the attacker.

While having the independence to defy adult authority or to run away may assist children in avoiding sexual attacks, these are not behaviors that are generally sanctioned in children. The same considerations that lead society to punish status offenses lead also to a systematic failure to reinforce behaviors in children that would contribute to successful avoidance of sexual abuse. Runaways are returned home. Physical and verbal challenges of adult authority are discouraged or punished. The father or stepfather is the abuser in a high proportion of cases. Devising an effective program to tell Daddy "no" and winning cooperation from families and schools to implement it present formidable problems at this point in time. Outcome data are needed for educational programs such as CAP in order to assess their preventive effectiveness.

Type 3

Proximal poststress interventions are targeted to assist individuals adjusting to the short-term effects of recent exposure to a stressful situation. Most of the interventions in the field of sexual child abuse are Type 3 interventions with identified victims. These include case monitoring, counseling, and outplacement— removal of the victim from the home. None of these interventions has been systematically evaluated. Case monitoring refers to the professional activity of systematic, periodic (weekly, monthly) contact, evaluation, and review of cases reported for abuse. Because repeated abuse extending over years is common in incest cases, the visible presence of a professional checking the status of the case through home visits and interviews with the child, parents, and teachers is believed to deter the abuser. Although common sense and anecdotal evidence support this view, there are no confirming empirical data. Counseling interventions include professional psychotherapies and crisis intervention methods as well as self-help groups. Giarretto's (1981) program in California involving court-ordered family, individual, and group therapy, reports a high degree of success in eliminating incest in families where the abuser is willing to admit culpability and cooperate in treatment. The use of self-help groups for abusers, victims, and other family members appears to be a major factor in the success of this program.

The enactment of federal and state child abuse and neglect legislation in the 1970s and the associated development of staff resources constitute a Type 3 intervention supported at the societal level. Supplementary legislation and related enforcement, professional training, and public education are logical follow-ups to this initial systems intervention. While the legislation cited mandates the reporting of cases of child abuse and neglect from a variety of professionals, the laws have rarely been enforced. As a result, reporting has been selective and sporadic (Finkelhor, 1984). Ironically, the barriers to enforcement lie not so much in lack of will as lack of resources. In isolated cases where professionals have been prosecuted for not reporting, the local child protective service system has typically been flooded with reports, overwhelming capacity to respond. Clearly, enforcement is tied to an expansion of resources. There are currently few professional health or mental health disciplines that include prevention and treatment of sexual child abuse as part of a formal educational curriculum. Establishing training programs in professionals schools as well as on the job could be expected to both increase the pool of professionals equipped to deal with these cases and stimulate reporting from those trained to recognize and treat the problem.

Type 4

Distal poststress interventions are targeted to persons suffering long-term problems in adjusting to previous crises. These interventions are appropriate for adolescents or adults still traumatized by childhood sexual victimization. The long lasting psychological effects of such experiences include phobias, multiple fears, depression, suicidal behavior and difficulties in establishing and maintaining intimate relationships (Herman & Hirschman, 1977; Lewis & Sarrel, 1969; Meiselman, 1978; Steele & Alexander, 1981; Silver, Boon, & Stones, 1983). The frequency and severity of these outcomes appear to vary according to three critical factors associated with the abuse: the amount of force used, the relationship between the abuser and the child, and the time period over which abuse occurs (Burgess & Holmstrom, 1974, 1980; Krasner, Meyer, & Carroll, 1977; Lewis & Sarrel, 1969). The more brutal the attack, the more likely the victim will be to exhibit disrupted functioning. The closer the relationship between the victim and the abuser, the higher the probability of dysfunction. The longer the time period over which the abuse occurs (weeks, months, years), the more frequent and severe the dysfunctional outcomes. Additional factors affecting outcome are the reactions of the victims (e.g., shame, guilt) and those of significant adults and peers. Silver et al. (1983) have documented the adult survivor's overwhelming preoccupation with a search for some meaning in the earlier incest victimization. For most the search is painful; for some it is fruitless. The authors suggest that interventions that teach these victims to block out or interrupt unwanted, obsessional thoughts could alleviate their distress. They suggest clinical techniques such as thought stopping, habituation training and cognitive restructuring. They also note that incest survivors who reported having a current confidant with whom they could discuss the incest experience were significantly more likely to report having made sense of the experience than survivors who reported having no current confidants.

The difficulties in developing Type 4 interventions are tied to the lack of a data base linking abuse to outcome. No systematic research has established what constitutes a "normal" adjustment period to a single or multiple childhood victimization experiences. Models of adult victims' postassault adjustment cannot be extrapolated to children, since a much higher proportion of reported adult victimization involves strangers. In addition, the adult victim's personality, knowledge of and attitudes about sexual activity, coping behavior, and support systems are substantially different. Empirical studies are needed assessing connections between the variables associated with childhood sexual abuse and health and mental health outcomes in adult life.

A TYPE 3 INTERVENTION: TRAINING THE PROFESSIONAL COMMUNITY IN THE IDENTIFICATION OF SEXUAL CHILD ABUSE

Auerbach, in discussing Type 3 interventions, notes that "observational data suggest that interveners might most productively invest their efforts in the initial poststress period with significant others, or those on the periphery, rather than directly with victims" (Chapter 1, this volume). This section reports on a Type 3 intervention in which the subjects of the intervention were professionals charged with identifying and treating sexually abused children, rather than the child victims themselves. The research was conducted by the author in Kansas City and surrounding areas over a period from 1976 to 1979. The study was supported by the National Institute of Mental Health through a grant from the National Center for the Prevention and Control of Rape (Grant #MH 29038-03).

SEXUAL ABUSE IN BOYS

Men who were sexually abused as children are overrepresented in the ranks of sexually abusing adult males (Goldstein, 1973; Groth, 1979; Serril, 1974; Swift, 1977, 1978). Thus prevention efforts directed toward identification of such cases, followed by early intervention and treatment, have the potential for reducing the incidence of sexual assaults. Identifying these cases is difficult, however, since sexually victimized boys report the abuse at a much lower rate than sexually victimized girls (Finkelhor, 1982; Landis, 1956). Victimized boys must cope with a double stigma, for their abuse violates not only the norm of sexual activity between consenting adults, but the heterosexual norm as well. Over 95 percent of reported sexual abusers are male. Social conditioning reinforces silence in young male victims. To report being abused is to admit failing in the duty of self-defense, a first-order priority of the male role. To report is to risk being labeled homosexual for participating in the censured sexual activity. Asssuming it were possible to elicit prompt, accurate reporting by young male victims it is likely that these reports would be met with inappropriate responses on the part of the adult community (Finkelhor, 1982; Swift, 1979). Therefore it is first desirable to change professional and public attitudes to create a climate of support and empathy, which would sanction equally reports of sexual victimization from both boys and girls.

A FOUR-STEP PREVENTION MODEL

Rationale and Objectives

The research project implemented the first step of a four-step prevention model. Steps one through three involve the education of professionals, parents, and children in the realities of sexual child abuse and means of prevention and treatment. The fourth step involves interventions with sexually abused boys. The underlying rationale of this model is that professionals in contact with sexually abused children and their families should be educated to the reality of sexual abuse of boys as well as girls, and trained to be receptive to taking such reports from children without further traumatizing the child for reporting the incident. Once the professional community is prepared to deal with these reports, parents should be educated to the fact that their male as well as their female children are at risk for sexual abuse. Following this, campaigns should be designed to encourage children themselves to report incidents of sexual abuse. Ultimately, early intervention and treatment of sexually abused boys would, hopefully, result in the prevention of sexual offenses by this population in later life.

The two primary objectives of the research project were to increase the reporting of sexual child abuse in selected agencies dealing with this problem in the metropolitan Kansas City area, with particular emphasis on increased reporting of sexual abuse of boys; and to build a data base of cases to permit an analysis of the ecology of sexual child abuse. It was recognized at the outset that the variables controlling the occurrence of sexual child abuse lie outside the control of the mental health professionals, school nurses and counselors, police officers, and child protective service workers targeted for training. However, the professionals involved are gatekeepers who have the power either to believe the reports of sexual child abuse that come to their attention, to process them through their official system, or to disbelieve or discount them. In the latter case, reports by individuals may not be entered into the official reporting system and thus may never surface to professional attention. Some professionals (school personnel, child protective service workers) are in direct contact with children in schools or in their work in investigating or assisting troubled families. An awareness of the physical and behavioral cues associated with sexual child abuse could result in increased direct identification of sexual abuse in the populations of children seen by these professionals. Baseline data taken by the project indicated that over 60 percent of the reported cases were initiated directly by individuals outside the agencies involved, with the balance referred by other agencies. One of the goals of the training intervention was to evaluate its effect on the numbers of cases entering the agencies' reporting system.

Definitions

Sexual child abuse cases considered in this study were those involving physical sexual abuse and use of children for pornography or prostitution. Adults were defined as persons 18 or over; persons under 18 were classified as children.* The general definition of sexual child abuse includes any act committed by an adult designed to stimulate a child sexually, or any act in which the child is used for the sexual stimulation of an adult. Physical sexual abuse of a child includes sexual intercourse—genital, oral, or anal, either attempted or completed; penetration of the vaginal or anal orifices with an object, or attempts to do so; touching the child's genitals, breasts, or nipples (other than in situations of routine care, such as in diapering and bathing infants, sterilizing and bandaging wounds, etc.); and having the child touch the genitals of an adult. Psychological sexual abuse of a child includes threatened physical sexual abuse from an adult; forcing children to witness sexual acts for the purpose of providing sexual gratification to adults; and preparing, training, or exhibiting children for abuse by other adults—as in pornography and prostitution.

*A set of data not included in this study is that in which the victim and perpetrator are both under the age of 18. While it is recognized that such events occur and that their incidence is unknown, the problems in eliciting systematic reporting of these cases in the various agencies in this study precluded including them. Professional attitudes about children "playing doctor," teenage sexual experimentation, and age of consent vary enormously. Behavior classified as sexual abuse by one professional is termed "just fooling around" by another when the parties involved are both minors. For these reasons data collection was limited to cases in which the victim was under 18 and the perpetrator was 18 or over. While data for girls who became pregnant while attending high school were gathered and included in summary form in the final report for this study, these data are not included here. This sample turned out to be significantly different on a variety of measures (e.g., no force used, consensual nature of sex, low incidence of incest). It was clear that these adolescent girls were involved in consensual sex with older boyfriends (Swift, 1983).

Subjects

Subjects for whom results are reported here were 315 professionals in the Kansas City area whose responsibilities involved the identification and/or treatment of cases of sexual child abuse. The total includes 52 officers from 2 police departments, 77 members of the clinical staff of 4 community mental health centers, 71 school professionals (64 nurses and 7 counselors) from 2 school systems and 124 child protective service workers from 5 county agencies in Kansas and Missouri.*

Instruments

Assessment instruments included a survey consisting of over 90 items for each case reported. Items covered characteristics in five categories: the victim and abuser, the incident itself, incest cases, and system response—the actions of the agencies involved in the case. For example, system response in police agencies included items on the crime classification, status of clearance of the case (e.g., cleared by arrest, waived, continued), and referral to medical/mental health services. System response in mental health centers included intake procedures and diagnosis, and treatment frequency and modality. In schools, system response items included the number of contacts with the child and family by various school personnel as well as referrals to other agencies. In child protective service agencies, information such as outplacement, severance of parental rights, ancillary services, recommendations to courts, and number of contacts were collected as part of system response. In police departments, these surveys were completed by reviewing agency files. In mental health centers, schools, and child protective service agencies, information in case files was supplemented by interviews with the personnel involved with the case. Case information for targeted agencies was collected across two time periods—the 12 months before training and the 12 months after training. A second set of surveys assessed professionals' knowledge about sexual child abuse. It was given to professional staff participating in the training intervention. This survey, administered both before and after training, was developed in both a long (48-item) and short (18-item) format for use in the training seminars (long form) and workshops (short form), which are described below. Items consisted of statements with which participants indicated their agreement or diagreement. A "don't know" option was also provided. Examples of items are: "Most sexually abused children are not acquainted with their abusers," "An incestuous father rarely victimizes more than one child," and "Boys who have been sexually abused are more likely to commit violent sexual acts later in life than other boys."

---

*Subsequent to contracting for the participation of child protective service agencies in Kansas City the author was contacted by other such agencies in the state of Missouri seeking to receive the training. As a result, an additional 83 protective service workers from 7 county agencies in Missouri also received the training intervention. However, their results are not included here, since most of these counties are rural, and their demographies differ from those of the urban area originally targeted for the experimental intervention.

Procedures

Experimental Design

Four types of agencies/institutions in the Kansas City area were selected to receive training based on their official roles in dealing with cases of sexual child abuse—either as part of the law enforcement process or the reporting/treatment process. The four agency/types targeted to receive training were police, mental health centers, schools, and child protective service agencies. To test the relative effectiveness of two models of training (see below), paired agencies (e.g., two police departments, two school systems) from each type targeted were selected to participate in a 22-week seminar. A third police agency in the metropolitan Kansas City area served as a no-training limited control group* for other police agencies. A unique research advantage offered by the Kansas City metropolitan area is that the city is really two adjacent cities located in two states, Kansas and Missouri. This made it possible to pair major agencies for the research purpose of establishing experimental and control groups. Within each of the four agency types (police, mental health centers, schools, and child protective services), one agency was assigned to receive the experimental training model and one was assigned the control training model. The third police agency was designated to receive no training.

Participating Agencies

One of the hazards of field research is that events and conditions cannot be controlled to the same degree as in the laboratory. The exigencies of the real world subsequently dictated a change in the length of training. Agencies in two (police and schools) of the four targeted institutions were unable to fulfill their original commitments of personnel to the 22-week seminar. Therefore, the training was adapted as a one-day workshop and administered to paired (experimental and control) agencies across the four targeted institutions.† In addition, the 22-week seminar was implemented with two mental health centers and two child protective service agencies as originally planned. (each with the experimental/ control split).

Training Models

The training included didactic presentations, small group exercises, case examples and films. Seven topics in the area of sexual child abuse were covered: (1) legal issues in reporting, (2) definitions, (3) identification of cases: physical and psychological indicators, (4) incidence and prevalence, (5) incest, (6) interview-

---

*While agencies were selected as no-training controls for the other three institutions as well, subsequent events (ranging from small Ns to administrative complications) make the inclusion of their data problematic.

†Police were an exception. Because of a variety of community crises (e.g., a once-every-100-years flood, school desegregation issues, reduced staffing and budgets), administrators were unable to commit personnel to more than a half-day workshop. Therefore police received a four-hour workshop, and participating schools, mental health centers, and protective service agencies received an eight-hour workshop.

ing the child victim and the family, and (7) follow-up: effects of victimization on short- and long-term adjustment. The case examples and small group exercises were designed to familiarize agency staff with the problems involved in interviewing sexually abused children and their families, and to desensitize them to the taboos associated with the issue. Small group exercises occurred in all groups except police, where time constraints prohibited their use. A female-male team presented the substantive material, except for the topic of legal issues. An attorney from Kansas and one from Missouri presented the material on legal issues and served as consultants throughout the project.

Two training models were developed, experimental and control. The experimental model was designed to expose agency personnel to the realities, risks, and treatment of cases of sexual child abuse of both male and female children. It was strategized that through such exposure the participants' skills in identifying and treating cases of sexual abuse of boys as well as girls would be increased. The control model followed the conventional approach of focusing only on girls as the principal targets of sexual abuse. Specific information about sexual abuse of young males was omitted.

Results and Discussion

Results will focus on the incidence of reported cases of sexual child abuse in targeted agencies before and after the intervention, changes in professionals' levels of knowledge and their attitudes about sexual child abuse, and changes in agency response to these cases. Information collected on the behavioral responses of the victim and the victim's mother to the crisis presented by the abuse will be described separately.

Incidence of Reported Cases

Overall, agencies receiving training increased the number of cases of sexual child abuse reported from the 12-month pre- to the 12-month posttraining period by 17 percent. However this finding did not hold across all agencies, as shown in Table 1. Three of the four participating institutions showed increases in cases reported while one showed a decrease. Schools increased the number of cases reported by 189 percent. Child protective service agencies increased their caseloads by 36 percent and mental health centers by 15 percent. The police agencies participating in the training logged 14 percent fewer cases in the year following than in the year preceding training—significantly fewer than the other agencies

Table 1 Number of cases of sexual child abuse identified by agencies in the 12 months before and the 12 months after training

	Cases		Change (in percent)
Agency	Before training	After training	
Protective services	152	207	+ 36
Mental health centers	53	61	+ 15
Police	198	170	− 14
Schools	19	55	+189
Total	420	493	+ 17

receiving training. The no-training police agency showed a 2 percent decrease in reported cases across the same period.

The overall incidence of reported male victimization showed no change following training. Reported incidence prior to the intervention was 15 percent of the 12-month data base of sexual child abuse cases, compared with 14 percent of the cases in the 12 months following the intervention. No significant differences in reported cases of male victimization were noted between the experimental and control groups overall, before and after training, or between those that received the training in workshop format. However, one finding suggests that length of training may be an important factor in the subsequent identification of male victims. The experimental groups receiving the 22-week seminar subsequently increased their identification of male victimization by 5 percent, while the control groups showed a 2 percent decrease.

Professionals' Knowledge of and Attitudes about Sexual Child Abuse in Boys

Professionals receiving the training scored significantly higher on posttests than on pretests of their knowledge and attitudes about sexual child abuse. The proportion of correct answers across all groups trained increased from 48 to 72 percent. Utilizing the test for differences between proportions (Mueller, Schuessler, & Costner, 1977), $z = 6.283$ ($p < .001$). Agency personnel who received the experimental training model scored significantly higher than those receiving the control training model. Overall, the proportion of correct answers for experimental groups increased by 25 percent following training, compared with a 20-percent increase for the control groups ($z = 1.8, p < .022$).

Agency Response

A number of changes in the types of cases reported and in agency response to reports following training will be noted here. In three of the four institutions there was an increase in the proportion of nonpenetrative acts of sexual child abuse reported. Cases identified by police in the 12 months following the training intervention reflected a significant increase (13 percent) in nonpenetrative acts ($\chi^2 = 5.81$, df = 1, $p < .025$). Increases in the same direction were noted in the child protective services data (7%) and the school data (5%) following training, but these changes did not reach significance. Professionals in protective service agencies tended to recommend removing the victim from the home less following training (12% decrease), although this trend was not significant.

Two other significant changes noted in police response following training merit attention here. The groups receiving training showed significantly more cases cleared by arrest than the no-training group. The categories of clearance are (1) cleared by arrest, (2) "exceptionally" cleared (cases judged as unfounded or waived), and (3) not cleared. The groups receiving training increased their clearance of cases by arrest by 17 percent in the 12 months following training, compared with an increase of 4 percent for the no-training group in the same period ($z = 2.725$, $p < .01$). In addition, the training groups showed significantly more cases cleared by arrest and significantly fewer cleared as unfounded, waived, or not cleared in the 12 months following than in the 12 months preceding training ($\chi^2 = 8.415$, df = 2, $p < .025$). The classification of the crimes in the categories of rape, sodomy, and other (molestation, exposure)* involved in sexual child abuse also showed significant changes ($\chi^2 = 14.12$, df = 2, $p < .005$). Following training 18 percent fewer rapes and attempted rapes were recorded. Sodomies increased by 6 percent and "other" sex acts increased by 12 percent.

Discussion

Increased Case Identification

It is not a part of the job responsibilities of many of the professionals involved to initiate reports of sexual child abuse. While police and mental health personnel make decisions about whether or not to process reports made to them by private individuals and professionals from other agencies they are rarely in positions to identify the phenomenon directly by observing victims' physical or behavioral cues. The significant increase in the number of cases identified by these professionals following training suggests that they were either more willing to believe the reports and log them into the official system, more sensitive or skilled in evaluating the reports, or both. The roles of professionals from schools and child protective services often place them in direct contact with children and families with a variety of social problems. They thus have opportunities to identify sexual child abuse directly and to initiate the official report themselves. For these groups of professionals, increased identification of cases suggests both an increased receptivity and skill in processing reports and an increased expertise in identifying cases and initiating reports.

Police

The decrease in cases logged by police following training was an unexpected result and is in contrast with the significant increase in the number of cases reported by the other three institutions receiving training. The reasons for this finding are not clear. Two factors are suggested as post-hoc explanations. The first has to do with the punitive role assigned to police in these cases. It is their function to arrest offenders and facilitate their prosecution. This contrasts with the helping role of the social service agencies. Mental health centers treat victims and their families with the goal of ensuring the child's safety, reducing the negative effects of abuse and restoring normal family functioning. Child protective service agencies are more likely to act as the child's advocate than to concern themselves with punishing the offender. The second factor has to do with community resources. The training included information and education about the services available in community agencies to treat sexually abused children and their families, as well as procedures for referral. It may be that the training sensitized police to the complexity of sexual child abuse—particularly intrafamilial abuse. An increased sensitivity to concerns of victims and their families and an increased awareness of alternative community resources may have resulted in police officers, in their gatekeeper role, opting to refer more cases to social service agencies as an alternative to processing them in the law enforcement system. This explanation is supported by the finding, in social service agency data, that police referrals increased by nine percent following training.

*None of these categories include incest cases.

Police have traditionally responded to incest as they have to spouse abuse. Confronted with the accusations of the child or wife and the denial of the male head of the house, they have characteristically admonished the participants and declined to process "domestic disputes" through the official reporting system. Taken together, the significant changes in police response might suggest that they were more sensitive to the occurrence of sexual child abuse following training, and that they considered the disposition of these cases more seriously.

Schools

Schools demonstrated the largest increase: Identified cases tripled following the training intervention. In addition to increased skill in case identification this probably reflects the fact that schools had a record of low reporting of these cases prior to training. A common response I encountered in the process of obtaining administrative permission to train school personnel was, "You won't find any cases in this school." In the course of training, many school nurses and counselors approached the instructors for advice about how to report cases directly to the state agency without risking their jobs. It seems that several schools had policies dictating that official reports of sexual child abuse were to be made by school administrators only. It may be that educating school staff about their legal responsibilities to report directly, and their options to report anonymously, led to the reporting of cases that had previously been suppressed. The training intervention in schools appeared to alter the political constraints that inhibited reporting. Unlike the other participating agencies, schools have no official role in enforcing sanctions or delivering treatment in cases of sexual child abuse. Therefore, while posttraining increases in the sexual child abuse caseloads of social service agencies reflect increased referrals to those agenices, referrals are not the source of the increase in school cases.

Child Protective Agencies

The 30 percent before/after increase in child protective agency caseloads appears to reflect two factors related to the training. First, the data suggest that professionals improved their skills in identifying cases encountered directly, including both new cases referred for other types of problems and cases already on agency caseloads. Following training the percentage of cases identified at the point of referral decreased by 11 percent and the percent identified as a result of investigation subsequent to referral increased by 11 percent. Second, referrals from other agencies increased slightly (5 percent overall).

Treatment "Dosage": Brief versus Extended Training

While the research was not originally designed to measure the "dose" effect of more versus less training, the expedient of providing workshops when seminars were not feasible offered the opportunity to look at the effects of such "doses." The results suggest that extended exposure to the evidence of male victimization in sexual child abuse may sensitize staff to the issue, and function to increase subsequent reporting. Social service agencies are microcosms within the macrocosm of societal values, attitudes, and shared wisdom. There is resistance to examining attitudes about taboo subjects. Changes in beliefs around emotionally charged issues come slowly. Brief exposure to new information that calls into question entrenched beliefs is not as powerful in effecting change as extended exposure.

The 5 percent increase in the identification of male victimization following training by the experimental groups receiving the 22-week seminar supports this suggestion.

Time has been documented as a significant variable in consultation success—especially in cases involving attitude change (Carner, 1982; Fairweather, Sanders, & Tornatzky, 1974; Lippitt, 1959; Newman & Bloomberg, 1982; Mannino & Shore, 1979; Tyler, 1971). The rationale of the extended (22-week) training was that studying a subject as taboo as sexual child abuse requires desensitization of strong feelings, establishment of trust and rapport with instructors and fellow students, continued exposure to the "facts" as revealed in current research, time to digest or integrate the material through discussion with peers in a supportive environment, and the opportunity to share cases and the feelings associated with these cases with professional peers. It seems reasonable that a one-day workshop focusing on such change would be less effective than a more extended training effort.

As noted earlier, the training was originally projected as a course that would meet weekly and extend for approximately six months. Only two of the targeted institutions were able to free up personnel for the 22-week commitment—the two social service agencies. While it is of value to learn that extended training may be effective, the professional contemplating Type 3 community training interventions is left with the problem of how to induce institutions that need training to receive it. In times of budget cuts and reductions in force, administrators—however persuaded they may be of the efficacy of training—are hard pressed to deliver the services required of them. Precious staff hours spent in training may be a luxury some agencies cannot afford. These issues suggest that such training should take place prior to the job—in schools of education, police training academies, professional schools of social work and psychology. Once in the field there may not be the opportunity for more than shotgun approaches for front-line agencies such as police and schools.

RESPONSES OF THE VICTIM AND FAMILY
TO THE CRISIS OF DISCLOSURE

While this chapter has reported a Type 3 community intervention targeting professionals, most interventions in this area are targeted to the victims and their families. Preliminary to designing Type 3 and 4 interventions with this population it is instructive to review their characteristic responses to the crisis situation. The remainder of this chapter draws on the data base from the Kansas City study to sketch a profile of the victims and their families and to review the behavior of the victim and mother in response to the crisis. The profile is based on 816 cases gathered from 15 county protective service agencies in Kansas and Missouri. This data base includes the cases collected from the Kansas City protective service agencies in connection with the experimental training intervention described earlier. It also includes cases from protective service agencies in two other urban areas, and six rural counties in Kansas and Missouri.* Protective service caseloads are currently the most accurate single source of data for these cases, since these

---

*These agencies requested to be a part of the project in order to receive the training. While their case data were added to the data base for purposes of epidemiologic analysis, their data were excluded from the impact analysis of the training intervention. Differences between the rural and urban cases of sexual child abuse are summarized elsewhere (Swift, 1983).

agencies are charged by law to receive all reports of child abuse and neglect, investigate these reports, and take appropriate action. In interpreting these data it should be kept in mind that 73 percent of the protective services sexual child abuse caseload was made up of incest cases.

Family Histories and Characteristics

Families in which sexual abuse occurs are often thought to be socially disrupted. According to this view they are subjected to a variety of stresses including frequent moves, isolation, spouse abuse, parental alcohol or drug abuse, and a parental history of child abuse. The Kansas City study supports most of these hypotheses. The picture that emerged was one of families afflicted with a greater than average share of social ills. One-fifth of the families had moved since the case was first opened. They tended to be more isolated from relatives and community activities than their neighbors; 40 percent were so categorized by the worker assigned to the case. Alcohol and drug abuse appeared to be major problems, afflicting 42 percent of the fathers and 17 percent of the mothers. The conventional wisdom that holds child abuse to be a repetitive factor across generations finds support here. In over one-third of these families, a parental history of abuse was reported. The mother was reportedly victimized in 49 percent of these cases, the father in 39 percent, and both in an additional 12 percent. Spouse abuse was not uncommon, reportedly occurring in one-fourth of the cases.

A large number of these families were poor. Forty-two percent were either currently receiving or had received financial assistance from a variety of state and federal programs. This finding is consistent with the results of the National Incidence Study (NCCAN, 1981), in which over three-fourths of the families had incomes under $15,000. The predominance of poor families in these two studies may reflect the higher likelihood of the crime being detected and reported when it occurs in this population rather than a higher incidence. Wealthier families presumably have access to a greater variety of options for concealing the abuse as well as for treating it.

Characteristics of the Sexual Abuse

Data from the social histories of victims support the conclusions that (1) most reports of sexual abuse occur only after multiple incidents of victimization, (2) the sexual abuse is often just one calamity in an extremely disrupted family situation, (3) sexual victimization by one abuser may place the victim at risk for subsequent victimization by others, and (4) sexual abuse of one child places siblings at high risk for abuse. Previous sexual victimization was reported for 90 percent of these victims. Seventeen percent had been victimized by more than one family member, or by a family member and someone outside the family. All combinations involved the father or stepfather. Fourteen percent of the victims were also found to be suffering from neglect and nine percent were physically as well as sexually abused by the perpetrator in the family. In one-third of the cases, one or more of the victim's siblings had also been victimized—again, most often (in almost 80 percent of these cases) by the father or stepfather.

An analysis of the sex acts involved utilizes the total sample of 1833 cases. In over one-half of the cases the children were subjected to sexual acts involving penetration. The most frequent was vaginal penetration (40%). Oral sexual acts by the victim occurred in 20 percent of the cases. The abuser performed oral acts in 16 percent of the cases and anal acts in 8 percent. The victim was forced to perform sexual acts on a person other than the identified abuser in 6 percent of the cases. Use of children for prostitution or pornography was relatively rare, occurring in 2 percent of the cases.

Child's Response to the Abuse

Why did these children not tell someone? The overwhelming number of cases in which previous victimization occurred—a measure of prevalence rather than incidence, is evidence of the strong forces that operate to silence these victims and immobilize the adults charged with their care. A major source of conflict lies in the relationship between the child and the abuser. In 95 percent of the cases the abuser was male. In almost two-thirds of the social service cases he was the parent. The confusion and divided loyalties victims experienced led to delays in reporting as well as to subsequent retractions of reports previously made. Roughly half of the children told their mothers about the most recent incident. Professionals—teachers, counselors, and nurses—were told almost as often as mothers. This study corroborates the finding of differential reporting by sex: 54 percent of the girls reportedly told their mothers compared with 36 percent of the boys. The primary obstacle to earlier reporting was fear of the consequences. The most common fear was that the abuser would physically hurt or punish them if they told. Many feared, realistically, that they would be removed from their homes. Another fear was that the public exposure entailed in seeking help would break up the family.

Roughly two-thirds of the children reportedly resisted the abuse. The most frequent means of resistance was physical (27%) followed by verbal resistance (24%) and attempts to escape (11%). Since three-fourths of the abusive acts occurred in either the victim's or the abuser's home (48% in their mutual home) escape was a poor option. A large proportion of sexually abused children turn up as runaways and prostitutes. In this study, 10 percent of the victims were reported to have run away at least once to avoid sexual abuse.

Role of the Mother

Assistance to the Child

The mother is a pivotal figure in determining the poststress response, both proximal and distal, to her child's crisis. She is the person the child is most likely to tell. If she believes her child's account and takes action, she has the capacity to mobilize an array of interventions from other persons and agencies. The literature yields little empirical data on the mother's response although a great deal has been written on the subject. As noted above in almost half the cases the children told their mothers of the incident that led to the report. The large majority of mothers (77%) were reported to have responded helpfully. Seventy-one percent sought professional help. Only 14 percent refused to believe the child or to discuss the incident. In the mental health center sample mothers reported over half (54%) of those agencies' cases of sexual child abuse reported by individuals—three times the proportion found in the protective services sample. Given the nonpunitive treatment orientation of mental health services this is not a surprising result. The power of protective services to remove the child from the home and sever parental rights may influence many mothers to seek a less disruptive solution.

What these data do not show is how many times the child told the mother or how many incidents occurred before the mother sought help. The high proportion of cases in which previous victimization occurred suggests that either the child had not told the mother before, or the mother did not accept or act on previous reports. A subsample of incest cases supports the latter interpretation. When mothers of incest victims were told of incidents occurring prior to the one that was finally reported they were over three times as likely (48%) to disbelieve the child or refuse to discuss the incident, and less than a third as likely (20%) to seek professional help.

Factors Influencing the Mother's Decision to Report the Abuse

Clearly, for many of these mothers, the incident that was finally reported was one in an extended series of incidents. Some condition or event triggered her decision to act. There are no studies that systematically assess the behavioral process these mothers go through from the time of their child's first report to their decision to "go public" and seek help. Her economic dependence, her traditional role as family arbiter, her conflicting loyalties to husband and child, and her commitment to keep the family together contribute to the mother's difficulty in acting effectively to protect her child (Meiselman, 1978; Walters, 1975). While the mother's dilemma may be alluded to she is usually cast as coconspirator.

Denial is the classic response attributed to mothers of incest victims. The Kansas City study supports the attribution of denial to the mother, as seen in the contrast between her reactions to earlier and later reports of abuse by the child. What the study also does is place the mother's initial denial into the larger context of a systems response to sexual child abuse. While the conventional analysis notes the mother's resistance to believing that her husband could be abusing their child sexually, it fails to note that resistance to believing the child is pervasive. The evidence of denial is widespread in the literature, as seen in both the paucity of documented cases until relatively recently (Gagnon, 1970) and the awkward explanations contrived to account for psychiatric patients' disclosures of childhood sexual victimization (Freud, 1966; Masson, 1984; Rush, 1977). In the Kansas City study evidence for denial at the systems level is found in the success of the training intervention. It is unlikely that the significantly larger number of cases identified by social service and school professionals after training was due to a sudden spurt in sexual child abuse in Kansas City. A more likely interpretation of the increase is that the training left these professionals less ready to deny and more ready to believe the reports of sexual child abuse coming to their attention.

Mother's Choice of the Referral Agency

Once the mother decides to report, what influences her choice of agency to receive the report? The evidence points to the degree of closeness between the victim and the abuser as the critical variable determining where the case is reported. Until the last decade the police department was the agency most likely to receive these reports. In the ten years since the enactment of mandatory reporting laws, child protective service agencies in each state have become the primary recipients.

This shift reflects the growing awareness of the high proportion of intrafamilial sexual abuse and the associated tendency to see the phenomenon as a social problem as well as—or rather than—a crime.

The likelihood of reporting to police appears to be inversely related to the degree of closeness between the child and the abuser. In the Kansas City study the natural father was the abuser in only one-tenth of the police cases compared with over one-third (39%) of the protective service cases. The discrepancy is reduced in abuse by stepfathers, which occurs in 14 percent of the police cases, compared with 24 percent of the protective service cases. Abuse by strangers occurred in one-third of the police cases compared with less than two percent of the cases found in the protective service caseload. The same pattern was found in the differential reporting of incest by agencies and private individuals. Private individuals initiated the police action by a ratio of 3:1 in incest cases, and by 15:1 in nonincest cases. For families with victimized children who sought to identify and punish the abuser the police were still the agency most often called. Requests for police action came primarily from individuals, not agencies, in the great majority of these cases (91%).

The pattern of reporting was reversed in the social service data. The closer the relationship between the child and the abuser, the more likely it was that the case was reported to mental health or protective services. Almost three-fourths of these agencies' sexual child abuse cases were incest. Roughly four-fifths of the abusers in these cases were either related to the child, or functioned in a pseudo-parent role (foster father, mother's boyfriend, etc.). This difference in reporting is not hard to understand. The purpose of mental health services is to prevent and treat mental illness. Families whose loyalties are divided between the child and the abuser, or those committed to staying together for whatever reasons, are more likely to seek treatment than criminal prosecution. Of the four institutions studied, mental health centers had the highest proportion of cases involving the natural father—40 percent of their sexual child abuse cases. Unlike police cases, which were primarily referred by individuals, less than one-fourth (23%) of the mental health cases entered the system this way. Of these, the mother or stepmother was the person most often (53%) requesting services for the case. The victim rarely self-referred (2.4% of the cases).

Implications for Future Programming

The results of this study, in the context of emerging research and literature in the field of sexual child abuse, suggest a multilevel program for prevention and treatment. Five broad areas of activity are needed: basic research, public education, changes in the criminal justice system's handling of sexual child abuse, training programs for professionals, and strategies for early identification, intervention, and treatment of cases.

Basic research is needed to identify the variables associated with abuse as well as the outcomes of abuse, both short and long term. Current models—such as child assault prevention training and Giarretto's treatment program—should be rigorously evaluated. Those with documented effectiveness should be replicated on as broad a scale as resources permit.

Public education is a vital component of prevention efforts. Since sexual child abuse is rooted in societal as well as situational variables, preventive approaches are appropriately directed to both. Public education promoting the elimination of sex role stereotyping in societal institutions such as the schools and the media would contribute to altering conditions that perpetuate the disproportionate sexual victimization of vulnerable populations. Such programs should include as fundamental the rights of persons—including vulnerable populations such as children, women, and incarcerated persons of both sexes—to control their own bodies. In addition, the education of the public to the social and emotional costs of sexual child abuse, its prevalence and possible means of prevention could mobilize public opinion to support programs for research and services. While individual community projects such as CAP training contribute to this goal, what is needed is a leveraging of such public education efforts through government sanction and funding on a society-wide level. While the data presented in this chapter provide information about a variety of responses of victims and community agencies to the crisis of sexual child abuse, they provide no estimate of the victimized children whose situations remain undiscovered. Interventions focusing on information and education campaigns could alert these children to supportive resources, or equip them with strategies of avoidance or escape.

Changes in the way the criminal justice system handles these cases could also contribute to prevention goals. Systematic and uniform enforcement of the laws prohibiting this crime could be expected to increase the certainty of punishment, which should ultimately result in a reduction in incidence (see below). A reduction in the practice of plea bargaining would contribute to the goal of educating the public to the true incidence of abuse. It would also result in more accurate labeling of offenders so they would have less success evading prosecution for subsequent offenses. Another change needed both in the criminal justice and social service systems is the development of uniform national reporting codes for acts of sexual child abuse. This would permit more accurate data collection and facilitate epidemiological analysis, a prerequisite to prevention efforts. Alternatives to mandatory court appearances should be developed to protect the victim-witness from the further trauma associated with providing testimony in court. Videotaping the testimony; greater use of expert witnesses (mental health professionals) in interpreting the child's behavior and testimony, as in Israel's use of the surrogate witness (Reifen, 1958), and taking testimony in the judge's chambers are some of the options to be explored. The development of a humane procedure for taking the testimony of child victims would increase the number of prosecutions of these crimes, since parents would be more likely to permit their child to participate in court proceedings.

From the perspective of system change, interventions involving legislation/ enforcement and education are paired. The primary power of legislation in reducing crime derives from the certainty of punishment (Andenaes, 1975; Erickson & Gibbs, 1973; Gibbs, 1968; Tittle, 1969). A secondary preventive effect of legislation is in the codification of cultural norms: "The legislation of one generation may become the morality of the next" (Walker, 1975). Currently, legislation prohibiting the crime of sexual child abuse and that mandating the reporting of abuse rarely result in convictions. In prevention terms, stepped-up enforcement of laws prohibiting sexual child abuse and mandating reporting would signal strong public sentiment that this crime is unacceptable.

Loh's (1981) discussion of the impact of rape reform legislation on the sexual assault of adults has parallels for sexual child abuse:

> The role of rape law as catalyst for attitude change may be greater than any im-
> mediate impact on the criminal justice system. The criminal law serves not only a general
> deterrent function. It also has a "moral or sociopedagogic" purpose to reflect and
> shape moral values and beliefs of society (citation omitted). The new rape law symbol-
> izes and reinforces newly emerging conceptions about the status of women and the
> right of self-determination in sexual conduct. Conviction of rape, rather than of some
> surrogate offense, is a dramatic lesson about society's disapprobation of the act, and
> helps to strengthen the public code. (p. 50)

The strong message of the research reported in this chapter is that training the
professionals whose responsibilities routinely bring them in contact with children
can increase professional skills in identifying cases of sexual child abuse, and
result in a larger proportion of victims receiving protection and treatment. The
evidence also suggests that such training leads to the earlier identification of these
cases in the abuse cycle, which should reduce the frequency and severity of
dysfunction associated with long-term abuse—especially incest. The education
of both the public and professionals to this problem should not only increase
receptivity to reports by children, but should reduce the pervasive denial—the
tendency to interpret warning cues in normal terms—that currently dominates
response to these reports.

A final direction for future programming is interventions with families in which
sexual abuse is identified. Since the topic is too broad to be covered here an
example is used to make the point. Interventions with the mother in incest cases
should focus on skill development in three areas. First, the channel of communication between mother and child must be kept open and active. The mother must
have the capacity to "think the unthinkable"—to identify behavioral cues that
signal sexual abuse and realistically evaluate her child's report. Second, she needs
the skills to confront her spouse. The incestuous father predictably denies his
involvement, further victimizing his child as a liar and placing the mother in the
position of having to choose between them. This sets up an extremely difficult
choice that too often immobilizes the mother. Confronted with conflicting
evidence, she quite literally cannot make sense of what she sees and hears. She
needs guidance in balancing her husband's words and actions against their child's
report. Third, the mother needs to know where to turn for help. Beyond dealing
with her husband and child she needs information about resources so that she can
insure the child's safety, express and explore her suspicions, and engage in problem
solving to resolve the situation. An empirical investigation of the behaviors and
role demands of the various family members should result in intervention strategies
designed to identify and arrest incipient or actual abuse, build the coping skills
of family members, and dilute the negative impact of the abuse situation.

SUMMARY

Most cases of sexual child abuse come to professional attention only after
repeated incidents of victimization. It is desirable to design interventions that
will permit identification of these cases as early as possible in the sequence of
abuse. Intervening before the abuse escalates in severity may prevent the trauma
associated with extensive victimization. A Type 3 community intervention was
reported in which professionals received training about sexual child abuse. The
results of the study suggest that such interventions can be effective in changing

the attitudes of professionals and improving their skills in identifying these cases. Survey data were presented dealing with the victims' behavior in resisting and reporting the abuse and with the mother's response to the crisis. Selected system responses of police, mental health centers, and child protective service agencies were also presented. Finally, the implications of this and associated research and literature for future programming were explored. It is hoped that the information in this chapter will help others in designing interventions for victimized children and their families.

REFERENCES

Andenaes, J. (1975). General prevention revisited: Research and policy implications. *Journal of Criminal Law and Criminology, 66*, 338-365.

Bart, P. (1981). A study of women who both were raped and avoided rape. *The Journal of Social Issues, 37*, 123-137.

Burgess, A., & Holmstrom, L. (1974). *Rape: Victims of crisis.* Bowie, MD: Robert J. Brady Co., Prentice-Hall.

Burgess, A., & Holmstrom, L. (1980). Sexual trauma of children and adolescents. In L. G. Schultz (Ed.), *The sexual victimology of youth.* Springfield, IL: Charles C Thomas.

Carner, L. (1982). Developing a consultative contract. In J. Alpert (Ed.), *Psychological consultation in educational settings.* San Francisco: Jossey-Bass.

Cooper, S., Lutter, Y., & Phelps, C. (1983). *Strategies for free children: A leader's guide to child assault prevention.* Youngstown, OH: Ink Well Press.

Erickson, M., & Gibbs, J. (1973). The deterrence question: Some alternative methods of analysis. *Social Science Quarterly, 54*, 534-551.

Fairweather, G., Sanders, D., & Tornatzky, L. (1974). *Creating change in mental health organizations.* Elmsford, NY: Pergamon.

Finkelhor, D. (1982). Sexual abuse of boys: The available data. In N. Groth (Ed.), *Sexual victimization of males, offenses, offenders and victims.* New York: Plenum.

Finkelhor, D. (1984). *Child sexual abuse: New theory and research.* New York: Free Press.

Finkelhor, D. (1985). Sexual abuse of boys. In A. Burgess (Ed.), *Rape and sexual assault: A research handbook.* New York: Garland.

Finkelhor, D., & Hotaling, G. (1983). Sexual abuse in the National Incidence Study of Child Abuse and Neglect (Final report, National Center on Child Abuse, Grant 90-CA840/01). Durham, NH. Family Violence Research Program, University of New Hampshire.

Freud, S. (1966). *The complete introductory lectures of psycho-analysis.* New York: W. W. Norton.

Gagnon, J. (1970). Female child victims of sex offenses. In A. Shiloh (Ed.), *Studies in human sexual behavior: The American Scene.* Springfield, IL: Charles C Thomas.

Giarretto, H. (1977). Humanistic treatment of father-daughter incest. *Child Abuse and Neglect, 1*, 411-426.

Giarretto, H. (1981). A comprehensive child sexual abuse treatment program. In P. Mrazek & C. Kempe (Eds.), *Sexually abused children and their families.* Elmsford, NY: Pergamon.

Gibbs, J. (1968). Crime, punishment and deterrence. *Social Science Quarterly, 28*, 515-530.

Goldstein, M. (1973). Exposure to erotic stimuli and sexual deviance. *Journal of Social Issues, 29*, 197-219.

Groth, N. (1979). *Men who rape: The psychology of the offender.* New York: Plenum.

Herman, J. (1982). *Father-daughter incest.* Cambridge, MA: Harvard University Press.

Herman, J., & Hirschman, L. (1977). Father-daughter incest. *Signs: Journal of Women in Culture and Society, 2*, 735-756.

James, J., Womack, W., & Strauss, F. (1978). Physician reporting of sexual abuse of children. *Journal of the American Medical Association, 240*, 1145-1146.

Kleven, S. (1981). *The touching problem.* Billingdam, WA: The Coalition for Child Advocacy.

Krasner, W., Meyer, L., & Carroll, N. (1977). *Victims of Rape* (DHEW Publication No. ADM 77-485). Washington, DC: U. S. Government Printing Office.

Landis, J. (1956). Experiences of 500 children with adult sexual deviation. *Psychiatric Quarterly Supplement, 30*, 91-109.

Lewis, M., & Sarrel, P. (1969). Some psychological aspects of seduction, incest and rape in childhood. *Journal of American Academy of Child Psychology, 8,* 606-619.

Lippitt, R. (1959). Dimensions of the consultant's job. *Journal of Social Issues, 15,* 5-12.

Loh, W. (1981). What has reform of rape legislation wrought? *Journal of Social Issues, 37,* 28-52.

Mannino, V., & Shore, M. (1979). Evaluation of consultation: Problems and prospects. *New Directions for Mental Health Services, 3,* 99-113.

Masson, J. (1984). *The assault on truth: Freud's suppression of the seduction theory.* New York: Farrar, Straus, & Giroux.

McIntyre, J. (1981). *Victim response to rape: Alternative outcomes.* (final report). Rockville, MD: National Center for the Prevention and Control of Rape, NIMH.

Meiselman, K. (1978). *Incest.* San Francicso: Jossey-Bass.

Mueller, J., Schuessler, K., & Costner, H. (1977). *Statistical reasoning in sociology.* Boston: Houghton Mifflin.

NCCAN (1981). *National study of the incidence and severity of child abuse and neglect.* (DHHS publication). Washington, DC: U. S. Government Printing Office.

Newman, R., & Bloomberg, C. (1982). Working with elementary school administrators. In J. Alpert (Ed.), *Psychological consultation in educational settings.* San Francisco: Jossey-Bass.

Raigrodski, E. (1983). *Annotated Bibliography on Sexual Victimization of Children.* Available from the National Center for the Prevention and Control of Rape, NIMH, 5600 Fishers Lane, Rockville, MD 20857.

Reifen, D. (1958). Protection of children involved in sexual offenses: A new method of investigation in Israel. *Journal of Criminal Law, Criminology and Police Science, 49,* 222-229.

Rush, F. (1977). The Freudian cover-up. *Chrysalis, 1,* 31-45.

Russell, D. (1984). Sexual exploitation: Rape, child sexual abuse, and workplace harassment. Beverly Hills, CA: Sage.

Serril. M. (1974). Treating sex offenders in New Jersey. *Corrections, 1,* 13-24.

Silver, R., Boon, C., & Stones, M. (1983). Searching for meaning in misfortune: Making sense of incest. *Journal of Social Issues, 39,* 81-101.

Sparks, C., & Bar On, B. (1982). A social change approach to the prevention of sexual violence toward women. Paper presented at the National Institute of Mental Health Staff College course, "Mental health services for women: Treatment and prevention," Washington, DC, July, 1982. Available from Community Living for Women, Box 265, Edgewater, MD 21037.

Steele, B., & Alexander, H. (1981). Long-term effects of sexual abuse in childhood. In P. Mrazek & C. Kempe (Eds.), *Sexually abused children and their families.* Elmsford, NY: Pergamon.

Swift, C. (1977). Sexual victimization of children: An urban mental health center survey. *Victimology: An International Journal, 2,* 322-327.

Swift, C. (1978). Sexual exploitation of children in the United States. In *Research into violent behavior: Overview and sexual assaults* (Hearings before the Subcommittee on Domestic and International Scientific Planning, Analysis and Cooperation of the Committee on Science and Technology, U. S. House of Representatives), No. 64, 323-366. Washington, DC: U. S. Govt. Printing Office.

Swift, C. (1979). The prevention of sexual child abuse: Focus on the perpetrator. *Journal of Clinical Child Psychology, 8,* 133-136.

Swift, C. (1983). Consultation in the area of sexual child abuse. *Final report,* Grant MH 29038-03). Rockville, MD: National Center for the Prevention and Control of Rape, NIMH.

Tittle, C. (1969). Crime rates and legal sanctions. *Social Problems, 16,* 409-423.

Tyler, M. (1971). A study of some selected parameters of school psychologist-teacher consultation. *Dissertation Abstracts International, 32,* 5626A. (University Microfilms No. 72-11, 721)

Walker, N. (1975). Quotation found in J. Andenaes: General prevention revisited: Research and policy implications. *Journal of Criminal Law and Criminology, 66,* 338-365.

Walters, F. (1975). *Physical and Sexual Abuse of Children: Causes and Treatment.* Bloomington, IN: Indiana University Press.

8

Coping in Siblings of Children with Serious Illness

Mary Jo Kupst
Children's Memorial Hospital
Northwestern University Medical School

Serious illness frequently disrupts normal family functioning as well as the functioning of individuals within the family. The impact can be particularly profound in siblings of the ill child (see reviews by McKeever, 1983, and Sourkes, 1980). An increasingly held view is that behavior problems in siblings result from illness-related demands and not from pre-existing psychopathological conditions (Cairns, Clark, Smith, & Lansky, 1979; Sourkes, 1980). They may be forced to deal with issues to which they might otherwise not be exposed, such as the cause and visibility of the illness, the treatment process and procedures, their own feelings of guilt about the illness, and increased attention paid to the child who is ill by other family members. Using the example of pediatric leukemia, this chapter will review relevant literature and describe an ongoing longitudinal study of families of pediatric leukemia patients. Special emphasis will be placed on specific issues relevant to siblings and the incidence of problems at different phases of treatment. An intervention strategy will also be described.

PEDIATRIC LEUKEMIA

Rather than constituting a single crisis, pediatric leukemia involves a series of stressors that depend on the stage of the illness and treatment, and the medical status of the patient. Five major stages of illness may be identified: prediagnosis, diagnosis and initial hospitalization, treatment, long-term remission, and death.

Prediagnosis

In some cases, there is little evidence of a problem, and leukemia is discovered "accidentally" when a battery of tests is conducted for another reason. Quite

The author wishes to thank Jerome L. Schulman, M.D., who was principal investigator of the Coping Project, for his leadership and knowledge in the areas of coping with serious illness. I am also grateful to those who worked on this project, including Lynne Tylke, M.A., Loy Thomas, M.A., Rhoda Kling, M.A., & Connie Stuetzer, M.A., who were the intervenors on the projects; and to research assistants Cathryn C. Richardson, Mary E. Mudd, Martha Schulman Stolberg, Ph.D., Betsy Gilpin, Ph.D., and Mary Fran Riley Maggio for their invaluable assistance. I also wish to thank volunteers Alice Saar and Di Cross for their help in data collection and analysis, and Cheryl Klaub for her help in rating of taped interviews.

This project was funded by the National Cancer Institute, Grant Number CA19344, and by the Margaret Etter Creche Learning Center.

often, however, some symptom or set of symptoms develops (fever, lassitude, bruising, etc.) that signals the existence of a potential problem. Appointments are made with the pediatrician, or the child may be taken to the hospital emergency room, after which referral is generally made to a pediatric hematologist/oncologist for diagnosis. At this time, siblings become aware of the emerging tension in the family as they await the diagnosis.

Diagnosis and Initial Hospitalization

Even when siblings do not understand what leukemia means, or are not informed of the diagnosis, they may realize that something is seriously wrong from the reactions of their parents. Suddenly, there is a flurry of activity to admit the child to the hospital and begin treatment. In many cases, arrangements must be made for care of the siblings while parents remain in the hospital, and siblings must adjust to living with relatives or friends. Parents are physically absent from the home for long periods of time, and when they are home, their thoughts are likely more directed toward the ill child. Thus, siblings may not get attention at a time when they are fearful and their needs for attention are high.

A related potential problem is poor communication within the family about the illness (McCarthy, 1975; McKeever, 1983; Townes & Wold, 1977). Siblings may wonder if their brother or sister will die, if they will catch the illness, and what will happen during treatment. If parents present a minimized or distorted version of the illness, siblings may develop fantasies about the cause of the illness. It is not uncommon for the children to think that they played a role in causing the illness by doing something "bad." Guilt may arise over previous negative interactions with the patient. If parents are unwilling to discuss the illness, the children learn that open questioning and revelation of their own fears and anxieties are not sanctioned, and they may stop talking about the illness altogether.

Treatment

Shortly after diagnosis, treatment is begun in order to induce remission. The view presented by the medical staff is generally optimistic, especially in cases of acute lymphocytic leukemia in which most children achieve remission. Emphasis is on the administration of medications and offsetting possible side-effects, on procedures such as bone marrow aspirations and lumbar punctures, and on the results of blood counts. The family routine is disrupted and most of the attention is placed on the ill child, who may look sicker as a result of treatment and who may experience pain and discomfort as a result of the procedures. Watching all of this, siblings worry more about the patient and are less able to concentrate in school, especially on days when the patient goes to the hospital.

Some siblings channel their worry into a kind of protectiveness of the ill child, taking on a nursing role which gives them a sense of mastery in being able to do something for the patient. Not all siblings, however, demonstrate such concern. Because of jealousy over attention, anger over the disruption of their lives, or anxiety that they cannot dispel, some siblings appear quite selfish and uncaring, immersing themselves in their own interests and activities.

Another common outgrowth of serious illness in a child is increased demands on siblings to assume more responsibilities, such as handling more chores and providing emotional support for other family members. There may also be increased financial strain due to high medical bills, and siblings are thus forced to make sacrifices. While the losses may be relatively small in the case of toys or new clothes, they can be significantly larger in the case of reduced leisure activities or even the loss of opportunity to attend private schools or colleges.

A subcategory of treatment involves bone marrow transplants. Siblings are often the best "match" and thus become donors. Frequently, because these centers are far from home, siblings may be uprooted from the very things that have provided support for them: home, school, friends, and familiar activities, which can be very difficult for them (McKeever, 1983). In most cases, as would be expected, donors feel responsible for the outcome of the transplant. If it works well, they may feel that it is partly due to their efforts, but if it does not, they may blame themselves. Some of the psychological issues regarding bone marrow transplants and their impact on the family have been described elsewhere (Brown & Kelly, 1976; Gardner, August, & Githens, 1977).

Long-Term Remission

Advances in treatment have enabled many pediatric leukemia patients to achieve long-term remission, which continues 5 to 10 years posttreatment or longer. The patient in remission and the family return to more normal lives. Visits to the hospital become less frequent and the illness recedes into the background. It is common to hear family members talk about the illness in the past tense. Often they do not want to spend much time talking about it but would rather focus on other concerns and activities. The family tends to relax more and siblings are better able to do the things they did before the illness occurred. More parental attention can also be focused on them.

The possibility of relapse still exists, however, and families differ in their ability to admit to this possibility. Some remain involved with other families from the hospital and in voluntary activities around the hospital, while others keep their contacts limited to clinic visits. A crucial time for the families is when the decision to end chemotherapy is made (currently two to three years after diagnosis). Since treatment was what kept the illness from recurring, it is difficult to give up the dependence on medications (Alby, 1980). Siblings may share these misgivings and worry about the outcome. A thorough examination of the issues surrounding long-term remission can be found in Koocher and O'Malley (1981).

Death

While many patients achieve long-term remission, death is still a strong possibility with acute leukemia, and if it occurs it is a devastating blow for the entire family. Cain, Fast, and Erikson (1964) have described grief responses following death of a sibling. These include crying, talking about the sibling, somatic complaints, depression, withdrawal, academic problems, guilt, and suicidal thoughts. Shrier (1980) also found acute reactions such as appetite loss, needing to talk about death, and stunned reactions, as well as chronic reactions such as nightmares, acting out, anxiety, guilt, learning disturbances, and distorted concepts of illness and death. It is clear that the death of a child has a profound impact on a sibling.

OVERVIEW OF RESEARCH

While there have been several extensive clinical reports, there have been few studies of siblings which document the incidence of problems using systematic data collection, standardized tests or scales, or adequate subject selection and design. In a study of families of children with leukemia, one year after diagnosis, Powazek, Schyving Payne, Goff, Paulson, & Stagner (1980) found that most of the siblings studied (74%) did not discuss the illness and that 19 out of 24 families had healthy siblings who developed a variety of problems, including school, somatic, and behavioral problems. Stehbens and Lascari (1974), in a follow-up study of families of children with leukemia, found that siblings were generally poorly informed, especially about the terminal nature of the illness, but noted a general lack of problems in siblings. In a study of 25 families of cancer patients who had died, Schyving Payne, Goff, and Paulson (1980) found that, according to parents, 36 percent of the siblings in a six-month postdeath group and 22 percent in a two-year group had developed psychosocial or academic problems after the death of a sibling, but that the rest did not.

The more rigorous research investigations not only suggest a somewhat lower incidence of psychological problems in siblings than indicated in clinical reports, but also note some positive aspects in their adaptation. Iles (1979) found that siblings of cancer patients became more compassionate, tolerant, empathetic, and appreciative of their own health. While McCarthy (1975) did not find appreciable behavioral commonalities among siblings of children with leukemia, some were found to be more mature and responsible as a result of the illness. Wold and Townes (1969) also found that siblings were more responsible, and that family communication actually improved in some cases.

Several variables have been found to be related to adjustment in siblings of children with serious illness. McKeever's (1983) review of the literature points to several factors, one being family size. Siblings in larger families were found to cope better than those in smaller families, because the expectations, responsibilities, and care were distributed among several children. Thus, one sibling in a large family would not have to bear the burden of responsibilities as much as an only sibling would. Socioeconomic level was another factor, with those in higher SES families tending to cope better perhaps because there would be fewer constraints related to finances placed upon them. Developmental level was a significant factor (Lindsay & McCarthy, 1974) as was maturity of the siblings (Weiner, 1970) with more mature siblings better able to cope. Lavigne and Ryan (1979) found preschool siblings to be more withdrawn and irritable, but older siblings demonstrated more acting-out behavior. They also found an interaction between age and sex, with younger (school age) females having more adjustment problems than males of the same age. Older (adolescent) females had fewer problems than older male siblings. Important variables noted by others include: honest and open communication within the family (Binger et al., 1969; Sourkes, 1980; McKeever, 1983; Weiner, 1970); the quality of the relationship with the ill child (Cain, Fast, & Erikson, 1964; Weiner, 1970), and the self-esteem of the sibling (Eiser, 1979).

Based on these findings, a preventive program involving siblings should include an initial assessment of family functioning and roles. Pertinent issues would include recognizing the sibling's needs for attention and information, facilitating open communication within the family about the illness, providing an outlet for sibling concerns, preparing parents for possible behavioral reactions to the illness and treatment, and preparing the siblings for the loss of the patient when death was imminent. Described below is a study that incorporated these strategies.

PRESENT STUDY

The data described herein were taken from a larger longitudinal study, the Coping Project, a long-term study of coping in families of children with leukemia (Kupst, Schulman, Honig, Maurer, Morgan, and Fochtman, 1982, Kupst, Schulman, Maurer, Morgan, Honig, & Fochtman, 1983; Kupst, Schulman, Maurer, Honig, Morgan, & Fochtman, 1984). The approach involved mutliple sources (parents, children, physicians, nurses, and psychosocial staff) and multiple methods (interviews, standardized tests, rating scales, systematic observation). In addition to collection of data on family coping, an intervention strategy was designed, which focused on salient issues at different periods in the illness process (Kupst, Tylke, et al., 1982).

METHOD

Subjects

Sixty-four families participated in the Coping Project. All new admissions over a two-year period were potential subjects, excluding patients treated previously for leukemia, those with multiple disorders, and families where language translation was necessary.

In 12 families, the patient was an only child. A total of 82 siblings from 52 families participated in the study. Twenty-two families had one sibling, 20 had two, 6 had 3, and 4 had 4 siblings. Twenty siblings were older brothers, 14 were younger brothers. Twenty-two were older sisters, 16 were younger sisters.

Apparatus

Family coping was rated by physicians, nurses and psychosocial staff using the Family Coping Scale, which was adapted from a scale by Hurwitz, Kaplan, and Kaiser (1962). Family members were rated on understanding, affective reactions, and behavioral indicators of coping, such as communication, support, participation in care, and ability to handle other responsibilities.

Parents also completed the Current Adjustment Rating Scale, a 12-item rating scale that has been used in psychotherapy research (Berzins, Bednar, and Severy, 1975) and that measures a person's self-reported adjustment to various aspects of life, such as work, leisure, children, spouse. Parents also completed the Summed Coping Scale (Joffe & Naditch, 1977) of the California Psychological Inventory (Gough, 1969) in the early outpatient phase, and at two years after diagnosis. The results of these assessments at various phases of treatment have been reported elsewhere.

Semistructured taped interviews were conducted with the family at diagnosis, early outpatient treatment, later outpatient treatment, and at home visits at six months, and one and two years after diagnosis. The topic of sibling reactions was discussed in these interviews.

Psychosocial staff also rated the families at one and two years postdiagnosis on several variables hypothesized to be related to coping: quality of marital/family relationships, adequacy of support systems, existence of concurrent stresses, existence of financial problems, and existence of sibling problems. For the first two categories, ratings ranged from $1 =$ poor, $2 =$ somewhat, $3 =$ adequate, $4 =$ very good. For the last three categories, a rating of 0 indicated absence of this variable, of 1 indicated somewhat present, and of 2 usually present in the family.

Most of the data on siblings are taken from parental reports of sibling behavior in the interviews, from their CARS responses to children and family adjustment, and less frequently, from sibling self-reports in the interviews.

Procedure

Families were asked for their written consent to participate (children over seven were also asked to sign a consent form). Based on a previously determined randomization, families were assigned to one of three intervention groups: total ($N = 22$), moderate ($N = 22$), or no intervention group ($N = 20$). While details appear elsewhere (Kupst, Tylke, et al., 1982), a brief description will be given with special reference to siblings.

The intervention provided in the study was designed to focus on the entire family and was based on our experiences as well as those of others (Kagen-Goodheart, 1977; Koch, Hermann, & Donaldson, 1974; Spinetta, Spinetta, Kung, & Schwartz, 1976). Goals were to aid family members in achieving an understanding of the realities and implications of the illness, to learn to manage emotional reactions, and to utilize available resources.

Diagnosis and Initial Week

After diagnosis, an initial conference was held with the hematologist and a clinical intervenor met with families who were in the total and moderate groups. (Clinical intervenor is a general term used here because it included people with master's degrees in social work or counseling.) This conference served to sanction the intervention, and introduction to the family by the hematologist conveyed that the intervention was part of the total treatment of the child. A research assistant met with those who were in the no-intervention group and explained the project to them in the same way the intervenors did. (This was really a "no project intervention group," since these families did receive the usual forms of support and care from physicians, nurses, child life workers, pastoral counsellors, volunteers, etc.)

In both intervention groups, families were seen throughout the same phases; inpatient, outpatient, readmissions, home visits, death, after death, and at a two-year assessment. In the no-intervention condition, a research assistant related to the families in a friendly, but nonintervening way, systematically observed patient behavior, and collected data on family coping from parents, children, and staff. This group was assessed during the same phases as the two intervention groups.

The differences between the two intervention groups reflected the degree of outreach and frequency of contacts. The total intervention group involved an intensive outreach approach with frequent contacts: daily in the hospital when the patient was an inpatient and at each visit to the outpatient clinic. After an initial period of relationship building (described below), intervenors made direct attempts to engage families in talking about their emotional reactions to the illness and treatment. The moderate approach involved less aggressive outreach. Intervenors were available to discuss psychological issues, but did not initiate such discussions. Families were seen for the same amount of time as the total group at diagnosis, but only about once a week in the early outpatient phase, and at an as needed basis in later phases, primarily leaving it up to families as to how often the intervention would occur.

There were several functions common to both groups. One was relationship formation, which involved an initial direct approach. Most families were not accustomed to a direct discussion of emotional issues in the same way that people seeking help for psychological problems might be. They tended to focus more on the medical details of treatment and procedures rather than on the possibilities of relapse and death. This type of denial was felt to be appropriate and intervenors made more progress in forming an alliance with the family when they discussed management issues: financial resources, travel to the hospital, juggling work and school commitments with clinic appointments, planning for care of siblings by others, information on reading materials related to leukemia, and housing arrangements for those who lived far from the hospital. We found that most of the families were quite stunned by the diagnosis, and while they could focus on specific management details, they did not appear to benefit from an intensive discussion of their psychological reactions. A more psychological focus had to be developed gradually, through frequent contacts with the family, and through a build-up of trust.

Another function of both groups was anticipation of possible problem areas during treatment, such as physical changes in the patient (hair loss, weight gain, weakness, etc.), what to tell other family members, how to manage time constraints, school-related issues. Intervenors also tried to prepare parents for siblings' reactions to the diagnosis. Parents were advised that not all siblings would behave the same way or have the same needs, but that there were some commonalities, such as their need for attention during treatment, their questions about the illness, their fears for the patient's health and for their own.

Treatment

After diagnosis and during early outpatient treatment (the first three months), intervenors worked in conjunction with the hematologist/oncologist to clarify any misconceptions, distortions, or misinformation family members might have about the illness and treatment. They also worked as a liaison between the family and hospital staff. At times families were reluctant to approach the physician with questions, but the intervenor sanctioned their need to do so, sometimes helping them to practice what they would ask.

Another early task was to assess the support systems within and outside of the family: Who could be counted upon to look after siblings, who provided emotional support for each member, how well family members supported each other. Families were encouraged to make use of available supports, and where these were lacking, the intervenor helped them seek additional sources, sometimes by using modeling and role-playing techniques. Sometimes family members, especially mothers tried to do everything themselves, giving the impression that they did not need help when they really did. Intervenors worked with them to help them see that they were taking on too much, that help was available (it usually was), and that they should take advantage of it.

During early outpatient treatment, interventions gradually became focused on facilitating expression and management of emotional reactions and on helping the family to maintain a sense of mastery. Once the initial shock was over, and the family began to adjust to the routine of clinic visits and treatments, it was common for emotional reactions to surface more readily. The intervenor sanctioned such reactions and advised parents to give siblings an opportunity to discuss any feelings they might have, such as jealousy, anger, guilt or fear. Many families brought siblings with them to the clinic, but in those cases where they did not, the intervenors encouraged them to do so, so that siblings could be exposed to the reality of treatment. During these visits, intervenors talked directly to siblings in front of parents, to get their reactions to the clinic: "Now that you've seen what goes on, what do you think about it?" or "Sometimes brothers or sisters tell us they feel really left out when . . .," or "Seeing your brother (or sister) go through this can be pretty scary at times."

In both early and later outpatient treatment, hospitalization of the patient or a lengthy wait in the clinic allowed the intervenor to spend time alone with the sibling, taking them for a walk outside or for a soft drink in the snack bar. Siblings frequently expressed thoughts and feelings that seemed to be inhibited in front of other family members, such as lack of attention, resentment about having to do more chores, worry about the patient, and reactions of friends and schoolmates. Again, the intervenor let them know that their fears and concerns were normal, and they encouraged siblings to be as open as possible with the parents and patient. They discussed what sources of support were available, such as family members, friends, teachers, and others, and how the sibling might make use of them. They also talked about what the sibling could do for the patient, to provide a sense of mastery, such as getting school assignments and helping with care at home

Sometimes siblings were included in an intervention with the patient. In one case, a previously athletic boy was diagnosed with leukemia. During his treatment, he appeared to become depressed over not being able to do anything. At the same time, his younger sister had been making open bids for attention from family and staff, frequently by negative behavior, which was becoming increasingly annoying to the family. The intervenor worked with the patient to help him learn basic photography, a subject in which he had shown an interest. Both the patient and his sister went with the intervenor to a nearby zoo to take pictures of animals, which they both enjoyed. After this trip, the family began to include the sister more in helping with the patient's care at home, and her negative behavior disappeared.

At other times, intervenors role-played possible problem situations with siblings, such as what to tell other schoolmates, and how to talk to parents about their feelings.

Remission

Once the patient was in remission, the interventions focused on helping the family to learn to live with the chronicity of the illness. At this time, the family typically returned to a more normal routine and parents could devote more attention to siblings. Intervenors remained in contact with the families and made home visits approximately six months after diagnosis to observe them in their own environments. Family members were encouraged to discuss any concerns they had regarding fears of relapse, school problems, changes at homes, etc. When the patient was due to end chemotherapy, the issues of ending treatment, fears of relapse and lack of support were common topics. Many families felt that more attention had been paid to them by staff in the beginning of treatment, but as the child progressed into long-term remission, they perceived staff as being more distant and unavailable.

The longer remission progressed, the more most families tended to think and talk less about leukemia. They came to clinic less often, sometimes at six-month intervals. Home visits made at one and two years after diagnosis tended to be more "social" and positive in focus with these families, who spoke mainly on topics not related to illness, such as school, vacations, home decorating, family leisure activities, and future plans. Some families were open in discussing the possibilities of relapse, while others viewed the illness as "ancient history."

Relapse

If relapse occurred, the intervenors dealt with reactivations of earlier emotional reactions to loss and possible death. Sometimes it was the first time that families really showed these emotions, since the activity during diagnosis and treatment had not permitted them time to do so. At this point, they appeared more able to discuss the possible death of the child. They also could share their anger stemming from the fact that the generally optimistic prognosis that had been presented to them did not hold for their child. Reinduction of remission (resumption of chemotherapy, sometimes with different drugs) was usually attempted again, but this time the family was more anxious and fearful.

Death

When a child was near death, the intervenor again reaffirmed her availability to the family, remained on call on a 24-hour basis, and often visited the family at odd hours. The intervention frequently involved sitting with the family in the child's room or in another quiet room, not talking a great deal but sharing the family's loss. While intervenors felt that they were not doing much during this time, parents later reported that they appreciated the support. The amount of involvement depended on the type of family and their expressed needs. Some welcomed the presence of the intervenor; others wished for more privacy. In general, their previous style of coping (seeking support or preferring to be alone) determined the way they dealt with the child's impending death.

During this time, involvement of the rest of the family, especially of the siblings was encouraged. Intervenors helped parents talk with siblings about their fears and worries, and encourage them to come to the hospital and be with the ill child. If, however, parents did not want to involve siblings at this time, their wishes were respected. Other functions of the intervention were to help the families work through issues of end stage treatment with the hematologist/oncologists, to be a liaison between staff and families, and to help them plan communication with other extended family members. Another important function was to help the family plan for specific postdeath tasks, such as burial and funeral arrangements.

After the death of the child, intervenors remained available to the families and usually attended services. Contacts were tailored to the needs of different families, but in general, home visits were made a few months later. It was clear that these families were more receptive to this intervention postdeath because the intervenors had been with them throughout the illness than if the intervention had begun at or after the death. These postdeath contacts often involved reminiscences about events during the child's treatment in which the intervenors had shared. Thus, while the intervention strategy was geared towards the whole family, there were several approaches which were found to be useful with siblings.

Assessments of family coping and of specific issues related to siblings were conducted at diagnosis, during treatment, after the death of the patient, and during long-term remission.

RESULTS

Outcome

In previously cited reports (Kupst, Schulman, et al., 1982, 1983, 1984) it was found that most of the families in the study coped well with the illness and treatment during diagnosis, treatment, and at one and two years after diagnosis. Outcome measures include physicians', nurses', and psychosocial staff's ratings of the family as well as parent self-reports on rating scales and tests and systematic time-sampling of observations. While these families showed a wide variety of coping reactions, most of them (51 of the 60 who completed the two-year assessment) were found to be coping well based on ratings by physicians, nurses, and psychosocial staff. Of the nine who were not coping well, a common variable was that of preexisting problems, such as marital, family, emotional, or financial problems.

Variables related to coping at one year included the quality of the marital and family relationships and the lack of other concurrent stresses. At two years, these included quality of the marital and family relationships, adequacy of support system, and lack of other concurrent stresses. Coping patterns which were related to good coping included open communication within the family and an attitude of living in the day-to-day present.

Issues and Stages

Some categories of reactions or areas of concern in relation to siblings were found to be especially salient at different stages of the illness. Commonly raised issues (38 siblings from 24 out of the 52 families with siblings) and the incidence of specific positive and negative behaviors are shown in Table 1. Siblings' needs for attention and their worries and concern about the patients were commonly noted issues at diagnosis, during treatment, and while the patient was in remission. Fear of the illness and concern about bone marrow transplants were also raised in a few families during diagnosis and treatment. While lower in frequency, several negative behaviors were noted. Somatic complaints emerged after the diagnosis, during treatment, after death, and in remission in a few siblings. Similarly, anger, school problems and overprotection were noted at diagnosis and in treatments

Table 1 Issues and behaviors of siblings of pediatric leukemia patients

Issue/Behavior	Diagnosis	Treatment	Postdeath	Remission
Issue				
Need for attention	5	6		3
Concern for patient	5	3		4
Fear of illness	3	2		
Transplant concerns	1	2		
Total issues	14	13		7
Negative behavior				
Somatic complaints	4	3	2	1
Anger	2	2		
Inability to discuss	2		3	
School problems	1	3		
Overprotecting patient	2	1		
Total behaviors	11	9	5	1
Postive behavior				
Supportive to patient				6
Closer to family				12
Better communication				5
Total behaviors				23

Note. These behaviors were noted at the time of the two-year follow-up and include siblings of children who had died as well as siblings of those in remission.

in some siblings. Somatic problems and inability to discuss the patient were noted after the death. Besides those shown in the table, less frequent issues raised included guilt, problems in living with relatives, the sibling's perception of the patient's distancing behavior, preoccupation with death, and the sibling's concern for his/her own needs.

While some commonalities in problems and issues were noted, the frequencies for specific issues are rather low. It is important to point out that no problems were noted during the first year in 44 siblings from 28/52 families (53.8%). By the two-year follow-up these siblings still had not developed problems. In cases where issues or problems were present in the first year (38 siblings), 10 still had problems by the two year follow-up assessment. Four were siblings of children who had died. Of these four, three were unwilling or found it very difficult to talk about the death of their sibling. In the case of four other siblings, the main concerns centered around somatic fears. Twenty-eight of the 38 who initially showed some problem or issues at one year, did not show problems by the time of the two-year follow-up assessment. Twenty-two of these 28 had been in families who received psychosocial intervention through the project.

In addition to lack of problems positive adaptation was shown in 23 siblings in terms of being able to communicate better within the family, being closer to the family and patient, and being more supportive. Among other indicants of positive adaptation were evidence of: physical health, school attendance, good scholastic performance, participation in usual activities and sports, and a good self-concept (based on clinical judgments of intervenors and project staff).

In analyzing differences between those who showed growth and those who still had problems by the time of the two-year follow-up, no significant differences were found for family size, socioeconomic status, or original position of the sibling. Males seemed to exhibit more problems (50% of the older males and 71% of the younger males presented issues or problems, whereas 36% of the older females and 31% of the younger females presented issues and problems). This may reflect common findings in more general child behavior research, in which males, especially school-age males, generally show more behavioral problems than females.

A significant difference was found between the support systems of the siblings, and between the quality of emotional supports both within and outside of the family, as rated by psychosocial staff. Siblings in the "growth" group had significantly better support systems ($\chi^2 = 7.14$; df $= 2$; $p < .05$) than those in the "problems" group. In addition, only three of the ten "problem" siblings had families where communication was judged by staff to be open, while all of the families in the "growth" group were judged to have at least moderately open communication. Six were judged as having very open communication about the illness.

It was also of interest that ten mothers became pregnant after the diagnosis and four did so after the death of the child. Five decided not to have any more children after diagnosis and had tubal ligations performed.

There were no significant differences among the three intervention groups at the one- and two-year follow-up assessments with regard to siblings' coping and incidence of problems. (An earlier article reported that intervention had been significant for mothers' coping in the early outpatient phase; Kupst, Schulman, et al., 1983). Intervention appeared to be a factor for those who had presented problems or issues in the beginning, since most of those who showed no problems at the end had been in families who received intervention.

In summary, most of the siblings were coping well by the time of the two-year assessment. Even where issues or problems were noted, most of these siblings were also doing well at two years, with a number of them showing positive adaptation.

DISCUSSION

The results showed that most of the problems and issues surfaced during the initial hospitalization and early treatment phases, and that nearly half of the siblings in the study demonstrated such behaviors and concerns. The problem areas were varied and the frequencies in each category relatively small, but key common areas appeared to be: need for attention, concern for the patient, fear of the illness, and transplant concerns. Negative behaviors included: somatic complaints, anger, school problems, overprotection of the patient, and problems in discussing the illness. By the two-year follow-up, however, only 10 or 12.3 percent of the siblings had problems noted. Besides the lower incidence of problems, 59.7 percent showed no problems and 28 percent showed some positive adaptation in terms of support, closer relationship with family members, improved communication. Thus, while the experience of serious illness in a brother or sister may present several upsetting and uncomfortable situations to a child, most of them appear able to cope with it, especially over time.

Concurrently, we found that most of the parents and patients tended to cope well during the same intervals, which probably had a positive effect on the siblings. Since intervention was found to be helpful to mothers in the early part of treatment, and since that was the point at which siblings' problems tended to emerge, perhaps there was an indirect effect on siblings in terms of mothers being better able to cope and thus attend to them as well. "Good" coping families were found to be open in their communication with each other in general and specifically about the illness and treatment. They were also mutually supportive and had good extrafamilial support systems as well. These variables could easily contribute to improving siblings' coping as well.

Clinically, it was felt that the effective efforts towards siblings in the early phases of treatment included those of the intervenors : detection of siblings who appeared to need intervention, provision of a climate that allowed them to express their thoughts and feelings; and modeling for parents by giving attention and encouraging open communication.

While this project was not designed specifically to be a preventive program for siblings, it suggests some areas to be incorporated into such a program. As close to diagnosis as possible, an early assessment of the family is important to determine those who might be at risk for coping poorly. In general, based on our previous findings, these at-risk families would include those with other serious stresses, such as marital, financial, or health problems; those where communication is poor or restricted and those where mutual and outside supports are minimal or lacking. If the present study were to be done again, even more attention would be paid to the support systems of the families, since support was a variable which differentiated the "growth" and "problems" groups. In cases where support was poor, the siblings could be viewed as at risk for development of problems.

In addition, with regard to siblings, special attention would be paid to sex (since males showed a somewhat higher incidence of problems), age, grade, and performance in school, and any behavioral problems prior to diagnosis. In general, the initial intervention would follow the format described earlier in terms of practical management issues. At this time, the intervenor would determine how the siblings would be cared for while the family spent time in the hospital.

During the early weeks of treatment, the family is primarily involved in the tests and procedures surrounding the patient, but they can be prepared for possible problems or concerns of the siblings, such as those found in this study. In a future study or program, we recommend stressing the needs for attention, especially in the initial and early treatment phases. Sometimes parents reported that siblings had unrealistic fantasies about what happened in the clinic and felt that they were missing out on something good. By bringing them to the clinic, parents allowed them to see what was really happening and also involved them in the process. Intervenors can suggest certain questions siblings might have about the cause of the illness, the future of the patient, and their own health, pointing out that they are not the only ones who have wondered about these things when a sibling is ill, and that it is all right to feel they way they do. Parents in turn can be prepared for their questions, as well as to look behind the questions for the sources of their fears.

During treatment, siblings, along with other family members, may feel helpless in terms of doing anything for the patient. When feasible, and if they want to do so, siblings can share in helping in the home care of the patient. They can work closely with parents and sometimes relieve them by giving medications, making the patient comfortable, cooking meals, and so on.

Parents sometimes asked project staff to talk with teachers, primarily for the patient, but for the siblings as well. School personnel can be made aware of potential problems, such as negative reactions by classmates, effects of frequent absences, and the tendency to single out these children as different. Knowing that the child is in treatment can also alert the teachers to sibling reactions, such as preoccupation when the patient is ill or is in the hospital that day.

Since intervention appeared to be most necessary in early treatment phases, we recommend that most of the effort be placed there. If the patient was in remission and doing well medically, most families tended to relax more and there were fewer worries and concerns. Some siblings, however, still remain worried about the patient and some still have attention problems. The intervenor can remain alert for these problems by remaining available to the family during remission and maintaining contact (once every couple of months or coinciding with clinic visits). The tone of these contacts is usually more "social", but they allow the intervenor to explore any changes in family functioning, and the development or cessation of problems. Our experience was that early problems tended to decline as remission progressed.

Occurrence of relapse is a crisis situation which often brings back earlier fears, anxieties, anger, and other expressions of impending loss. Again the focus returns to the patient, and again siblings may experience similar reactions to those they had at diagnosis. These are also appropriate times to spend some time along with the siblings, especially when the prognosis worsens, since they may be reluctant to show their fears in front of the rest of the family. Parents should be encouraged to be honest with them and to keep them informed of changes in the patient's condition. Sometimes remission is achieved again, and the family can maintain hope that the patient will remain illness free, but sometimes patients do not achieve remission, or they begin to have remission/relapse cycles of lessening time intervals. When treatment no longer appears warranted and the patient's prognosis is poor, the family will have to decide how to tell the siblings, who generally already suspect the severity of the situation. Much depends on the family style, age and personality of the sibling, and the relationship with the patient, but many of the siblings of children who were dying wanted to and were able to say goodbye to their brother or sister in their own way. This leave-taking was felt to be an important step in the grieving process.

Since some problems were found in siblings of patients who died, the intervenor could watch them closely during the postdeath contacts with the family, and where needed, see them separately to talk about their reactions. We found no serious pathological reactions, however, even at two years after diagnosis. Some children appeared quite willing and able to talk about the child who had died, while others chose not to do so. Interestingly, these opposite reactions sometimes occurred in the same family, and appeared to depend upon the typical coping style of the child. Some families found it helpful to have their children participate in a sibling group of Compassionate Friends, a self-help organization for families who have lost a child. While the Coping Project did not provide such groups, they could be beneficial in a preventive program, especially with older siblings.

In planning preventive efforts towards siblings, one must first look both at the incidence and severity of problems. A number of studies have noted a relatively high incidence of problems in siblings, but more recent studies are showing a somewhat lower incidence. One reason, especially in the case of more clinical reports, is that frequently the only siblings brought to the attention of a clinician were those who had developed problems, and one might be inclined to infer that these problems were characteristic of all siblings of children with serious illness.

Another reason lies in the assessment of problems. If one is only measuring pathology, one will only find pathology, as in cases where siblings can have only a greater or fewer number of problems based on a checklist. In studies where a sibling (or other family members) has the room to grow or to cope well, the incidence of problems is lower. Part of the concern is in the definition of what constitutes pathology. In terms of severity, our study divided responses into issues and behaviors. The issues (e.g., attention, concern for the patient, fear of the illness) all pertain to normal concerns given the sibling's situation, and are not considered evidence of pathology. Thus, while we can say that nearly half of the siblings showed reactions in the categories listed, the number is much less when one considers degree of severity. Similarly, negative behaviors, such as anger and overprotection of the patient seem to be normal responses to the crisis of diagnosis. Somatic complaints can also be seen as reflecting the need for attention and concern for one's own health. School problems and difficulty in discussing the issues are more serious, but also understandable in the beginning stages of the illness.

A third consideration is the need to view the siblings' coping longitudinally, as part of a process of learning to deal with the crises of the illness. Our sample did show a fair incidence of issues and negative behaviors in the early stages of treatment, but most of the problems were not enduring nor were they severely pathological. We found no evidence of seriously disturbed behavior in the siblings who participated in the project.

This is not to say that problems do not exist in siblings of children with serious illness. They do. Nor should it be said that because the incidence of problems seems lower that efforts not be made to intervene with siblings (of those siblings who had problems initially, those who had received intervention tended to show no problems later on). But in terms of planning a preventive program, the incidence of very serious problems is quite small to begin with, and it would be very difficult to demonstrate the efficacy of a program designed to prevent serious mental health problems. It would make more sense to include the siblings as part of an all-out effort to improve total family coping (especially since the coping of parents, patients, and siblings appears to be related).

Realistically, unless outside funding were available, most hospitals or institutions do not have adequate funding for a preventive program directed solely towards siblings of children with serious illness. Some of the strategies described here, however, could be included in ongoing clinical intervention with families. If, however, such funding could be obtained, we would recommend a similar approach to that described here, with more focus on the siblings, and perhaps more direct psychological assessment, using instruments which were not available to us when the project was conducted, such as the Family Coping Inventory (McCubbin, Boss, Wilson & Dahl, 1979); and the Impact on Family Scale (Stein & Riessman, 1980).

Also realistically, a family intervention will center around the child with leukemia and his/her parents, especially the mother, who is usually most directly involved in treatment. But the intervention can and should assess sibling needs and issues and attempt to enhance their coping as well. Ideally, the intervention program should begin at diagnosis and follow the family through the treatment process with the same intervenor working with the family.

The intervenor should be a psychosocial professional with experience in the area of pediatric cancer, and who has already worked out his/her own issues in relation to the illness and death. We have found that even experienced mental health professionals may respond with intense reactions to loss, dying, death, and helplessness in the face of the illness. Ongoing supervision and an informal support group composed of project staff were helpful in trying to work through these issues.

It is preferable for the intervention program to be integrated into the medical treatment program so that the intervenor may work closely with the medical and nursing staff throughout treatment. We found that it is essential to achieve a strong working relationship with the hematology/oncology staff. Their support of the project enabled families to see the intervention and assessment as an integral part of their child's treatment.

Again, I stress the need to look at coping as well as pathology. Coping took many diverse and sometimes opposite forms in these family members (Kupst, Schulman, et al., 1984). Coping is a long-term process that can involve struggles, emotional upsets, and use of defensive behavior in efforts to adjust to difficult situations. Coping did not mean absence of suffering. These families learned, sometimes in a long and slow process, how to manage their pain and to live their lives in the best way they could. And they coped remarkably well.

REFERENCES

Alby, N. (1980). Ending the chemotherapy of acute leukemia: A period of difficult weaning. In J. L. Schulman & M. J. Kupst (Eds.), *The child with cancer: Clinical approaches to psychological care—research in psychological aspects.* Springfield, IL: Charles C Thomas, pp. 175–182.

Berzins, J. I., Bednar, R. L., & Severy, L. J. (1975). The problems of intersource consensus in measuring therapeutic outcomes: New data and multivariate perspectives. *Journal of Abnormal Psychology, 84*(1), 10–19.

Binger, C. M., Ablin, A. R., Feuerstein, R. C., Kushner, J. H., Zoger, S., & Mikkelson, C. (1969). Childhood leukemia: Emotional impact on patient and family. *New England Journal of Medicine, 280*(8), 414–418.

Brown, N. N., & Kelly, M. J. (1976). Stages of bone marrow transplantation: A psychiatric perspective *Psychosomatic Medicine, 38*(6), 439–446.

Cain, A., Fast, I., & Erickson, M. (1964). Children's disturbed reactions to the death of a sibling. *American Journal of Orthopsychiatry, 34,* 741–752.

Cairns, N. U., Clark, G. M., Smith, S. D., & Lansky, S. (1979). Adaptation of siblings to childhood malignancy. *Journal of Pediatrics, 95,* 484–487.

Eiser, C. (1979). Psychological development of the child with leukemia: A review. *Journal of Behavioral Medicine, 2*(2), 141–157.

Gardner, G. G., August, C. S., & Githens, J. (1977). Psychological issues in bone marrow transplantation. *Pediatrics, 60*(4), 625–631.

Gough, H. (1969). *The California psychological inventory manual* (Rev. ed.). Palo Alto, CA: Consulting Psychologists Press.

Hurwitz, J. I., Kaplan, D. M., & Kaiser, E. (1962). Designing an instrument to assess parental coping mechanisms. *Social Casework, 10,* 527–532.

Iles, J. (1979). Children with cancer: Healthy siblings' perceptions during the illness experience. *Cancer Nursing, 2*(5), 371–377.

Joffe, P., & Naditch, M. P. (1977). Paper and pencil measures of coping and defense processes. In N. Haan (Ed.), *Coping and defending: Processes of self-environment organization.* New York: Academic.

Kagen-Goodheart, L. (1977). Reentry: Living with childhood cancer. *American Journal of Orthopsychiatry, 47*(4), 651–658.

Koch, C., Hermann, J., & Donaldson, M. (1974). Supportive care of the child with cancer and his family. *Seminars in Oncology, 1*(1).

Koocher, G. P., & O'Malley, J. E. (1981). (Eds.). *The Damocles syndrome: Psychological consequences of surviving childhood cancer.* New York: McGraw-Hill.
Kupst, M. J., Schulman, J. L., Honig, G., Maurer, H., Morgan, E., & Fochtman, D. (1982). Family coping with childhood leukemia: One year after diagnosis. *Journal of Pediatric Psychology, 7,* 157–174.
Kupst, M. J., Schulman, J. L., Maurer, H., Honig, G., Morgan, E., & Fochtman, D. (1984). Coping with pediatric leukeumia: A two year follow-up. *Journal of Pediatric Psychology.*
Kupst, M. J., Schulman, J. L., Maurer, H., Morgan, E., Honig, G., & Fochtman, D. (1983). Psychosocial aspects of pediatric leukemia: From diagnosis through the first six months of treatment. *Medical and Pediatric Oncology, 11,* (4), 269–278.
Kupst, M. J., Tylke, L., Thomas, L., Mudd, M. E., Richardson, C., & Schulman, J. L. (1982). Strategies of intervention with families of pediatric leukemia patients: A longitudinal perspective. *Social Work in Health Care, 8*(2), 31–47.
Lavigne, J. V., & Ryan, M. (1979). Psychologic adjustment of siblings of children with chronic illness. *Pediatrics, 63,* 616–627.
Lindsay, M., & McCarthy, D. (1974). Caring for the brothers and sisters of a dying child. In L. Burton (Ed.), *Care of the child facing death.* London: Routledge & Kegan Paul, pp. 189–206.
McCarthy, M. (1975). Social aspects of treatment in childhood leukemia. *Social Science in Medicine, 9,* 263–269.
McCubbin, H. I., Boss, P. G., Wilson, L. R., & Dahl, B. B. (1979). *The family coping inventory.* St. Paul, MN: University of Minnesota Family Social Science.
McKeever, P. (1983). Siblings of chronically ill children: A literature review with implications for research and practice. *American Journal of Orthopsychiatry, 53*(2), 209–218.
Powazek, M., Schyving Payne, J., Goff, J. R., Paulson, M. A., & Stagner, S. (1980). Psychosocial ramifications of childhood leukemia: One year post-diagnosis. In J. L. Schulman & M. J. Kupst (Eds.), *The child with cancer: Clinical approaches to psychosocial care–research in psychosocial aspects.* Springfield, IL: Charles C Thomas, pp. 143–155.
Schyving Payne, J., Goff, J. E., & Paulson, M. A. (1980). Psychosocial adjustment of families following the death of a child. In J. L. Schulman & M. J. Kupst (Eds.), *The child with cancer: Clinical approaches to psychosocial care–research in psychosocial aspects.* Springfield, IL: Charles C Thomas, pp. 183–193.
Shrier, D. K. (1980). The dying child and surviving family members. *Developmental and Behavioral Pediatrics, 1*(4), 152–157.
Sourkes, B. M. (1980). Siblings of the pediatric cancer patient. In J. Kellerman (Ed.), *Psychological aspects of childhood cancer.* Springfield, IL: Charles C Thomas, pp. 47–60.
Spinetta, J. J. (1982). Psychosocial issues in childhood cancer. In M. Wolraich & D. Routh (Eds.), *Advances in developmental and behavioral pediatrics* (Vol. 3). Greenwich, CT: JAI Press, Inc., pp. 51–72.
Spinetta, J. J., Spinetta, P., Kung, P., & Schwartz, D. (1976). *Emotional aspects of childhood cancer and leukemia: A handbook for parents.* San Diego, CA: Leukemia Society of America.
Stehbens, J. A., & Lascari, A. D. (1974). Psychological follow-up of families with childhood leukemia. *Journal of Clinical Psychology, 30,* 394–397.
Stein, R. E. K., & Riessman, C. K. (1980). The development of an Impact-on-Family Scale: Preliminary findings. *Medical Care, 18*(4), 465–472.
Townes, B., & Wold, D. (1977). Childhood leukemia. In E. Patterson (Ed.), *The experiences of dying.* Englewood Cliffs, NJ: Prentice-Hall, pp. 138–143.
Weiner, J. (1970). Reaction of the family to the fatal illness of a child. In B. Schoenberg, A. Carr, D. Peretz, & A. Kutscher, (Eds.), *Loss and grief: Psychological management in medical practice.* New York: Columbia University Press, pp. 87–101.
Wold, D. A., & Townes, B. D. (1969). The adjustment of siblings to childhood leukemia. *Family Coordinator, 18,* 155–160.

9

Crisis Intervention with Children Exposed to Natural Disasters

Stephen M. Auerbach
Virginia Commonwealth University

Anthony Spirito
Rhode Island Hospital/Brown University Program
in Medicine

Disasters have been a part of human existence since man has inhabited this planet. The term disaster subsumes both naturally occurring (e.g., tornadoes, floods, volcanoes) and manmade (e.g., coal mining or nuclear fuel disasters) destructive events that impact large numbers of persons. Almost all research on disaster behavior is based on response to natural disasters (Perry & Mushkatel, 1984) and thus they will be the focus of this chapter.

In general, disaster agents which are of low predictability, minimal controllability, rapid speed of onset, little forewarning, extended duration, broad scope of impact and great destructive potential are most likely to produce a crisis (Wenger, 1978). But, as with other potentially stressful events, disasters are classified as crises only if they are perceived as such by those who are affected. Thus floods inundating unpopulated plains, underground nuclear bomb explosions, or earthquakes on the floor of the ocean are generally not crisis-inducing events. The degree to which disasters produce crisis-level behavior, and the effectiveness with which they are coped, are very much a function of the nature of the society and the persons that are impacted. In communities that have a history of exposure to given disaster agents and thus are prepared for them organizationally and psychologically, the probability of adverse consequences and crisis-level disruptions are lessened.

The recent upsurge in behavioral research on natural disasters has focused on assessing the factors that help explain differences in the ability of individuals and communities to cope with disasters, and on the development of procedures to help people prepare for impending disasters and recover from their effects. In this chapter we will: a) briefly outline some general behavioral phenomena which have been found to be characteristic of persons and communities exposed to natural disasters, b) review the research on the emotional impact of disasters on children and families, c) give a brief overview of general trends in mental service delivery in disasters, and d) review prevention and intervention procedures used with children exposed to disaster. In the last section we present an adaptation of stress inoculation training as a postdisaster intervention technique to minimize emotional distress in children exposed to disaster.

GENERAL BEHAVIORAL PHENOMENA

Disasters, by definition, occur in a social context. Among the behaviors regularly observed in the aftermath of disasters are expressions of altruism, sharing, and community solidarity. Private property is voluntarily allocated for communal use and normative social caste distinctions dissolve. Victims are readily taken into the homes of strangers (Prince, 1920); in the aftermath of a tornado striking Mississippi communities in the 1950s, black children were not only cared for by relatives who came far distances to provide needed support, but also by white families who would not normally socialize with them (Perry & Perry, 1959; Perry, Silber, & Bloch, 1956). Prestige and leadership roles accrue to persons with specific disaster-relevant skills. As the salience of the emergency declines, however, the traditional values of wealth, status and comfort reemerge as guides to behavior (Dynes, 1978).

Contrary to popular opinion, rioting, looting, or panic are rarely observed in the wake of natural disasters (Chapman, 1962; Taylor, Ross, & Quarantelli, 1976). The question of the degree to which severe psychological disturbance is an outgrowth of exposure to disaster has been a matter of some controversy, and revolves in part around the differing perspectives of social scientists and mental health professionals on the psychiatric "disease" model. Available data clearly indicate that though the prevalence and severity of severe psychopathology after exposure to disaster has been exaggerated, under certain circumstances natural disaster may produce high levels of social disruption and longer term psychological disturbance (see Auerbach, Chapter 1, this volume). and thus there is clearly a need for postdisaster social and psychologically related services.

EMOTIONAL IMPACT OF DISASTERS ON CHILDREN AND FAMILIES

A number of investigators have studied the psychological impact of natural disasters on children and families. Most of these reports are based on subjective observations, interviews, and, in some cases, psychological test data. Because natural disasters are largely unanticipated events and would be avoided if they could be predicted efficiently and since large scale pretesting of disaster-prone communities is impractical, predisaster baseline data are rarely collected, and conclusions are based on postdisaster observations made on selected individuals. One widely-held belief derived from such data is that "heavily impacted families often tend to be psychologically better off in the long run than comparable non-victim families" (Taylor et al., 1976). This compelling notion, which relates to the idea that successful coping with stress is inherently a growth process that produces a generalized sense of mastery as well as specific coping skills (see Auerbach, Chapter 1) remains unvalidated.

Several research reports have focused on evaluating the severity and nature of emotional disturbances that are evident in children after a disaster. Newman (1976) concluded on the basis of interviews and projective testing of 224 children survivors of the Buffalo Creek (West Virginia) flood that "most were . . . significantly or severely emotionally impaired by their experiences" (p. 306), and exhibited "increased vulnerability to future stresses" (p. 12). Harshbarger (1976) reported that over a year after the flood, children at Buffalo Creek exhibited phobic responses to rain. Similar fears were reported by Kliman (1976) in children who had been exposed to a flood disaster (particularly for those who had to undergo a major readjustment such as evacuating their homes) and by Ollendick and Hoffman (1982). Blaufarb and Levine (1972) reported that among 300 families who contacted a child guidance clinic after the 1971 Los Angeles earthquake the most common problem for children was a fear of going to sleep in their own rooms away from their parents. Children between the ages of three and six were also afraid to be alone or leave their mothers to play with other children. The authors concluded that these behaviors were indicants of separation anxiety and an attempt "to maintain contact with parents who provide safety and security" (p. 18).

Blaufarb and Levine's observations are consistent with those of several other investigators who noted the crucial role that parents play in determining children's reactions and emotional adjustment in the wake of disaster. Along with Blaufarb and Levine, Hansen (1971; cited in Fraser, 1973), and Crawshaw (1963) found that children's reactions (especially anxiety levels) tended to reflect parents' psychological status.

The first and one of the most thorough analyses of children's emotional reactions to disaster and the role of parental behaviors in influencing these reactions was conducted in studies of the impact of tornadoes which struck Mississippi in the mid-1950s (Perry & Perry, 1959; Perry et al., 1956). The Vicksburg tornado (Perry et al., 1956) struck a community that, despite the prevalence of tornadoes in the general area, many people thought would never be hit because of the hills surrounding much of the city. The main target was a motion picture theater filled with children. Virtually all of the injured and dead were white and urban middle class in background. Eighty-eight families were selected for interviews two months after the tornado. Emotional disturbance (defined as overt anxiety and symptom formation) was judged on the basis of psychiatric interviews. Of 185 children evaluated, 32 were judged to be exhibiting mild signs of emotional disturbance and 24 were rated as severely emotionally disturbed. Regressive behaviors such as enuresis and directly disaster-related fears such as sensitivity to loud noises, nightmares, and apprehension about building safety were particularly noted. A significant association was found between presence of emotional disturbance and personal injury or death and injury in the immediate family [These findings are consistent with Newman's (1976) findings with child survivors of Buffalo Creek.] Significantly, the parents' immediate response to the tornado in the presence of the child seemed to play a very important role in the child's response. One particularly destructive type of parent response, in which the parent–child roles were reversed, was labeled the "dissociative-demanding" reaction. Parents who behaved in this way demanded attention and support from the child, or fainted or engaged in disorganized motor behavior (the "dissociative" aspect); and the child had to look after the parent. Eight of the nine children in the sample with such experiences were judged to be emotionally disturbed.

Perry and Perry (1959) evaluated the effects of tornadoes that struck two Mississippi schoolhouses and killed a number of children who were in class at the time. In contrast to the victims of the Vicksburg tornado, both schoolhouses served rural communities and virtually all of the families affected were black. Thus an excellent opportunity was afforded to test the generality of the Vicksburg findings.

In the wake of the schoolhouse disasters, similar indicants of emotional distress were displayed as in the Vicksburg children. However, the symptoms were judged to be less severe and characteristic of a smaller proportion of the children. Contrary to expectation, a high incidence of hysterical, physiological expression of maladjustment was found among parents. But this parental behavior was a pattern that had been well established before the tornado, and was a recognized, acceptable way of expressing psychological problems in these communities. Thus it was likely viewed as a less unusual event by a rural than an urban child. In addition, despite these hysterical expressions, parents quickly shifted roles to meet the emergency needs of their children when necessary.

Other differences contributed to the superior adjustment of the schoolhouse children versus the Vicksburg victims. The schoolhouse disasters affected virtually the entire communities whereas in Vicksburg, victim families tended to be isolated from those which had not undergone trauma. As a result, in the rural families there was more frequent communication and working through of the fears and losses associated with the experience. In addition, the overall social support base was stronger and more flexible in the rural communities. Children could readily move in with kin outside the nuclear household and relatives came in from outside to provide support and affection. Also, the child's place in these rural black families differed from that of the typical urban middle-class Vicksburg child. The loss of a child in a rural family meant new, often more prestigeful duties for the remaining children. Thus children were given the opportunity for active involvement and perhaps a sense of control and enhanced self-esteem in an uncertain situation which had produced helplessness and despair.

The studies by Perry and his colleagues established the importance not only of the immediate parental response in affecting children's adjustment after a disaster, but also of the broader family and community context in which it occurs. As demonstrated many years later at Buffalo Creek, once stripped of community support and a meaningful social context, it is very difficult for disaster victims to marshall personal resources (see Erickson, 1976). In addition, establishing a supportive, flexible environment where any new demands are a logical extension of previous roles appears to be important in facilitating postdisaster adjustment.

In summary, it is difficult to draw firm conclusions about the prevalence and severity of emotional disturbance in children after exposure to natural disaster since (of necessity) data consist of post hoc behavioral observations or self-reports, and in some cases important conclusions and recommendations are based on cumulative impressions rather than statistical analyses. However, there appears to be sufficient concordance in the results of available studies to conclude that a fair proportion of children exposed to a disaster will experience circumscribed, time-limited fears or behavioral problems. The severity of a child's reaction appears to be a function of how directly the child or a family member was observed to be affected by the event, immediate parental reactions, and the family and community context during the postdisaster period.

In the next section overall trends in the delivery of mental health services in disasters are outlined. In the last section, prevention and treatment strategies for emotional problems in children of disaster are described.

MENTAL HEALTH SERVICES IN DISASTERS

Taylor et al. (1976) outline the history of the delivery of mental health services in disasters. They note that despite widely held beliefs that disasters occasioned widespread psychopathology, prior to the 1970s intervention efforts were almost totally geared toward providing food, clothing, and shelter, and rebuilding the "physical" aspects of the community. Little attention was paid to the emotional needs of victims. Systematic efforts to provide large-scale mental health services began only after a series of major disasters, notably the Wilkes-Barre (Pennsylvania) flood of 1972. Section 413 of the Federal Disaster Law of 1974 gave formal impetus to the delivery of such services, mandating that "training and services in relief of mental health problems in major disasters" be provided under the auspices of the National Institute of Mental Health (Farberow & Frederick, 1978c, p. 1). Project Outreach (Heffron, 1977), through which mobile crisis intervention services were provided by specially trained local residents to victims of the Wilkes-Barre flood, was one of the first programs funded under this law. Baisden and Quarantelli (1981) sought to clarify the current status of organized delivery of mental health services in disasters through a comprehensive survey of relevant communities, key government officials and offices, service delivery agencies, and disaster victims. Among their conclusions were that from the standpoint of formal mental health services a "social service delivery" model appeared more appropriate and practical than a "medical treatment" model, since most disaster-related difficulties tend to be transient "problems in living" that do not seriously impair social functioning, and there is an absence of demand for traditional mental health services. Mental health relevant services are provided by voluntary groups as well as established agencies which are staffed primarily by nonprofessionals. Though children are among those targeted for attention, especially by projects funded under the Federal Disaster Law, they are not among the most likely recipients of mental health services.

INTERVENTION WITH CHILDREN OF DISASTER

In this section we review intervention procedures and recommendations for parental behavior with children exposed to disaster. The section is organized around the temporal model presented in Chapter 1 of this volume, with emphasis on type 3 postcrisis interventions. Included here is a description of how to apply stress inoculation training to children who have developed disaster-related fears.

Type 1 interventions refer to activities that are designed to minimize the possibility that individuals will be exposed to crisis-inducing events, or to limit damage sustained if exposure does occur. Since danger is not imminent during this precrisis period, it is often difficult to motivate such preventive behavior, and it often takes repetitive experiences with a given disaster agent for communities to begin to systematically prepare for the next occurrence. In some cases, "disaster subcultures" emerge. That is, communities "as a part of their cultural development have evolved arrangements which routinely prepare them for (repetitive) emergencies" (Kreps, 1978). For example, in southern Manitoba, where there is repeated flooding, there is constant monitoring of flood prediction devices, permanent structures have been built to mitigate the potential harmful effects of high water, and highly defined relationships have been established among organizations and agencies participating in flood control (Hannigan & Kueneman, 1978).

Consistent with historical trends in the provision of services in disasters, as noted above, precautionary efforts at dealing with potential mental health problems are not nearly as prevalent as those focused on averting the disaster itself or dealing with the physical needs of the community or its inhabitants. This state of affairs seems to be largely the result of the disinterest and perhaps active avoidance by most persons of explicitly labeled disaster-related mental health services (Baisden & Quarantelli, 1981), rather than any practical problems in implementation (see Hartsough, 1982).

Research with children suggests some relatively nonintrusive preventive activities which could help avert some of the short-term emotional problems that have been observed in at least a substantial minority of those exposed to a disaster. Perhaps most importantly, parents need to be informed beforehand about stress responses they might expect in their children and opportunities for help that are available in the community. The National Institute of Mental Health (NIMH) has suggested a 75-second media release that would be very helpful in this regard:

> Disasters frequently have a significant impact on your children, upsetting them emotionally. For them, the disaster feels like an unknown, fearful force which has shaken their world and made them feel less secure. When this happens, some children begin to show signs of regression, or behavior of a more childish sort which they have already outgrown. For the young child this may show in a variety of ways, such as a loss of toilet control, night terrors, whining and clinging, or being unwilling to leave Mother out of sight. For the school child, it may appear as refusal to attend school, withdrawal, loss of interest, irritability, or unusual fears.
>
> Parents need to understand that these symptoms have resulted from the disruption of the child's world and to help the child rebuild his sense of security. This may mean extra time spent with the child, abundant reassurances, and talking about the child's fears and bringing them out into the open. Some children are helped by making up games about the disaster.
>
> If problems persist, however, it may be advisable to get expert help. Call   between the hours of   and   . Remember, help is available if and when you need it. (Farberow & Frederick, 1978b, p. 6)

A more detailed though concise summary of potential behavioral reactions of children to disaster and suggested responses for them, grouped by age categories from preschool through adolescent, is available in two other NIMH pamphlets (Farberow & Frederick, 1978a, 1978c; also see Farberow & Gordon, 1981). This information would be most useful if made available to parents in disaster-prone areas prior to the onset of a disaster. Parents should also be made aware that during the impact periods and those immediately after impact, children need family support—and if separated should be united as soon as possible (Blaufarb & Levine, 1972; Kafrissen, Heffron, & Zusman, 1975). Maternal commitment to the community represents misplaced loyalty if it is at the expense of family needs (especially those of preadolescent children) in the immediate postdisaster weeks (Perry et al., 1956). Parents should also be prepared to avoid discussing their own anxieties about the disaster with children. The appropriate audience is other adults (Perry et al., 1956).

Type 2 interventions involve precrisis preparatory activities undertaken with the knowledge that the stressor will make its impact shortly. In the case of natural disasters, if accurate warnings are delivered early enough and in such a fashion that people believe them, then the disaster agent may sometimes be avoided or its impact minimized if appropriate behaviors are undertaken. Perry and Mushkatel (1984) have outlined some of the variables that influence whether a warning message will be believed and acted on effectively. Since a common response to a disaster warning is disbelief, an effective warning message supplies sufficient relevant information to assess the reality of the threat, including information on location and timing of impact as well as the probable extent of damage. Family relationships are important in that warnings conveyed through the mass media are often not believed or acted on until they are confirmed by friends or family members. Children, of course, depend on adults to accurately assess warning messages and take appropriate action. Though many natural disaster agents are difficult to predict, parents should apprise older children for whom adult guidance may not be available how to best assess and confirm different danger cues and of appropriate avoidance behaviors to maximize their safety.

Type 3 interventions are targeted toward short-term reactions occurring during the immediate (first weeks and months) postdisaster period. A number of useful strategies that are extensions of Type 1 recommendations and that do not require mental health expertise are indicated in the literature. For example, parents' meetings during the postdisaster period would provide a forum for appropriate expression of parental fears (instead of placing this burden on children) and for an exchange of information on common problems and solutions (Perry et al., 1956). Tuckman (1973) used the parent meeting in a way similar to a hotline by describing normal child responses and answering questions. Blaufarb and Levine (1972) actually set up a parent telephone hotline after the Los Angeles earthquake and noted that most of the 800 parents who called simply needed reassurance that they were acting properly. Many parents need to be encouraged to permit children to talk about the disaster, but instructed not to *insist* that they do so—the goal being to help the child integrate the experience, but at his or her own speed. Kliman (1976) argues that not dealing with children's questions forces them into "affective isolation just at the time they most need open communication and support" (p. 332).

Working with the schools is also a potentially effective way of dealing with children's response to disaster, especially when families are disrupted, living in temporary quarters, and/or separated. Kliman (1976) recommends incorporating the disaster experience into the teaching plan via plays, drawings, and essays about the disaster. Perry et al. (1956) similarly recommend that expressive activities (e.g., working with paint or clay, or through impromptu stories or plays) are more likely to provide an opportunity for meaningful integration of the disaster experience than intellectual activities during the first week after a disaster. Most important, according to Perry et al., is to reestablish school as quickly as possible since it allows the child to talk to friends about the disaster, reestablishes a familiar structured activity, and usually provides an adult atmosphere more conducive than the family for discussing the disaster experience.

As noted earlier in this chapter, there appear to be a fair minority of children who develop sleep disturbances, somatic complaints and various circumscribed stress-related fears which would seem to merit professional attention. Though some writers (Blaufarb & Levine, 1972; Fraser, 1973) have described how traditional psychotherapy might be useful treatments, more focalized short-term behaviorally-oriented techniques would seem to be more appropriate and conservative approaches given the situational basis of the problem. However, there has only been one report of the application of a behavioral technique (a variant of desensitization) for this purpose. Church (1974) treated a 12-year-old boy who survived the Buffalo Creek flood disaster but who, as a result, manifested somatic complaints, was fearful of thunder and rain and of the noise of passing trains. After eight sessions during which the therapist played checkers with the child while listening to a tape recording of a thunderstorm that was increased in volume by small increments, the child's symptoms vanished. In the following section, a broader-based cognitive-behavioral approach designed to diminish disaster-related fears and also to provide the child with specific cognitive coping skills is described.

A STRESS INOCULATION PROGRAM FOR TREATING POSTDISASTER FEARS IN CHILDREN

Stress inoculation is based upon a cognitive model of self control developed by Meichenbaum (1975). In this approach, the child is taught a number of coping skills that allow for the management of small amounts of stress and that "provide 'inoculation' against greater intensities of threat" (Meichenbaum, 1977, p. 149). Both cognitive and behavioral coping skills are taught and then practiced under regulated stress conditions so that the child is able to deal with actual stressors. According to this cognitive model, behavioral change results from a sequential process in which alteration of the client's internal dialogue is the crucial variable. As conceptualized by Meichenbaum (1977), stress inoculation consists of three phases: education, rehearsal, and application training.

Educational Phase

In this phase, the nature of the child's response to stress is explained, so that the child becomes aware of his or her maladaptive behaviors, cognitions, and emotions. The explanation must be phrased in such a way that it is plausible and understandable to the child, and will lead to an acceptance of the specific cognitive and behavioral coping techniques that follow. In discussing the basis of anxiety with the child, it often helps to explain that he or she is not alone in this problem, though at the same time it is important to personalize and individual-ize the conceptualization. Thus, it is important to have the child explore in detail the thoughts and feelings that occurred during the disaster or afterward when reminded of it. An effective technique is to have the child "run a movie" through his or her head of reactions felt during the most recent anxiety-provoking situation (Spirito & Finch, 1980). This procedure not only serves to help the child begin to experience and confront his reactions in a benign context, but also allows the therapist to key in on relevant self-statements that will be useful in the subsequent treatment phase.

Rehearsal Phase

In this phase the child is provided with the specific techniques to employ during the coping process. Stress inoculation procedures incorporate different combina-tions of behavioral and cognitive techniques (e.g., self-monitoring, problem-solving, didactic training, modeling, rehearsal, etc.) depending upon the needs of the child and the problem at hand. The two key components of stress inoculation training for anxiety control are relaxation training and cognitive methods (self-instructional training).

Relaxation Training

Since high levels of anxiety are frequently seen in children following a natural disaster, relaxation training should be useful with this population. There are four main types of relaxation techniques: progressive muscle relaxation (Jacobsen, 1938), mediative breathing (Benson, 1975), autogenics (Luthe, 1969), and imagery-based techniques. *Deep muscle relaxation training* involves teaching the child to alternate tensing and relaxing of various muscle groups throughout the body to reduce stress and produce relaxation. A particularly useful variation designed expressly for children has been developed by Koeppen (1974) who uses fantasy in her instructions in such a way that several muscle groups can be relaxed with little noticeable gross motor movement. *Mediative breathing* emphasizes inhalation and exhalation. *Autogenic training* involves passive concentration on certain words or phrases such as "relax" or "I feel calm."

Imagery procedures can be a particularly effective way of teaching relaxation to a child. Children are often more open to suggestion than adults and readily adopt imaginary situations. A typical visual image might be of a favorite place that suggests a happy experience or secure feeling. Imagining all the details of such a place (e.g., vacation spots, a grandparent's house, special or secret locations, or a favorite chair for television viewing) and the activities associated with the scene typically serves to deepen feelings of relaxation.

The exact procedure or combination of procedures employed will vary according to the age of the child, his expectations for treatment, motivation, imaginativeness, and other pertinent characteristics. For example, a fidgety child, one with a short attention span or limited imagination, may have difficulty using passive imagery techniques but will respond to the concrete, step-by-step approach afforded by systematically tensing and relaxing muscles via progressive muscle relaxation.

Cognitive Methods

Cognitive methods, which consist primarily of verbal self-instructions, are a particularly unusual aspect of stress inoculation training. These methods are an essential treatment component because from a cognitive self-control standpoint, altering how a child construes a situation, and what he tells himself about it, is an essential precursor of behavioral change and the success of this process will determine its duration and generalizability. Changing self-talk influences the child's attentional direction, his interpretation and experience of his physiological state, and thereby plays a direct role in behavior change (Meichenbaum, 1977).

The self-instructions are related to the specific presenting problems of the child, which are modeled by the therapist and then rehearsed by the child. The following steps are involved (Meichenbaum and Goodman, 1971): *Cognitive modeling*—therapist models the task while talking aloud to self; *Overt, external guidance*—child performs the task while talking aloud to self, with therapist instructing her or him; *Overt self-guidance*—child performs the task while talking aloud to self; *Faded, overt self-guidance*—child whispers the instructions to self while performing the task; and *Covert self-instruction*—child performs the task silently.

When applying stress inoculation procedures with children, the therapist first needs to elicit those negative self-statements that interfere with a child's functioning and increase his or her anxiety. For example, in the case of a hurricane, maladaptive self-statements might include "My parents could have died in this hurricane," "If it happens again, I might never see my family," "When I hear heavy rain, I know another hurricane is coming," or "If I go to sleep at night, another hurricane will come and kill me and my family."

After the negative statements have been elicited, the child is taught a number of adaptive self-statements designed to lessen anxiety. The verbalizations modeled by the therapist and rehearsed by the child are generally of four types: problem definition ("What is it I should do in this situation?"), focusing of attention ("I have to concentrate and do what I'm supposed to do"), coping statements ("I'm starting to feel nervous, I've got to take a deep breath and relax"), and self-reinforcement ("Great! I did it.").

The actual training format and the contents of each session will not be presented here. Representative training programs that provide the focus from which a specific program geared toward coping with disaster might be developed include Spirito and Finch (1980) and Kendall and Braswell (1984). For example, adaptive self-statements might include: "Hurricanes are dangerous, but I'll be okay if I'm in a safe place," "My parents and family know where to go to safety so they'll be okay," "Bad hurricanes are rare so plain old rain doesn't necessarily mean a hurricane is coming," or "If a hurricane does come while I'm asleep, there'll be plenty of time to reach a safe place." A videotape and/or audiotape of a hurricane for background effect might also be added to facilitate training.

Application Training

Once the child has become proficient in the skills taught in the rehearsal phase, he is placed in a stressful situation other than the actual anxiety-provoking one so that he can practice his coping skills. Application training serves to consolidate the coping techniques acquired during the rehearsal phase. Generalization and efficacy may be enhanced by teaching the training package to the child's family and friends so they may assist and support the child (Spirito & Finch, 1980), or by having the child train another child with a similar problem in the stress inoculation procedure (Meichenbaum, 1977).

Conclusions

A stress inoculation approach appears suitable for disaster-induced fears since it is a problem-solving approach emphasizing coping. The procedure could be delivered in groups at school and thus avoid the stigma of the "mental health" label. In addition, some children who need services but who ordinarily would not receive them would be reached in the school setting. Teachers could also be trained to administer the program and would therefore be able to provide additional situational support. In short, the stress inoculation program provides for the main emotional needs of children exposed to disaster: "human company, physical closeness, information, and, later, a chance to question and discuss the experience" (Fraser, 1973, p. 80). In addition, specific techniques for reducing anxiety are taught and coping skills are enhanced. As the child's anxiety level decreases and coping abilities increase, it also seems likely that his perception of personal control will be enhanced and he will feel to a lesser degree at the mercy of the unpredictable and uncontrollable forces of nature.

Cognitive-behavioral programs have shown promise in dealing with a range of stress-related problems in children, such as fears associated with chronic illness (Spirito, Russo, & Masek, 1984). However, many specialized applications, such as the stress inoculation program for disaster victims outlined here, have not been adequately tested. The same may be said with greater emphasis of the other intervention suggestions made in this chapter, which derive largely from survey research and careful clinical observations. These suggestions have face validity, but from the most rigorous standpoint they should be considered hyptheses that await validation through systematic research.

REFERENCES

Baisden, B., & Quarantelli, E. L. (1981). The delivery of mental health services in community disasters: An outline of research findings. *Journal of Community Psychology, 9,* 195–203.

Benson, H. (1975). *The relaxation response.* New York: William Morrow.

Blaufarb, H., & Levine, J. (1972). Crisis intervention in an earthquake. *Social Work, 17,* 16–19.

Chapman, D. W. (1962). A brief introduction to contemporary disaster research. In G. W. Baker & D. W. Chapman (Eds.), *Man and society in disaster.* New York: Basic Books.

Church, J. S. (1974). The Buffalo Creek disaster: Extent and range of emotional and/or behavioral problems. *Omega, 5,* 61–63.

Crawshaw, R. (1963). Reactions to a disaster. *Archives of General Psychiatry, 9,* 157–162.

Dynes, R. R. (1978). Interorganizational relations in communities under stress. In E. L. Quarantelli (Ed.), *Disasters: Theory and research.* Beverly Hills, CA: Sage Press.

Erickson, K. (1976). Loss of communality at Buffalo Creek. *American Journal of Psychiatry, 133,* 302–305.

Farberow, N. C., & Frederick, C. J. (1978a). *Field manual for human service workers in major disasters.* DHEW Publication No. (ADM) 78-537. Rockville, MD: National Institute of Mental Health.

Farberow, N. C., & Frederick, C. J. (1978b). *The media in a disaster.* DHEW Publication No. (ADM) 78-540. Rockville, MD: National Institute of Mental Health.

Farberow, N. L., & Frederick, C. J. (1978c). *Training manual for human service workers in major disasters.* DHEW Publication No. (ADM) 77-538. Rockville, MD: National Institute of Mental Health.

Farberow, N. L., & Gordon, N. S. (1981). *Manual for child health workers in major disasters.* DHHS Publication No. (ADM) 81-1070. Rockville, MD: National Institute of Mental Health.

Fraser, M. (1973). *Children in conflict.* New York: Basic Books.

Hannigan, J. A., & Kueneman, R. M. (1978). Anticipating flood emergencies: A case study of a Canadian disaster subculture. In E. L. Quarantelli (Ed.), *Disasters: Theory and research.* Beverly Hills, CA: Sage Press.

Hansen, H. (1971). *Psychiatric aspects of hospitalized children in disaster: The California earthquake, 1971.* Paper presented at the American Association of Psychiatric Services for Children, Los Angeles, CA.

Harshberger, D. (1976). An ecologic perspective on disaster intervention. In H. J. Parad, H. L. Resnik, & L. G. Parad (Eds.), *Emergency and disaster management.* Bowie, MD: Charles Press.

Hartsough, D. M. (1982). Planning for disaster: A new community outreach program for mental health centers. *Journal of Community Psychology, 10,* 255–264.

Heffron, E. F. (1977). Project outreach: Crisis intervention following natural disaster. *Journal of Community Psychology, 5,* 103–111.

Jacobsen, E. (1938). *Progressive relaxation.* Chicago, IL: University of Chicago Press.

Kafrissen, S. R., Heffron, E. F., & Zusman, J. (1975). Mental health problems in environmental disasters. In H. L. Resnik & H. L. Reuben (Eds.), *Emergency psychiatric care: The management of mental health crises.* Bowie, MD: Charles Press.

Kendall, P. C., & Braswell, L. (1984). *Cognitive-behavioral therapy for impulsive children.* New York: Guilford Press.

Kliman, A. S. (1976). The Corning Flood Project: Psychological first aid following a natural disaster. In H. J. Parad, H. L. Resnik, & L. G. Parad (Eds.), *Emergency and disaster management.* Bowie, MD: Charles Press.

Koeppen, A. S. (1974). Relaxation training for children. *Elementary School Guidance and Counseling,* Oct. 14–21.

Kreps, G. (1978). The organization of disaster response. In E. L. Quarantelli (Ed.), *Disaster: Theory and research.* Beverly Hills, CA: Sage Press.

Luthe, W. (1969). *Autogenic training.* New York: Grune and Stratton.

Meichenbaum, D. (1975). Toward a cognitive theory of self-control. In G. Schwartz & D. Shapiro (Eds.), *Consciousness and self-regulation: Advances in research.* New York: Plenum.

Meichenbaum, D. (1977). *Cognitive-behavior modification: An integrative approach.* New York: Plenum.

Meichenbaum, D., & Goodman, J. (1971). Training impulsive children to talk to themselves: A means of developing self-control. *Journal of Abnormal Psychology,* 115–126.

Newman, C. J. (1976). Children of disaster: Clinical observations at Buffalo Creek. *American Journal of Psychiatry, 133,* 306–312.

Ollendick, D., & Hoffman, M. (1982). Assessment of psychological reactions in disaster victims. *Journal of Community Psychology, 10,* 157–167.

Perry, H. S., & Perry, S. E. (1959). The schoolhouse disasters: Family and community as determinants of the child's response to disaster (Disaster Study No. 11, Publication 554). Washington, DC: National Academy of Sciences–National Research Council.

Perry, R. W., & Mushkatel, A. H. (1984). *Disaster management: Warning response and community relocation.* Westport: Quorum Books.

Perry, S. E., Silber, E., & Bloch, D. A. (1956). The child and his family in disaster: A study of the 1953 Vicksburg tornado (Disaster Study No. 5, Publication 394). Washington, DC: National Academy of Sciences–National Research Council.

Prince, S. H. (1920) *Catastrophe and social change.* New York: Columbia University Press.

Spirito, A., & Finch, A. (1980). A stress inoculation manual for anxiety in children. Unpublished manuscript, Virginia Commonwealth University, Richmond, VA.

Spirito, A., Russo, D. C., & Masek, B. J. (1984). Behavioral interventions and stress management training for hospitalized adolescents and young adults with cystic fibrosis. *General Hospital Psychiatry, 6,* 211–218.

Taylor, V. A., Ross, G. A., & Quarantelli, E. L. (1976). *Delivery of mental health services in disasters: The Xenia tornado and some implications* (Book and Monograph Series No. 11). Columbus, OH: Ohio State University, Disaster Research Center.

Tuckman, A. J. (1973). Disaster and mental health intervention. *Community Mental Health Journal, 9,* 151–157.

Wenger, D. E. (1978). Community response to disaster: Functional and structural alterations. In E. L. Quarantelli (Ed.), *Disasters: Theory and research.* Beverly Hills, CA: Sage Press.

10

On Being Different

Children with Physical Disabilities

Nancy Kerr
Arizona State University

It is easy to assume that a child with a physical handicap is under stress. When ordinary people, unfamiliar with the coping adjustments that come with experience, close their eyes, plug their ears, or even imagine being unable to walk, they almost always feel hopeless, helpless, or frightened, and they conclude that to be permanently blind, deaf, or crippled means a life of frustration, uncertainty, fear, and distress. It is a popular notion, even among some professionals who work with disabled persons, that such people are so limited and dependent that they must necessarily feel anger, failure, despair, and constant stress. These beliefs are so strong, that when the person with a disability appears happy, thriving, and content, an onlooker may speak of bravery and courage on the one hand or "denial" on the other hand. The insistence of many that people with disabilities must be miserable has been described by Dembo, Leviton, and Wright (1975) as "The Requirement of Mourning."

Certainly the child, or the adult for that matter, who becomes disabled or grows up in our society with a congenital disability is likely to experience more than his or her share of problems. It is a rare person indeed who escapes a sizable number of the physical, social, and emotional problems associated with disability. Problems can be described and discussed as if they are immutable and unsolvable ("Isn't it sad? Isn't it awful?"), or they can form simply the background for sketching some constructive solutions that ameliorate or remove unnecessary stress.

Although the problems presented by living with a physical disability can be difficult and intense, they are solvable. Children with a permanent disability can thrive with physical and psychological comfort. Our task as parents, teachers, and professional helpers is to understand and implement the conditions under which a child who is physically different can avoid, cope with, and overcome stressful situations.

STATUS OF RESEARCH FINDINGS

In comparison with many other disability topics, there is very little research available on stress or crisis intervention and physically disabled children. The

The author is deeply indebted to Lee Meyerson of Arizona State University for his guidance throughout the years and for his assistance in developing this chapter.

studies that do exist are not very helpful either in understanding the relationships between stress and physique or in suggesting how stress can be alleviated. A computer search of Psychological Abstracts in 20 disability categories revealed only 27 articles published since 1967. Many of those were discussion papers that were not based on data or theory. O'Brien's (1975) description of a model program of services for visually impaired children and their parents is one example of this type of paper.

Several articles describe the authors' theories about how physically disabled children or their parents ought to feel and then give one or more clinical examples that support the authors' ideas. For example, Spink (1976) described parents of hearing impaired children in terms of denial, rationalization, shock, grief, helplessness, guilt, anger, and overidentification. Parks (1977) produced a similar document to describe all parents of handicapped children. Some authors recognize that all people do not manifest the syndrome described, and they make considerable effort to explain the absence of the hypothesized anger and guilt that ought to be present in terms of such defense mechanisms as intellectualization, identification with staff, idiosyncratic rituals, humor, and repression (Galdston & Gamble, 1969; Geist, 1979). Similarly, Gogan, Koocher, Foster, and O'Malley (1977) interviewed sibs of children with leukemia and, in their less than systematic discussion of the results, also devoted considerable attention to speculating about why they failed to discover the feelings of abandonment and anger that sibs are supposed to experience. The most refreshing article on parental reactions appeared in a special education newsletter, in which an anonymous parent made a very tactful, but earnest plea to the professionals to stop telling parents how they are *supposed* to feel (Lloyd, 1983).

Another type of research, containing data, is based on the theoretical assumption that disability per se is a cause of psychological distress, and therefore disability, or severity of disability is used as an independent variable or a correlational variable. In a typical design, a group of handicapped children or their parents is compared to a nonhandicapped group and the average of scores on some measure of stress is generally found to be higher for the disabled group (Bedell, Giordani, Amour, Tavormina, & Boll, 1977; Bradshaw & Lawton, 1978; Friedrich and Friedrich, 1981; Tavormina, Boll, Dunn, Luscomb & Taylor, 1981).

These findings replicate the conclusions drawn from reviews of the literature more than 30 years ago (Barker, Wright, Meyerson, & Gonick, 1953; Meyerson, 1955). At that time, Meyerson (1955) stated, "The evidence at one point is clear. Children who have disabilities, as a group, tend to have more frequent and more severe psychological problems than others" (p. 16). He then went on to argue that this finding was not universal or inevitable as a direct consequence of physical disability. It reflects primarily some unfavorable social psychological life conditions that disability helps to create for the child. The important task for the psychologist is to understand the conditions under which distress may or may not be present and to determine how to alleviate it even though the disability cannot be changed.

When severity of disability is correlated with amount of stress experienced by child or parent, the findings also replicate those reported 30 years ago. Little, if any, correlation is found (Bradshaw & Lawton, 1978; Friedrich and Friedrich, 1981). In fact, it sometimes is found that people with less severe "marginal" disabilities experience more stress than severely disabled people (Wright, 1983). Other studies show a higher incidence of other stresses, such as financial problems, in families with a disabled child (Kalnins, Churchill, & Terry, 1980; Beckman-Bell, 1981). Such studies leave unanswered questions of *how* disability and other stresses may be related and what effect each variable may have on the stress scores obtained. Katz, Kellerman, and Siegel (1980) found that every child experienced stress at the moment of undergoing a painful bone marrow biopsy, but even in this condition there was wide variation in the amount of stress experienced.

In addition to numerous methodological flaws in the studies cited, the criticisms of theory and research method made in the now classic works published three decades ago (Barker et al., 1953; Meyerson, 1955) and more recently (Meyerson & Kerr, 1979), still apply. If, as the data show, the relationships between physique, emotion, and behavior are not direct ones, then it would be useful to design studies to tease out what those indirect relationships are. The primary task of the theoretician and researcher is to ask, "Under what conditions will a person with a disability experience high or low stress?" If it is desirable to solve problems, instead of merely "understanding" them, then a second critical question is, "Under what conditions can stress be reduced?"

The following three studies, although vulnerable to criticism because of some methodological flaws and unsupported interpretations, are valuable in that they illustrate approaches for answering these two important questions.

Tyler and Kogan (1977) reported successful use of behavior modification instruction sessions to reduce stress. Using videotapes and "bug-in-the-ear" feedback to mothers as they interacted with their handicapped children, the investigators were able to reduce the frequency of stressful negative interactions between the two. Most of that reduction was still present nine months after the intervention. The study showed, therefore, one procedure for reducing stress. This study represents one of the first efforts to employ behavior modification principles to the study of stress between mothers and physically handicapped children. In view of the success of behavior modification procedures with a myriad of other behaviors, it seems only a matter of time before they will be employed more widely in stress management and crisis intervention.

After comparing the norms for able-bodied children with stress scores of children who had a variety of handicaps, and finding more stress among the disabled, Bedell et al. (1977) divided the handicapped group into high and low stress groups. In doing so, the investigators discovered that the mean age for the two groups did not differ and that type of disability was irrelevant. Each of several types of handicaps was represented in the high and in the low stress groups. The group with low life stress was found to have more positive attitudes toward themselves, better self-concepts, and fewer instances of illness or injury during the period of the study. Thus they demonstrated that disability per se does not cause high life stress, and that it is the interaction of the person with the psychosocial environment that produces stress or comfort. The finding that some disabled children had higher than average stress scores when compared with the norms was interpreted to mean that children with disabilities may be at higher risk for stress, and that special attention should be given to insure that the psychosocial environment is optimal.

Tavormina et al. (1981) studied stress in parents of handicapped children. As in many studies, they found that the stress scores, as a group, exceeded the average norms for parents of ordinary children, and that they were lower than scores obtained from parents of emotionally disturbed children. Assessment of coping skills showed that although the parents experienced more stress they were coping well, though with some strain. The conclusion was that parents needed support to enable them to cope comfortably with the added demands that may be made by children who need special care.

In summary, all of the research indicates that children with physical handicaps and their families may experience an added measure of stress. The relationship between disability and stress is by no means a necessary or direct one, and the results of research designed to study the indirect relationship indicate that the quality of the psychosocial environment is the crucial variable in determining the degree of stress that will occur.

The remainder of this chapter is devoted, therefore, to an analysis of how the child and the environment may interact to produce stress or comfort in everyday living. We will attempt to show some of the practical applications of these ideas. Other applications are readily derivable by insightful application of these theoretical concepts to any stressful situation that may be of concern.

FIELD THEORY AS A WAY OF THINKING
ABOUT CRISIS AND STRESS

According to Kurt Lewin's Field Theory (1935), *behavior* is a function of the *person* interacting with the *environment* [B = f(P, E)]. Although most psychologists agree with this formula, dynamically oriented professionals tend to emphasize the crucial attributes "in" the *person* and attempt to demonstrate that behavior is caused by an individual's personality characteristics, intelligence, or physical characteristics. They are likely to lean toward thinking and acting as if behavior is a function of the personalities. Behavioral and social psychologists, on the other hand, emphasize the ways the *environment* controls the behavior and are likely to highlight those situations in which behavior is a function of the environmental variables.

In Field Theory, the major emphasis is not on the person nor the environment alone, but squarely on the *interaction* between the two. Any change in the person or environment changes the interaction and thus changes behavior. A field theorist is more likely to study and explain the interaction than to focus on the person or environment alone.

For example, suppose three psychologists are asked why Johnny is doing poorly in arithmetic. An extremely dynamic psychologist might propose giving Johnny a battery of tests to determine what deficits he may have, such as poor eyesight, or what emotional or motivational problems may exist. The effort would be to account for his client's poor performance in terms of one or more characteristics of the person.

An extremely behavioral psychologist might look for the problem only in the environment by studying the reinforcing contingencies of the classroom, and analyzing the discriminative stimuli of the curriculum. A behaviorist might easily conclude that Johnny's lack of progress is caused by a bad or poorly designed educational system.

A field theorist's approach would focus on the interaction between Johnny and his school: If Johnny is having a problem with arithmetic, there must be a mismatch between him and his educational system. Both Johnny (person) and the school (environment) need to be studied in the effort to bring about a better "fit" or interaction between the two.

Dynamic and behavioral psychologists have a long history of fighting with one another about which approach to solving human problems is more successful. Field theory, on the other hand, is not "anti" either approach. Instead, it provides a framework in which formulations from both systems can be employed to alter an interaction that is crucial for solving a problem.

A good match in Johnny's case might be achieved by strengthening Johnny in a variety of ways to enable him to cope with the school system as he finds it, or by altering the school system to accommodate Johnny as he is. Frequently, the easiest and most practical way to solve this problem is to facilitate some changes in both Johnny and the curriculum.

The same principle of focusing on interactions holds for those who have physical rather than learning problems. Suppose Susie uses a wheelchair and has a problem entering the school through a heavy door that has a bumpy threshold. Therapy to strengthen Susie's arms may enable her to manage the task with no environmental change. Altering the threshold and installing an automatic door opener may allow her easy access, although her arms remain weak. Or a combination of some strengthening of her arms and some minor alterations of the entrance may also solve the problem. Whether Susie experiences stress every time she tries to enter the school depends neither on her nor the doorway. Instead, stress or comfort depends on whether she has easy access to the building. Whether that access is made possible by changing her or the door is of little import. It is the *interaction* between her and the door that determines whether she will be under stress.

So far we have considered primarily overt behaviors—doing arithmetic or entering a building. People also have feelings and emotions, however, and some psychologists believe that how people feel about what they are doing may be as important or more important than the behavior itself. Here, again, psychologists of different persuasions employ different approaches. Some behaviorists prefer to ignore feelings and deal only with overt behavior. Other behaviorists predict that people will be happy or unhappy, stressed or comfortable, about what they are doing depending on whether they are behaving under positive or negative reinforcing contingencies. Dynamically oriented psychologists are more likely to attribute states of happiness or unhappiness to personality characteristics of the person. They may offer such explanations as "She's an optimistic person" or "He has a passive-aggressive personality."

Field theorists do not try to account for feelings solely in terms of personal characteristics or environmental events. They believe that both objective behavior and subjective emotions are determined by how a situation is perceived. Technically, this perception is called the *psychological situation* (PS). The PS is a way of describing how people perceive themselves interacting with their environments.

Understanding some principles of psychological situations will allow us to determine when a person is in a stressful or crisis situation and suggest what can be done to prevent and/or remediate stress.

For field theorists no environmental event, such as a hurricane, school starting, or parents divorcing, necessarily or unilaterally creates stress. Nor can any personal characteristic such as a physical or mental disability by itself cause psychological stress. Whether or not a person feels stress or experiences a crisis depends solely and completely on his or her psychological situation. The psychological state of stress is only indirectly related to the objective reality of personal characteristics or environmental events.

In order to understand the indirect relationships between physical disability and possibility of stress, some of the rules governing psychological situations may be helpful.

BASIC ASSUMPTIONS ABOUT PSYCHOLOGICAL SITUATIONS

As already noted, the PS is a hypothetical construct that describes how a person perceives his or her situation at any given moment. The PS is not a tangible entity that exists somewhere in the brain. It is simply a way of drawing a diagram or map to represent how the person sees himself or herself in relation to the environment. Figure 1 shows examples of these diagrams. Some of the rules governing these relationships are as follows:

1. The PS always contains the person's perception of himself or herself (P) and his or her perception of the environment (goals).

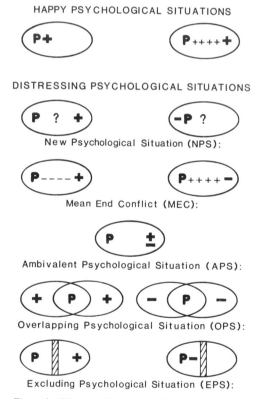

Figure 1 Diagram of happy and distressing psychological situations, in which P represents person, pluses and minuses represent valences of goals, question mark represents uncertainty, and striped area represents barrier.

2. The goals always have some degree of attractiveness or aversiveness (+ or – valences).
   a. By definition, a goal cannot be neutral. If it were, it would not be perceived at all. Therefore, goals are represented as pluses or minuses.
   b. Few goals for which one might strive are totally + or –. Most goals have advantages and disadvantages and for purposes of this theory, the + or – that is assigned to a goal is actually an algebraic sum of the + and – aspects of the goal. For example, if the attractiveness of a goal greatly outweighs the aversive aspects, it is assigned a +.
   c. Goals can range from mildly + or – to very strongly + or –. The strength or potency of a goal depends on a combination of (1) the needs and knowledge of the person, (2) the characteristics of the goal, and (3) the conditions of the field.
3. The field describes the "space" surrounding the person and the goal.
   a. Some goals may be seen as close by; others seem remote. All other things being equal, more distant goals are less potent than immediate ones.
   b. The pathway to the goal may seem unclear or it may be well structured. The steps that one must take to reach a goal may be perceived as + or –.
   c. Perceived barriers to reaching a goal may be present or absent. They may seem penetrable or impenetrable. All other things being equal, a penetrable barrier may increase the attractiveness of a goal.
   d. The field may contain several possible goals that may be equally or differentially attractive.
4. Any diagram of a PS represents the person's *present* perception of a situation. The PS can change from moment to moment, but it also has some durability. The real world forces attention to some activities or problems and each time thoughts of a particular situation recur, they will appear with the same constellation of pluses and minuses until something reorganizes the pattern.

The theory, then, as it is used here, creates a system of pluses and minuses with rules about their relationships that apply to all people. It is the translation of a wide diversity of phenotypic details about people and environmental events to a pattern of valences that allows a genotypic set of rules to be applied universally.

Putting It All Together

Using the theoretical concepts and the ground rules just described, we can understand, predict, and facilitate change in the behavior and feelings of ourselves and others.

Mapping the Field

By observing and talking with a person, it is possible to obtain information about his or her specific concerns that can be translated into pluses and minuses that allow us to *hypothesize* the person's PS.

Understanding Behavior and Feelings

The map allows us to understand what the person is trying to do. The relationship among the pluses and minuses helps us to understand what conflicts or uncertainties may be creating distress.

Predicting Behavior and Feelings

We can predict that the person will continue the same pattern of behavior and continue to experience happiness or distress until something changes the pattern of valences in the psychological situation.

Solving Problems

A person has a problem when in a *distressing psychological situation* (DPS). Application of the theory suggests what must be changed to what in order to turn DPS into a *happy psychological situation* (HPS) where behavior will be purposeful and well directed, and the person will enjoy what she or he is doing.

PSYCHOLOGICAL SITUATIONS

Happy Psychological Situations

There are two types of happy psychological situations. In the first, the person is in a positive goal region as shown in Figure 1. It represents consummatory behavior such as a person—either ordinary or disabled—actually eating and savoring a good meal; or glowing with the joy of gaining admission to a favorite school; or sitting in front of a fireplace, enjoying the comfort of the fire. Such situations probably are relatively short lived, however. Before long, one of three things will happen: The person will become satiated (good food is no longer attractive after one has eaten to satiety), the ecstacy of high emotion will subside (the person will eventually tire of "celebrating" good fortune), or something will have to be done to maintain the comfortable position (sooner or later the fire will have to be tended). Although the consummatory moment spent in a positive goal region may represent the epitome of joy, it is likely that most people spend only a relatively small proportion of time in such situations.

A second happy psychological situation in which a person is comfortable is also shown in Figure 1. The person perceives a positive goal and sees a clear pathway of steps leading to that goal. The same "map" can be applied to whatever situation the person is considering at a given moment. For example, if a child wants to go on a picnic (positive goal) and enjoys helping to prepare the food, load the family car, and take the trip to the picnic site (pathway steps), the child is in a happy psychological situation. Whenever a person perceives a positive goal with positive steps leading to it, in a situation free from other competing goals, this person will "feel good." Behavior will be adaptive and well organized.

Distressing Psychological Situations

New Psychological Situations (NPS)

The person has a goal and does not know how to reach it. There is no clear pathway. The distress associated with an NPS results from uncertainty about whether an action leads toward or away from the goal. Unless the person structures a pathway that will lead to the goal, the distress will continue, or he or she will leave the field. The newness is not in the physical environment. In fact, a person may enter the same reality situation many times, but until a path to the goal is structured, the situation will remain psychologically new. For example, a blind child may want to know what the teacher is writing on the blackboard, but until the child finds a reliable way of retrieving the material before the teacher erases it, he or she will be in an NPS every time the teacher applies the chalk to the blackboard.

Those with physical disabilities, especially at the onset of disability, may face many NPSs. Getting from one room to another, or heating a can of soup suddenly may become an NPS for a newly blinded person. A person who becomes deaf may have difficulty in maintaining verbal communication.

Figure 1 shows a schematic description of a new psychological situation. The diagram also shows the same "newness" with respect to moving away from an aversive situation. A person may be in the presence of an aversive stimulus and simply not know the steps to resolve it or to move from it. A child may suffer from the teasing of classmates, and is in an NPS if she or he does not know how to stop them or how to retreat from the setting.

Means/End Conflicts (MEC)

Sometimes a person knows exactly what must be done to reach a positive goal. There is no uncertainty. However, the steps that must be taken are negative and unpleasant. Such situations are common in everyday life. Some students want to receive good grades, but they do not want to study or take exams. People who become ill or disabled frequently are in situations that require distasteful medical treatment, or painful surgery for later better health or function.

A counterpart situation is one in which the immediate consequences are positive (the pathway behaviors are fun), but they lead to a bad end. To the extent that the person sees the negative end result, the person will be disturbed because he or she continues the path. Overeating, watching TV instead of doing homework, staying out too late are common examples. Young children are less likely to perceive the long-term consequences of their behavior, and, being controlled more by the immediate situation, probably experience fewer MECs than older children and adults.

Ambivalent Psychological Situations (APS)

The ambivalent situation is one in which the person considers only one option and cannot proceed toward or away from it because the valence of the goal is both plus and minus and potency is equally balanced. The child who asks "Should I go over to John's house or not?" and finds that the advantages and disadvantages are equally balanced may take a long time to decide, or will be in distress because one action is not clearly better than its opposite. The person who becomes disabled may find that some situations, previously positive, may become ambivalent. For example, an activity that was pleasurable may become much more difficult to accomplish from a wheelchair. If, following disability, fellow students and teachers devalue a child, she or he may have more mixed feelings about going to school even though school was highly attractive before the disability.

Overlapping Psychological Situations (OPS)

The figure shows the well-known approach-approach and avoidance-avoidance situations. When people play numerous roles in life, there are likely to be instances in which two roles, equally desired, are incompatible. Those roles may be *interfering* or *antagonistic*.

A simple interfering OPS is one in which the person cannot do two things at the same time. A child may be unable to play in the school band and go camping with the Boy Scouts simultaneously. In an antagonistic OPS, the very action of playing one role well requires that the other role be played poorly. For example, an eighth grader may want to please the teacher by being a model student and at the same time gain acceptance from his peers by joining in the gang's misconduct in school. In addition to the OPSs experienced by able-bodied people who play many roles, the person with a disability may have an additional conflict between playing the disabled role or a "normal" role. Of course, in the central area of overlap are the options that are common to both roles (the compatibility between the roles). However, the disabled person often has to make a choice of doing something in an easier, safer, "disabled" way, or trying to appear "normal" at the cost of greater energy, ineptitude, and risk of failure. For example, some people must choose between walking easily with a cane or crutches and walking more precariously without any support. A hearing-impaired child may have to choose between communicating reasonably well with a hearing aid or understanding speech poorly without one.

Excluding Psychological Situations (EPS)

As Figure 1 shows, the most positive goal for a person may lie beyond a physical, social, or emotional barrier. In the person's perception, the barrier is the only impediment to reaching the goal. An ordinary child may experience an EPS if not invited to a friend's birthday party, fails to win a contest, or loses a favorite pet. Children with disabilities may experience an extra share of excluding situations because more areas, open to most other people, may be closed to them. An architectural barrier places people with disabilities in an EPS. Discrimination in school does the same.

The second EPS in Figure 1 shows the situation in which the person is trapped in an aversive situation. The only difference between this EPS and the corresponding NPS is that the person knows exactly what bars passage, but cannot remove the barrier. In the NPS, the person simply does not know where the exit is. A person lost in a forest may not know whether he or she is walking deeper into the wilderness or toward safety. In the EPS, on the other hand, a child accidentally locked out of the house may know exactly what is needed to remove the barrier: a key—but the child does not have one.

Summary of Distressing Psychological Situations

As has been stated in previous discussions of these schematic life spaces (Kerr, 1976; Meyerson, 1971), if people with disabilities are exposed more frequently than others, and for longer periods of time, to one or more of these distressing psychological situations, it is not surprising that they more frequently experience crisis and stress than those not so exposed. The significant variable is not that they have disabilities but the frequency and duration of exposure to distressing psychological situations.

Depending on the intensity of the distressing situation, the person may be under mild stress or an intense crisis. In addition, if a person experiences fewer and fewer of these distressing situations while reorganizing life in order to live with a disability, and if parents and teachers intervene to avoid or alleviate some of the distressing situations, the common tendency for "maladjustment" to be more severe at the time of onset of disability is understandable. Finally, when two people have the same kind and degree of physical disability and one seems happy and the other does not, we can account for that difference if the first person has resolved many of the distress situations while the second person has resolved few.

If these psychological situations represent *all* situations of human distress, then, clearly, the twofold task of helpers is to aid people in avoiding such situations and to help them change those distressing psychological situations that do occur into happy psychological situations. These concepts, which state what must be changed to what in order to change distress to comfort, can be viewed as a way of thinking about crisis intervention and stress reduction.

RELATIONSHIP OF FIELD THEORY TO OTHER THEORIES OF CRISIS

These formulations provide a way of understanding stress that is somewhat different from other theoretical approaches.

Dynamic Theories

It is obvious that field theory would not lead one to study reactions to stress as a function of personality characteristics, ego strength, or intelligence. It would not suggest looking for individual differences in coping with stress. Nor would it suggest that any personal characteristic, such as physical disability, need produce stress. Instead, the major question would be: In what ways does the person, whatever his or her physical condition, interact with the environment—whatever it may be—to produce stressful PSs? A second major question would be: What can be done, either to the person or the environment to change the stressful PSs to comfortable, happy situations? People that dynamically oriented psychologists would call maladjusted would be seen by the field theorist simply as people who spend large amounts of time in distressing PSs. People who are deemed well adjusted spend considerable time in happy PSs.

Environmental Theories

Likewise, field theory suggests that no environmental event necessarily causes stress or crisis. The topics of the chapters in this text simply describe events that may throw large numbers of people into an increased number of new, excluding, or other stressful PSs. The theory would not lead an investigator to construct scales that attempt to measure the amount of stress people have experienced by asking them about what events have occurred in their lives. A divorce in one family may be a blessing; in another, a catastrophe. Nevertheless, it is helpful to know what kinds of distressing PSs may arise in association with major life changes.

Temporal Model of Crisis Intervention

The model described by Auerbach (Chapter 1, this volume) postulates that different types of intervention are needed depending on the temporal position of the intervention in relation to the crisis. Interventions to prepare people for an impending stressor may differ from those given during or after a crisis.

An analysis of the temporal model from a field-theory point of view would agree that preparation for a potential stress would involve giving the person both instructions for coping with a strange set of circumstances and whatever assurances are realistic that the event need not result in personal disaster. Anticipation of strange events (hurricane, school, divorce, illness, or disability), according to field theory, may put people in new psychological situations, and the effort would be to prevent or reduce the "newness" by providing the person with a structured pathway to a successful survival of the experience. Therefore, both models suggest similar interventions. However, we would suggest that effective interventions may be determined more by the kind of PS the person is in than by the temporal relationship between the crisis and the intervention.

One convenience of the field-theory model is that organizing our thoughts around one specific crisis is not necessary. We do not conceptualize a hurricane, divorce, illness, or disability as a finite event that has a before and an after. Rather, what appears to be a single event may become a set of experiences that involves one crisis after another. Even a circumscribed event like a tornado may produce a variety of PSs. At one point, people may be in NPSs trying to determine how to protect themselves from danger, later they may be in another NPS trying to determine how to protect themselves from inclement weather, hunger, and disease after their homes have been destroyed. Some may experience an NPS whenever storm clouds gather and may need more education about what to do when a tornado warning comes, as well as desensitization procedures to help them know when to worry and when not to. At the same time, other people may find themselves in EPSs if they cannot obtain loans to rebuild their homes. Finally, people who were previously dissatisfied with their homes may experience little or no stress. They may be in the happy psychological situation of having found shelter in a very safe place during the storm; they may have reasonably adequate interim living quarters, and their insurance money will allow them to build the kind of house they really wanted all along.

Field theorists would view the major task of the helper as one of determining what PS the person is in and seeking an intervention to change the stressful PS to a happy PS. Nevertheless, they would strongly support the development of preparation and orientation programs prior to likely stress as a way of preventing or reducing psychological newness.

Preparation for Stress

It is doubtful that children should be given highly specific "precrisis" interventions to prepare them for every possible bad thing that could happen to them. There are, however, some child-rearing practices that may help the child to learn to cope with whatever stresses may arise. In fact, few children go through a day without experiencing a distressing psychological situation; Johnny gets "lost" for a minute or two in the supermarket (new PS), Mary does not know if she wants to jump into the wading pool or not (ambivalent PS), Susie wants to go out with her parents, but does not want to get cleaned up first (means/end conflict), Tommy must choose between a cupcake and the cookies (overlapping PS), and Jane doesn't get invited to her friend's party (excluding PS).

These "minicrises" provide fertile ground for parents and teachers to teach children to cope with and/or avoid distressing psychological situations. It is helpful to recognize that everyone feels bad sometimes; that they can tell someone about their troubles, that the bad times usually get better; and that they can discover things they can do to relieve the distress. If children learn that life is a series of little "ups and downs" and develop skills for solving problems that do arise, they are less likely to be overwhelmed if really serious problems come their way.

There is a strength to be derived from gaining confidence in one's survival skills. There are literally hundreds of opportunities for parents to teach children that no matter what happens we will muddle through; that if you want to do something, give it a try—it is no sin to fail; that, to call on John Wayne's old adage, "When the going gets tough, the tough get going." If children do not expect to live in a just and perfect world where they will lead a pampered life on a bed of roses, they can derive great confidence from the belief and knowledge that they can "play under pressure" and that they need not fear hard times. President Roosevelt said it well: "We have nothing to fear but fear itself."

Of course we are not advocating throwing roadblocks into children's paths simply to help them acquire these skills. Children should also learn to enjoy the good times to the hilt. Hopefully, they can experience a preponderance of happy psychological situations. However, learning how to turn the distressing PSs into happy ones is a valuable lesson that can be taught in the ordinary course of growing up.

Preparation for Physical Disability

Again, it would be ridiculous to prepare children specifically for a multitude of dire circumstances that probably will not happen. However, some general attitudes about people with various physical impairments can certainly be helpful if a child should happen to become disabled; and the same kinds of attitudes would seem desirable in helping all children to cope with the fact that we are all only human.

The philosophy that everyone has strong points and weak points, and that we all ought to try to capitalize on our assets and minimize our liabilities can be useful. Also, children can learn that there are many ways to reach a goal. If you cannot get there one way—improvise. If people want to go to the store, some ride in cars; some ride bikes, some walk, some ride in wheelchairs. Some people find their way to a store by looking at where they are going; some get their bearings by tapping a white cane and listening, others use a guide dog. Children can learn to value their ability to discover new ways to reach a goal when a conventional path is blocked—it is called resourcefulness. Parents can place a premium on being like everyone else and encourage their children to emulate the "average person." Alternatively, they can teach children that everyone is unique, and that it is more important to develop your own unique talents than to "keep up with the Joneses." The latter value is more likely to teach children that being different is not bad.

Preparation for Imminent Stress

When a specific set of unexpected circumstances is about to occur, it is, of course, advantageous to try to prepare the child for that occurrence by explaining what is going to happen and how the child and others will cope with the situation, and above all, by reassuring the child that she or he is not alone—that those who love the child will be there through the difficulty—be it a hurricane, divorce, illness, or disability.

With respect to disability, it is sometimes clear ahead of time that a child is about to become permanently disabled, as when an amputation is required. More often, there is uncertainty about the outcome of an illness or accident. In either case, it is more helpful to reassure the child that he or she is loved and that things eventually will work out all right regardless of the physical outcome than to tell the child that he or she will be physically whole again. It is also helpful to let a child know that it is healthy and natural for both parent and child to mourn a loss and at the same time offer reassurances that the sadness will not last forever. Finally, it is helpful to remember that, when facing such a possibility, the parent may be more fearful of how the child will face life with a disability and the child is more likely to have more immediate concerns about having to stay in a hospital all night. The orientation programs to prepare children for medical procedures obviously are helpful. Equally important is remembering to find out from the child exactly what is on his or her mind. The whole idea of preparing specific interventions for particular events carries with it the danger that the adults may presume to know what the child is upset about. Many are familiar with the story about the little boy who anxiously asked his mother "Where did *I* come from;" After the mother gave him a long lesson about sex and reproduction, the boy said, "Gee, Bobby says he came from New York."

Intervention during a Crisis

When a person is undergoing a strange new experience, it helps to tell the person what is happening. A sudden illness or injury from accident may be difficult to comprehend. It is common for the people to act as if nothing were happening and show great concern for the delay in doing whatever they were doing before the sudden change in their lives. Or the person may be in a state of total confusion. Here, simple explanations of what is happening and assurances that whatever they were about to do is taken care of probably are the most helpful ways to structure an intense new PS. For example, one moment a young lady driving her car turned left into the university to attend classes. The next moment, as she regained consciousness, she was lying almost upside down in an overturned car, with a broken windshield scattered along the length of her body, and a priest leaning into the car to administer the last rites. She later described how she first made sense of the confusion by concluding that it must be a dream. After all, if that glass were real, she would be cut and bleeding and she was not (the windshield broke into harmless rounded pieces); and she did not need the last rites because she was not a Catholic. However, she could not wake up from the dream. As soon as she opened her eyes again, the priest did about the most helpful thing one could do. He begain explaining to her that she was in an overturned car; there had been an accident, a car hit her and her car rolled on its side. Please lie still, an ambulance is on the way. Was she in pain? *No.* Could she move her fingers and toes? *Yes.* He replied, "Fine, just lie still and let them get you out without hurting you; they will take you to the hospital and check you over."

He repeated the message until in a few moments she was fully aware of what was occurring. She fussed about being late for class; she was assured that her professors were being notified. She wanted to take her books and notes on the stretcher to the hospital, a student offered to gather up her belongings and keep them safe for her. She was upset about leaving her car in the middle of an intersection; a policeman told her they would remove it and notify her where it was. The explanations of what was happening to her, and the fact that the bystanders took her relatively unimportant concerns about books, classes, and the car seriously, were the keys to helping her structure her new PS and to putting the crisis of the accident behind her. Thus she was free to enter and cope with the several more distressing PSs that were to occur before she fully recovered. Her comment in the emergency room was "Well, I survived the accident. Now let's see if I can survive the treatment."

Summary of Early Interventions

Preparing people for events that may or may not occur, or for a possible imminent crisis, can be considered theoretically as a task of reducing "newness." If contemplating an event that has not yet occurred puts people in new PSs, the suggestions just described can help to structure the situation. Likewise, the interventions suggested during a crisis are purely efforts to structure a new psychological situation.

INTERVENTIONS TO CREATE HAPPY PSYCHOLOGICAL SITUATIONS

Unlike some of the crises described in other chapters, physical disability is not a temporally confined event that occurs and then disappears. Children growing up with a disability may continue to face possibly stressful situations that are rare or unknown to their able-bodied counterparts. The following suggestions are but a few of the ways parents and teachers can help children to avoid or change common distressing psychological situations into happy ones. The basic question is always: "How can we create an environment in which the child, regardless of disability, finds a clear positive pathway to a desired goal?"

Be Creative! There Are Many Ways to Reach a Goal

Often we feel that a disabled child is limited and is unable to do many things because we assume that there is only one way to reach a goal: If Johnny cannot participate in the *same way* that other children do, then he must be excluded.

For example, a third-grade teacher wanted her students to get experience in talking to the class and made an assignment that required each pupil to give an oral report. She was in a quandary when Johnny who had a severe speech impairment joined the class. She did not want to embarrass Johnny and wondered if she should just forget about that assignment for the current semester. However, it seemed to unfair to deprive the whole class of a valuable experience just because of one child. Perhaps she should go ahead with the rest of the class and simply excuse Johnny, or have him submit something in writing. That didn't seem right because it might also put Johnny in an unfavorable light. Still, she knew that everyone would have great difficulty understanding him, and it seemed so cruel to force him into a situation where he would perform so poorly.

Then she realized that her real objective in making a class presentation assignment was to help the children strengthen their communication skills. If the goal was communication, there may be many ways to reach it. She then saw many possible pathways a child could use to reach the goal. Some messages can be communicated more effectively with a demonstration than by trying to explain something verbally. Pantomime can at times be an interesting and effective way to communicate. Visual illustrations also may communicate at one glance information that verbally might require a thousand words. A child could use slides, drawings, photographs, or even videotapes. A group could dramatize a message by acting it out.

She discussed the possibilities with the whole class, and all wanted the opportunity to develop a unique way of presenting their reports. What had traditionally been a series of oral reports of little interest to most of the children now became an exciting class project.

Johnny could do just what the rest of the class was doing—discovering and presenting his message in an effective way. Intelligible speech was only one of many suitable ways of fulfilling the assignment.

In addition, the class discussed how some people draw better than others. Some like to talk, others would rather demonstrate a skill. They decided that planning their presentations so as to use their best individual talents was a smart thing to do. They also decided that because this was school, where kids can try out and learn new things, this project would also provide a chance to try some things they might not be so good at—it would be a chance to practice. One student who thought she could not draw tried her hand at a graph to accompany her oral presentation. Johnny relied heavily on his visual aids to send his message. But in the atmosphere that had been established, he also chose to speak a little, and performed better than anyone had expected.

The teacher, who had previously resisted "mainstreaming" exceptional children into her classroom, used the principle of creating many pathways to a goal on many subsequent occasions—always to the benefit of the entire class.

Do Not Make a Child's Disability a Taboo Subject

Often adults communicate to children, directly or by example, the idea that one should not take notice of an obvious disability. Nothing makes for more awkward situations than trying to pretend a visible disabilty doesn't exist. Children are curious, and they ask questions about the lady they see in a wheelchair just as surely as they ask about other things that they do not understand. Often mothers look embarrassed when a child comments on a disabled person they encounter, shush them and tell them not to look. The child may learn by that experience that there is something very bad about people with disabilities, and that they are to be avoided. Also, the fact that they should not peek makes them all the more curious about the person.

More appropriately, some mothers respond to their children's questions by treating the presence of a disabled person as a perfectly natural event with a comment like, "Oh yes, that's a wheelchair. Some people ride in them instead of walking." When mother gives a casual matter-of-fact answer, the child is generally satisfied.

When a disabled child joins a class, it is rather natural for the students to want to know about him or her. With the disabled child's permission, of course, it generally is best to explain, or let the child explain, the disability. It is also helpful to emphasize how the child does function rather than portraying him or her as someone who cannot do a number of things.

A classroom policy of open discussion has merit in its own right. Here it not only has the effect of minimizing concern and curiosity, but also it allows others to learn or to recognize the considerable skills that many children have acquired in functioning with a disability.

Make Some Rules

Whether a teacher wants to structure a class in an autocratic manner or to develop more democratic guidelines is not an issue here. Every group needs some rules about how it will function and how problems will be resolved.

Even after children's curiosity is laid to rest in a matter-of-fact way, and a disabled student is no longer presenting a new PS to others, there are likely to be occasions when students tease or ridicule a child who is different. Parents and teachers are sometimes rendered so helpless by such occurrences that they seek to reduce distress by removing the victim from the group. A common reason given for excluding exceptional children is, "Susie really wouldn't be happy in the group. The other children would laugh at her awkwardness. You know how cruel children can be." It is ironic, with so many people's concern about the "helplessness" of the disabled, that in this situation the adults handle their own helplessness by expelling the victim from the group. There are more appropriate ways of creating a happier classroom environment. One is a hard line approach that assumes that the adult is responsible for establishing some rules or guidelines about what is acceptable behavior. If a teacher sits back and allows children to beat each other physically, she is not likely to have her contract renewed. It is not possible to discuss here the many strategies that can be used in dealing with discipline problems, but it is clear that an adult supervisor of a group must find a way to prohibit physical violence. It seems reasonable that the adult can be just as firm in insuring that verbal abuse toward anyone will not be tolerated. If adults will actively teach youngsters what is acceptable and unacceptable, children are more likely to learn to behave themselves in civilized ways.

Increase Understanding of People with Disabilities

A common way that adults use to attempt to persuade children to be nice to one another is to say, "Now don't tease Johnny. He can't help it that he walks funny. How would you feel if you only had one leg?"

This sort of plea is damaging in at least three ways. First, it implies that it would be all right to ridicule Johnny if he had two good legs. Second it suggests that Johnny is already feeling bad because of his disability, when, in fact, he may be feeling bad only because the other kid is harrassing him. Third, it asks the able-bodied offender to identify with Johnny in a way that is quite foreign to his or her own experience. Asking anyone who takes a normal body for granted to imagine how it feels to have a part missing is an invitation to conjure up stereotyped visions that probably are unrelated to reality.

In the Lewinian tradition, Beatrice Wright (1983) has shown a way to deal with psychological "feelings" by considering psychological rather than physical situations. Instead of asking children how they would feel if they were physically disabled, she asks, "Has anyone ever been teased by someone?" Almost everyone has, and youngsters begin to describe their own experiences (often with a sibling) with considerable emotion. It is not difficult to identify with the psychological situation of the disabled child. Further questions are: "How do you feel when someone pokes fun at you?" "How do you feel about the person who's teasing you?" and "What can you do about it?" Such discussions generally result in youngsters understanding each other better and treating each other with a bit more kindness. This kind of discussion sends three different messages. First, it shows that everyone, not just the physically handicapped, finds ridicule offensive. Second it places the problem where it belongs—in the social interaction—not in Johnny's wooden leg. Third, it provides the ordinary and the exceptional child a common base of experience from which mutual understanding can grow.

Teach Cooperation as Well as Independence

A common notion in rehabilitation circles that deserves to be challenged is that the person with a disability should be as independent as possible. Such a philosophy can be damaging. If the disability is of a sort that makes physical independence totally impossible in all situations, for example, the person is asked to set a goal that cannot be achieved. For individuals who have less than total physical dependence, there are occasions when a task can be completed only with time-consuming and unnecessary labor that delays the progress of the rest of the group. It might be better all around to accept a bit of help and allow the whole group to proceed.

Of course it is sometimes desirable to test the limits and allow a child to learn what she or he can do totally alone. However, it is also useful to recognize that mature people often help each other. In any social group, be it a family, a place of employment, a school, or a recreational group, people count on and help each other. The undesirable kinds of dependency that many fear that the person with a disability may develop do not result from receiving help. They may develop if all the help flows in one direction. Teachers and parents can do much to insure that the disabled child gives help as well as receives it. The life of one high schooler in a wheelchair was much easier and less stressful because her fellow students were quite willing to give her a push, help her over curbs, and run occasional errands for her. It happened that she was an excellent student who was quite willing to help her friends with solving perplexing homework assignments. Their meetings outside school to study or work on projects provided the opportunity for forming social and recreational liaisons. Had she been unwilling to accept the convenience of their help, they might have been embarrassed to seek her help.

Hints about Help

People are often uncertain about whether to offer help to a person with a disability. Some disabled persons are offended if others do not perceive their need and offer help; others are offended if people try to give help that is unneeded or unwanted. The confusion about when to offer help does much to create social distance that is quite unnecessary. Ladieu, Hanfmann, and Dembo's (1947) classic advice still holds true: The best thing an onlooker can do is to say, "Can I help?" and allow the person to instruct the helper about what to do and how to do it. A helper should be willing to take "No" for an answer. There are many reasons why the person may not want help. It may be important to the person to demonstrate the ability to do the thing alone (e.g., when the person is surrounded with people who hold the belief that disabled people are poor helpless creatures). It almost seems at times that nondisabled people need to push help on a person with a disability in order to avoid challenging their beliefs about the helplessness of such people. A person sometimes may refuse help because it is easier to do the task alone than to teach someone else how to help. A child may appear to struggle with locking a brace, but has found it easier to do it himself than to explain it and wait while the helper bungles and does it poorly. A hostess may decline to let a guest prepare the salad because she knows the guest makes soggy salads. A child who is blind may want to pour his or her own milk so as to gain skill from practice. Occasionally disabled people do not want help simply because they do not want anyone to know what they are up to!

The person with a disability also bears responsibility for facilitating smooth helping relationships, and children can gradually be taught several ways to assume that responsibility. First, they can be helped to recognize that, as Ladieu et al. (1947) found, able-bodied people are likely to offer help when they see it as expedient, and do not necessarily mean to imply that the recipient is incompetent or helpless. Second, they can learn to make their wants and needs known to others, instead of assuming that others are mind readers or experts on the needs of people with disabilities. Third, they can learn to respect the needs of others by evaluating how much they will inconvenience others when asking for help and weighing that consideration against the intensity of their own need or want. Fourth, the disabled child can learn to take "No" for an answer to a request for help without offense and can learn socially acceptable ways of refusing unwanted help.

Teach Children to Share Responsibility

One of the most important lessons to be learned in school is to function as a member of a group. As adults, most people have to be able to participate and carry their share of the load in family, work, and community settings if they are to lead satisfactory lives and if the society is to survive.

As children, the classroom provides an ideal opportunity for children to learn to work together with a peer group. Hopefully, the exceptional child can be a full-fledged participant in group activities. This means that she or he must share the responsibilities as well as the rewards of the group. Too often, the disabled child is excused from her or his share of the work. In group activities, different people have different skills to bring to a project. For example, when planning a party, someone who can cook, bakes the cookies; someone who can draw, makes the posters; someone with a telephone, calls the guests; and someone with a bicycle may run the errands. Such sharing of responsibilities allows the child with a disability also to contribute her or his best skills to an endeavor.

A Girl Scout leader allowed a 10-year-old deaf girl to enroll in a regular day-camp. The child had been in special education classes, had never been in a group with hearing children, and she had no camping experience. There were great fears on the part of many, that under these stresses she would not be able to cope, or that she would keep the rest of the girls from enjoying their usual activities. The leader did a number of things already described in earlier sections. On the first day of camp, she introduced Mary; announced that she was deaf, and would not hear a thing that was said, but that she could read lips sometimes; and demonstrated with Mary the importance of making eye contact before starting to talk.

She and the child also demonstrated other ways to communicate through gesture signs and finger spelling.

The first handicraft project for the group was to make note pads that could be attached along with a pencil to each camper's belt. Of course, as soon as the youngsters had made note pads they wanted to write notes. Mary was deaf, not uneducated. She could read and write. For a day or two a popular means of communication was note writing. As the camp progressed, even the skeptics discovered that not a lot of oral communication is required to show a new camper how to build a fire or peel a potato. Most of the camp activities were naturally more visual than auditory. However, Mary's full participation in every activity was still not possible. She was polite but bored during the daily songfest. Also, there was nothing special that Mary was contributing to the camp—she was always the follower, never the leader. The leader then solved both problems by making Mary the chief trail blazer and sending her out along with a couple of other kids who did not like the music to lay a trail for the others to find and follow after the songfest each day. Mary with her years of experience in responding to subtle visual cues found ingenious ways of creating markers from the materials in the woods. Previously, trails had been marked with mundane and obvious rocks piled to form an arrow. Her trails provided clear but challenging subtle cues that led to the day's treasure. She was able to teach the other Scouts creative trail blazing and became a contributing member of the group instead of being just the deaf kid who managed to survive in a hearing daycamp.

Teach the Golden Rule—Especially to the Exceptional Child

If children with disabilities are to grow up to take their rightful places in the world "just like regular people," it is important that they learn to "do unto others as you would have them do unto you." Much is discussed in professional circles about the special needs of the exceptional child. There is perhaps too much emphasis on worrying about what we must do to help the "poor, unfortunate" devalued members of our society. On the one hand, it is not uncommon in classrooms for the child with a disability to be excused for whatever problems the child may create for others.

On the other hand, it is also not uncommon for teachers to complain about unacceptable aggressiveness, stating, for instance, "These kids think the world owes them a living just because they have a disability; they're obnoxious, demanding, and then cry 'prejudice' if people don't like them; I don't like the way they try to exploit other people." Of course, if such comments are made with reference to "all disabled people," they represent the same kind of stereotyping that occurs when disabled people as a group are labeled passive, pitiful, unfortunate people. Certainly some people who are disabled are overly aggressive and some are overly passive. Children are not born demanding or self-effacing. Throughout childhood, in home and school, they gradually learn to be considerate of others' needs and viewpoints as well as their own. The over-solicitous attitude of some adults toward people with disabilities may represent another form of devaluation—one that says that these people are too incompetent to be expected to behave like mature human beings. Whatever the motives, patting the child on the head or making excuses for his or her mistreatment of others deprives that child of the opportunity to learn important lessons that everyone needs to know.

These comments should not be interpreted to mean that a child should never express anger or make demands. All people can be as obnoxious as they want to be—so long as they are prepared to take the consequences. Sometimes, it becomes necessary for people to stand up for their rights in ways that irritate others. Whether considering situations in everyday living, or times of confrontation and dispute, disabled children are quite capable of learning and caring about how they affect others as well as how others affect them.

Failure Is Not a Sin

Nowhere is it written in stone, "Thou shalt not fail." Yet as adults, we try very hard to protect children from failure. Somehow, it becomes critical to some that a child with a disability enter only those situations in which success is guaranteed. Such a philosophy can impose more stress and more limitations than any physical disability ever could. Children are forever asking parents, "Can I do this or that?" and parents' answers are often guided more by their fear of failure than by more realistic considerations. The problem is compounded in disability cases, because it is often more difficult to predict how successful a child will be.

For example, the parents of a mentally retarded adolescent were upset when their son insisted that he wanted to drive a car. The parents did not want to be overprotective, but had grave misgivings about his ability to drive safely. They sought the advice of a psychologist, who thought that a retarded person should not be allowed to drive. The young man persisted in his pleas, so the parents took him for a second opinion and a more optimistic psychologist gave the parents a lecture on "normalization" and expressed confidence that he could drive. The parents still had misgivings and finally visited a third psychologist, who said, after patiently listening to all the pros and cons given by the first two, "Why not let him try? If he passes both the written and field portions of the driver's license test, let him drive."

A young woman, three feet tall, described how her parents helped her as she grew up as a dwarf. She was always asking them what she could do. "Can I climb up and get the cookies?" "Can I reach the water faucet?" "Can I get on the bus?" To thousands of questions, their answer was "Go ahead and try. That's the best way to find out." For her, the value was placed on trying—not necessarily on succeeding. For her, failure was not a personal catastrophe—it simply provided her with information to guide her future activities.

The same principle applies to all children. Many teachers ask students to put homework problems, in math for example, on the blackboard. Those who do not know how to do a problem or who have errors in their work frequently are criticized. In one class, however, the teacher made it clear that if the students already knew how to do algebra, they would not need to take the course. Putting homework problems on the board, errors and all, provided an opportunity to learn. When going through a problem, instead of commenting on the student's general bungling, or "dumb" mistakes, she would say things like, "Ah, there's your problem. Good, now I see what's confusing," or "Oh, you've got the basic idea all right. It's only a computation error." The students did not dread being called on and the achievement of the class was high.

One may wonder how trying and failing can be considered one of this chapter's happy psychological situations. First, it is possible to value oneself as a person who is willing to take a chance and discover one's own talents and limitations.

This view is an alternative to feeling like a worthwhile person only when successful. Second, it is fortunate that people who try a variety of activities are likely to succeed at some of them, and—to borrow a concept from behavior theory—find themselves on an intermittent schedule of reinforcement. Third, if someone keeps trying the same activity, the chances of improved skills may increase with more practice. Fourth, success and failure are not an all-or-none dichotomy. People often find that they enjoy an activity even though they are not highly skilled at it. For every outstanding major league ball player, there are thousands of less-able folks who enjoy a game of softball on a Sunday afternoon. Finally, people who value trying perhaps agree with the old adage, "Better to have loved and lost than never to have loved at all." Even if the young man had been unable to pass the driver's test (he did pass), he would have felt better than to have been denied the opportunity to try because he was retarded.

Summary of Happy Interventions

The above suggestions describe some ways in which helpers can aid in changing common distressing psychological situations frequently encountered by children with disabilities into happy psychological situations. Children reared in environments where there are many acceptable ways to reach a goal, where it is permissible to talk about one's weaknesses as well as strengths, where adults set reasonable rules, and where people refrain from verbally abusing one another and learn to cooperate, to give and receive help freely, to share responsibility, to respect each others' rights and needs, and to value trying more than succeeding are likely to thrive psychologically, even though their physical bodies may be less than perfect.

SUMMARY

Following the tenets of Kurt Lewin's field theory, this chapter has attempted to show that crisis or stress cannot be defined in terms of objective environmental events or physical characteristics of a person. Instead, stress occurs when a person is in a distressing psychological situation and is ameliorated when the person's psychological situation changes to a happy one. Specific suggestions have been made about how these theoretical concepts can be applied to help better the lives of children with physical disabilities.

REFERENCES

Barker, R. G., Wright, B. A., Meyerson, L., & Gonick, M. R. (1953). *Adjustment to physical handicap: A survey of the social psychology of physique and disability.* New York: Social Science Research Council.

Beckman-Bell, P. (1981). Child related stress in families of handicapped children. *Topics in Early Childhood Special Education, 1,* 45–53.

Bedell, J. R., Giordani, B., Amour, J. L., Tavormina, J., & Boll, T. (1977). Life stress and the psychological and medical adjustment of chronically ill children. *Journal of Psychosomatic Research, 21,* 237–242.

Bradshaw, J., & Lawton, D. (1978). Tracing the causes of stress in families with handicapped children. *British Journal of Social Work, 8,* 181–192.

Dembo, T., Leviton, G., & Wright, B. (1975). Adjustment to misfortune: A problem of social psychological rehabilitation. *Rehabilitation Psychology, 22,* iii–100.

Friedrich, W. N., & Friedrich, W. L. (1981). Psychosocial assets of parents of handicapped and nonhandicapped children. *American Journal of Mental Deficiency, 85,* 551–553.

Galdston, R., & Gamble, W. J. (1969). On borrowed time: Observations on children with implanted cardiac pacemakers and their families. *American Journal of Psychiatry, 126,* 104–108.

Geist, R. A. (1979). Onset of chronic illness in children and adolescents: Psychotherapeutic and consultative interventions. *American Journal of Orthopsychiatry, 49,* 4–23.

Gogan, J., Koocher, G. R., Foster, D. J., & O'Malley, J. E. (1977). Impact of childhood cancer on siblings. *Health and Social Work, 2,* 42–57.

Kalnins, I. B., Churchill, M. P., & Terry, G. E. (1980). Concurrent stresses in families with a leukemic child. *Journal of Pediatric Psychology, 5,* 81–92.

Katz, E. R., Kellerman, J., & Siegel, S. E. (1980). Behavioral distress in children with cancer undergoing medical procedures: Developmental considerations. *Journal of Consulting and Clinical Psychology, 48,* 356–365.

Kerr, N. (1976). Field theory and behavior modification in rehabilitation: Tools for twin tasks. *Rehabiliation Psychology, 23,* 97–108.

Ladieu, G., Hanfmann, E., & Dembo, T. (1947). Studies in adjustment to visible injury: Evaluation of help by the injured. *Journal of Abnormal and Social Psychology, 42,* 169–192.

Lewin, K. (1935). *A dynamic theory of personality: Selected papers.* New York: McGraw-Hill.

Lloyd, J. (Ed.) (1983, December). Parent's corner. *Special Education Today,* p. 7.

Meyerson, L. (1955; 1971). Somatopsychology of physical disability. In W. Cruikshank (Ed.), *Psychology of exceptional children and youth.* Englewood Cliffs, NJ: Prentice-Hall.

Meyerson, L., & Kerr, N. (1979). Research strategies for meaningful rehabilitation research. *Rehabilitation Psychology, 26,* 228–238.

O'Brien, R. (1975). Early childhood services for visually impaired children: A model program. *New Outlook for the Blind, 69,* 201–204.

Parks, R. M. (1977). Parents' reactions to the birth of a handicapped child. *Health and Social Work, 2,* 51–66.

Spink, D. (1976). Crisis intervention for parents of the deaf child. *Health and Social Work, 1,* 140–160.

Tavormina, J. B., Boll, T. J., Dunn, N. J., Luscomb, R. L., & Taylor, J. R. (1981). Psychosocial effects on parents of raising a physically handicapped child. *Journal of Abnormal Child Psychology, 9,* 121–131.

Tyler, N. B., & Kogan, K. L. (1977). Reduction of stress between mothers and their handicapped children. *American Journal of Occupational Therapy, 31,* 151–155.

Wright, B. A. (1983). *Physical disability: A psychosocial approach.* New York: Harper & Row.

11

Effects of the Holocaust on Survivors and Their Families

Norman Goldwasser
Virginia Commonwealth University

THE CHILDREN OF SURVIVORS PLEDGE

With love and respect, we pay tribute to the miracle of your survival. The term "survivors" does not do you justice. You did more than just survive. You resisted the Nazi Final Solution both spiritually and physically. Battered by war, you built new lives for yourselves in an unfamiliar land. And when it may have been reasonable to surrender to life's hardships, you brought forth a new generation of Jewish sons and daughters. Our very existence is proof of your faith and courage. We pledge to commit our lives to actions that flow from your memories. We vow to join together in local and international groups of Children of Survivors, to carry on the responsibility of remembering.

David Kupfer,
Co-Chairman, Yom Hashoah
Tidewater Children
of Holocaust Survivors

The Holocaust of World War II was undoubtedly one of the darkest periods in the history of mankind. Six million Jews were killed, millions of non-Jews perished, and many of those who lived to tell the unspeakable horrors of their experiences are now, 40 years after their liberation, still affected by the scars and the nightmares of the war. The following is an effort to gain a better understanding of the Holocaust survivor family, with emphasis placed on the psychopathology that seems to be common among survivors and their children. Following a brief introduction that includes a historical perspective of the Jews' experiences during the war, a description of the symptomatology that is common in what has been referred to as the "concentration camp syndrome" will be presented. Psychological and political issues related to the survivors' postwar experience will be discussed, as will issues concerning psychotherapy with survivors. Then, the cross-generational effects of the Holocaust will be examined in terms of how the children of these survivors are being affected by their parents' trauma and postwar behavior.

INTRODUCTION

As in the United States, which was experiencing a period of prosperity during the "Roaring 20s," Germany was also in the midst of an economic and political high point when it was suddenly thrust into a deep depression. Life had become

227

quite bitter for Germans who had become accustomed to "the good life," and they eagerly sought out strong leadership that would lift their country out of its misery. Adolf Hitler gave Germans pride and some desperately needed hope for the future. He also provided them with a reason for their economic woes by singling out the Jews of Germany as the culprits. Jews were prominent politically and in some areas economically in pre-Depression Germany, and were a natural target for a German people hungry for a scapegoat. With Hitler's rise to power came increasingly harsh restrictions for German Jews. They were removed from all public offices and were boycotted in the business world. No effort was made to protect the rights of Jews, and in fact it was apparent that the government was directly responsible for these actions.

On November 7, 1938, in response to the assassination of a German official in Paris by a crazed Jew, a wave of violence and destruction erupted against Jewish businesses, homes, and places of worship throughout Germany on a night that is now referred to as "Kristalnacht" or "The Night of the Broken Glass." Jews throughout the now-expanded Nazi Germany were arrested, taken from their homes, and deported to concentration camps. When they arrived, they faced a German official, usually a physician, who selected them for either a hard labor camp or immediate extermination. Families were mercilessly separated as young men and women who were chosen for labor watched helplessly as their parents sisters, brothers, and even children were taken away, never to be seen again.

Life in the camps was unbearable, to say the least. Prisoners were severely malnourished, poorly dressed, and were forced to work 16 to 20 hours a day. Those who did not succumb to the extreme somatic stress and pain suffered emotionally as they watched campmates die. What was worse than the torture was the uncertainty of what was to happen next. The total lack of control and knowledge about the future paralyzed some with fear, whereas others found some meaning in the madness of the camps and faced the future day by day (Frankl, 1962). People suddenly found themselves in a situation of utter helplessness and despair. The world inside the camp, its values and stimuli, had no connection to any reality outside of it. The indescribable conditions in which the prisoners lived was a persistent source of physical and psychological stress. The stench of burning flesh from nearby crematoria was almost continual, and most prisoners wondered when it would be their turn.

Toward the end of the war, the Nazis retreated, and prisoners were taken on death marches that would last in some cases for weeks with little or no food and rest. Any prisoner that would sway from the road or away from the group would be shot on the spot. Several marches ended with mass shooting in ditches along the road after weeks of marching. Other inmates in camps closer to Germany remained in the camps until the war was actually over, after which they were liberated by Allied soldiers. Nearly dead, they were brought to Displaced Persons (DP) camps from where they would eventually be resettled in countries such as England, France, Canada, Argentina, the U. S., and Israel.

Many survivors were fiercely intent on putting their horrible past behind them and immediately began to rebuild their lives in their new countries. Some worked in factories while others started small businesses. Others, however, were unable to function adequately—the scars were too deep. They were experiencing the "concentration camp syndrome," a constellation of psychopathological symptoms that resulted from their prolonged trauma. Although those who had poured themselves into rebuilding their lives had functioned relatively well during the early postwar years, they too began to experience similar aftereffects of their wartime experiences.

SYMPTOMATOLOGY OF THE CONCENTRATION CAMP SYNDROME

Eitinger (1972) studied a large group of Holocaust survivors and found that many cognitive, behavioral, psychological, and social problems were common among these individuals. As opposed to those who spent the years during World War II in hiding or serving in the military, these survivors were all concentration camp prisoners. Most of them experienced significant fatigue, restlessness, irritability, and nervousness. Many had difficulty retrieving both short-term and long-term material and had problems in concentration as well. Psychopathology symptoms including dysphoria, mood disorders, anxiety, and phobias were commonly seen, as were feelings of insufficiency and lack of initiative. Heightened suspiciousness and paranoia often resulted in social withdrawal and subsequent isolation. Pathological expressions of mourning related to survival guilt also prevented many of the survivors from functioning effectively. Finally, environmental stimuli such as an image or symbol reminiscent of the camps (i.e., barbed wire, smokestacks, trains, German shepherds, etc.) would elicit sudden flashbacks, resulting in panic and severe anxiety.

The regularity with which these symptoms seemed to occur among the subjects of this study was striking. Consequently, the use of the term *syndrome* to describe this phenomenon was justified on the basis of the consistency and universality of the constellation of symptoms. Numerous other investigators have found similar commonalities in the symptomatology of concentration camp survivors (Chodoff, 1970; Luchterhand, 1970; Niederland, 1961).

A question that was raised by Nathan, Eitinger, and Winnik (1964) challenged the uniqueness of the survivor. Specifically, they proposed that any form of extreme stress could produce the same effects as described above, and that the concentration camp experience per se is not unique. To test this hypothesis, they compared two groups of survivors, one of which was interned in German camps and the other consisting of individuals who spent the war years either hiding from the Nazis or in Soviet detention centers. The two groups were fairly comparable in terms of age, prewar socioecnomic and cultural backgrounds, and postwar experiences (e.g., DP camps, emigration to Israel). The results showed that the concentration camp group showed more prolonged, chronic CCS cases than did the noncamp group, and that the camp survivors had significantly more atypical disorders as well as chronic depressive and anxiety disorders. They also had more social and family disturbances, and less paranoid and psychotic disturbances than their noncamp counterparts. Thus, it was demonstrated that CCS did represent a distinct phenomenon different from the disorders found in other survivors.

Another issue raised by Eitinger (1972) concerned differences in the effects of incarceration upon camp survivors of different religions or nationalities, and for whom the circumstances leading up to internment were different. Specifically, it was noted that non-Jewish Norwegian survivors suffered more neurological and physiological damage than Jewish survivors, for whom psychological damage seemed more prominent. The author noted that non-Jewish camp inmates were primarily political prisoners, usually arrested for resistance, treason, or smuggling. Their hardships consisted primarily of torture during interrogations, resulting in head trauma, and severe malnutrition and recurrent somatic diseases. Obviously, the mental stresses to which they were subjected were severe, but compared to the continual threat of death that faced the Jewish prisoners, their degree of traumatization was relatively moderate.

Klein (1973, 1981) also compared the post-war level of adjustment of Jewish survivors in Israel and in the U. S., and observed that those who emigrated to Israel after the war seemed to have less severe psychopathology and were better assimilated into their new culture than their American survivor counterparts. It was noted that although this may be due, to some extent, to the sheer numbers of survivors that made their way to Israel, another factor may have been that the new nation of Israel provided many opportunities for survivors to feel like productive, valuable citizens, and helped to give meaning to their suffering. Sociopolitical factors such as community life in the kibbutz, Holocaust memorials, and national days of remembrance were all seen as important in facilitating the reintegration of psychic structure in Israeli survivors. In contrast, those who came to the U. S. were treated more as refugees and were given less opportunities to feel useful and productive, thus opening the door for the development of psychopathology. However, these were purely observations on the part of the author; no empirical research has been done to validate these cross-cultural differences.

PSYCHOTHERAPY WITH SURVIVORS

Despite the severity of their symptoms, survivors suffering from CCS are generally reluctant to seek help from a therapist. Various reasons have been offered to explain this phenomenon. First, West German reparation agreements do not provide funds for psychological treatment, only for the treatment of physical illnesses related to their internment. This is in accord with the argument set forth by the German government following World War II that a normal, healthy person can adequately manage severe stress. Thus, any person requiring psychotherapy, according to this view, was never healthy or normal. This restriction often serves as a deterrent in keeping a survivor from seeking help from a psychologist or psychiatrist, especially since there is the fear that their restitution payments would be jeopardized should an attempt be made to undergo therapy (Chodoff, 1980).

Klein, Zellermayer, & Sharan (1963) noted that by becoming a psychiatric patient, a survivor is deprived of his or her unique status as a heroic witness or brave survivor of the Holocaust, only to become a "mental patient." This preservation of self-concept often prevents a severely maladjusted individual from receiving much-needed help. Chodoff (1970) also suggested that psychiatrists are often reluctant to undertake cases involving survivors because of the difficulties that they inevitably encounter. Furthermore, an assumption that is present among psychoanalytically oriented therapists is that the etiology of all psychopathology can be traced to intrapsychic crises in early childhood. These cases do not fit easily into such a theoretical model. For a survivor whose life was nearly destroyed in his or her late teens or early 20s, it indeed seems futile to focus solely on what was experienced at age 5.

For those who do seek treatment, the obstacles inherent in such a difficult therapeutic encounter are innumerable. Trautman (1971) maintains that, in spite of all efforts to achieve a therapeutic effect, alleviation of a patient's suffering is nearly impossible because a "survivor cannot forgive or forget" (p. 125). This is to imply that such anger, guilt, and profound feelings of loss cannot simply be talked through and alleviated. Furthermore, survivors tend to view the therapist as an authority figure and thereby create complex transference issues that complicate the therapeutic process (Chodoff, 1980). Depending on their style of coping in the camps, survivors may be passive-aggressive, overly compliant, withdrawn, or completely resistant to the therapist and to his or her efforts to establish rapport and a therapeutic relationship.

Klein et al. (1963) found that disturbances in survivors are so severe that they can only be dealt with through an intense, long-term psychotherapeutic process, often on an inpatient basis. In addition, Klein et al. maintain that therapists should accept limited objectives with survivors because of their delicate psyches and that the emphasis in therapy should be on strengthening defenses to facilitate functioning, rather than on analyzing them. Although these seem to be sound recommendations, no data are presented to support their validity. Chodoff (1980) explains this emphasis on the strengthening of defenses and limited objectives by maintaining that the effects of persecution, especially in younger persons, may be nearly irreversible, because the psychological and physical deprivation may have disrupted normal maturation to a point of no return. Even without the tragic losses, unspeakable atrocities, and brutalities, the survivor suffered interference in nurturance, companionship, and education, and was instead immersed in an atmosphere of fear and suspicion rather than one of trust. This is often referred to as the "missed adolescence syndrome"; crucial formative years spent this way would likely result in maladaptive behavior patterns so inextricably bound into the personality structure that, in later years, psychotherapy could be expected to have only limited impact.

COMMON ISSUES IN PSYCHOTHERAPY WITH SURVIVORS

Distrust

The initial goal of most models analyzing the therapeutic process is the development of rapport or the initial "hooking stage." To achieve this goal, however, the individual must be willing and able to trust. The experiences of survivors during the war had a shattering effect on whatever degree of trust they had beforehand. Thus, an initial goal of therapy may be to facilitate the development of trust and to help the individual feel a sense of intimacy with another person—an ability that many survivors completely lost as a result of the war. Although the issue of trust and rapport must be dealt with initially, it may continue to be an issue throughout therapy, regardless of the quality of the initial rapport that had been established.

Guilt

A particularly strong element influencing the behavior of survivors is the pervasive feeling of guilt. This guilt could be a result of actual behavior or actions that were done for the sake of survival, such as the "kapos" who were selected by the

Nazis to oversee their fellow inmates. Most who experience guilt, however, relate it to more existential factors; the feeling of having survived when so many others were lost, most of whom were, in the minds of the survivors, more worthy and deserving of life than they were. Regardless of the etiology of guilt, its behavioral and emotional ramifications often prove to be an intractable problem in psychotherapy. It is the contention of many that the best way of dealing with guilt is to help the individual to understand his feelings and learn to live with them, rather than to try to change something that may be unalterable (Chodoff, 1980).

Body Image

The ability to feel comfortable and at ease with one's body was often severely challenged by the disturbances of body image that took place in the camps. This was primarily due to the devastating effects of severe malnutrition, but also to bodily changes from illness and injury. Such body image disturbances may have a profound and longlasting effect on the individual's ability to function, as well as his or her personality structure. Powers (1983) has suggested that the use of Gestalt techniques can help women who have lost dramatic amounts of weight to cope with and understand the changes that have taken place in their body image. This method may be useful in therapy with survivors for whom body image disturbances presents as a problem.

Culture Shock

Many survivors were born and raised in small Eastern European villages where strict adherence to religious and social values was emphasized. Most of the survivors, except for those who were from the larger German cities, were from rural, backward areas where the lifestyle was basic and simple. When, after liberation, the survivors found themsevles resettled in large metropolitan areas such as New York, Montreal, and Buenos Aires, the culture shock was nearly universal. The value systems and the religious frameworks around which their lives had been centered were no longer adaptive in the more open Western world. Further, they were totally unprepared to deal with the fast pace of the inner city and the crowded conditions. For some, the severe effects of this culture shock prevented them from healthily adjusting and assimilating into their new environments. Many fiercely resisted any attempts to change their lifestyle, whereas others could not change fast enough in an effort to completely Americanize themselves. Both reactions to the culture shock were maladaptive, as the former individuals were attempting to disassociate themselves from the realities of the present, whereas the latter individuals were trying to cut themselves off from the harsh realities of the past.

Countertransference

Therapists who attempt to treat survivors must be prepared to come to terms with profound and disturbing emotional reactions in themselves. Feelings of horror and disgust in response to the almost unbearable stories of torture and persecution are not uncommon. Thus, countertransferences that interfere with the empathy and understanding that is so crucial to the therapeutic relationship are especially likely to occur in cases as emotionally charged as these.

Dimsdale (1980) suggested that guilt is almost omnipresent in these situations as the therapist tends to feel guilty for not having been subjected to the brutalities that the survivor was forced to endure. Indeed, it is not difficult to imagine the enormous guilt that would arise as a therapist compares her or his activities and whereabouts during the war to those of the survivor client: college football games, high school, family vacations, and so on. He further states that a failure to surmount these countertransferences makes an already difficult situation an impossible one. He feels that in order to offer a survivor the most hopeful possibility of productive change, the therapist must not only be aware of and control these reactions, but also be able to provide an emotional atmosphere with a delicate balance of firmness and consistency in addition to empathy and compassion.

CHILDREN OF SURVIVORS: CROSS-GENERATIONAL EFFECTS OF THE HOLOCAUST

Although the understanding and treatment of Holocaust survivors remains a matter of vital importance today, there appears to be a definite shift in the focus of Holocaust literature toward its effects on the children of survivors. The severe deprivation and trauma experienced by survivors may have caused sufficient psychological and physical dysfunction to render them incapable of providing the emotional fortitude and insight that is necessary for the healthy upbringing of a child. Much research has attempted to investigate whether trauma-produced alterations in parental behavior had psychopathological consequences for their children. It was Trossman's (1968) opinion that children of survivors must be adversely affected by their parents' chronic anxiety, depression, and somatization. He described several types of disordered parent-child interactions, which he posited as being the underlying factors involved in the psychological problems he encountered with survivor families at the McGill Mental Health Clinic in Montreal. The first pattern was characterized by excessively overprotective parents, resulting in moderately phobic children or those locked in with their parents. The next problematic family situation was depicted as one in which children had often become an involuntary audience to their parents' relentless recounting of their horrible experiences, resulting in depressive pathology and feelings of guilt in these children. A third type of interaction involved parents who responded with anger and suspicion to the Gentile world and who expected their children to do so as well. Their children either rebelled against their parents' paranoia or become equally mistrustful. Another pattern, which Trossman describes as the most deleterious, is one in which children were pressured to provide meaning for their parents' empty lives and to redeem their past suffering. Their parents place unrealistic demands upon them causing many to either "give up in despair or seethingly rebel" (p. 122).

As opposed to what has appeared to be a clear-cut, uniform "survivor syndrome" in first-generation survivors, Simitis (1981) noted that the clinical picture in the second generation appears to be more diverse and less prevalent. She suggested that the traumatic experiences of survivor parents had an effect on the psyches of their children as a "cumulative trauma." It was proposed that the existence and severity of psychopathology in the children was directly propor-

tionate to the extent of traumatization of their parents during the war. A prominent variable that was mentioned as being especially associated with pathology
in the children were parents who were both survivors of extermination camps and
had lost children in the Holocaust. Another significant variable was the parents'
inability to discuss their experiences with their children without excessive emotionality or alternatively blunting of affect.

Freyberg (1980) identifies conflicts in the rapprochement stage in the development of a survivor child as a key factor in later intrapsychic impediments in
developing autonomy. In this critical period during which strong impulses towards
exploration and self-initiated action emerge in the child, the mother's love, support,
and encouragement are crucial for the normal development of autonomy. This
process of becoming autonomous becomes impaired when the survivor mother,
who is depressed, grieving, and withdrawn, is unable to give the child the desired
support. A further impediment in the child's progress toward autonomy is that
the child's striving for independence as well as her or his anger over the mother's
withdrawal of love are threatening to the survivor mother who has already suffered
innumerable losses. The result in later years is an adult filled with anger, with weak
ego boundaries, and a poorly differentiated sense of identity.

Axelrod, Schnipper, and Rau (1980) suggested that the size of the extended
survivor family is negatively correlated with degree of pathology in the children.
Additionally, as a result of studying female inpatient children of survivors, support
was found for the "anniversary hypothesis"; a relationship seemed to exist between
the age of many of the children upon admission and their parents' age when
interned or age when they experienced a highly significant trauma during the war.
This phenomenon, however, needs further analysis before any conclusions can be
made.

More empirically based studies using control groups have been designed to
determine whether different stressful circumstances would produce distorted
family relationships and ultimately a common set of behavior disorders among
the children. DeGraaf (1975), cited in Solkoff (1981) attempted to separate the
direct effects of having lost relatives, but without having been in a camp, in
determining whether these experiences differentially affected the survivors'
children. From a sample that had been referred to a military outpatient clinic
in Israel, three groups of soldiers, both male and female, were delineated. One
consisted of those whose parents survived the camps or spent at least a year in a
ghetto during World War II. A second consisted of those whose parents lost relatives
but themselves were not victims of Nazi persecution, having emigrated to Palestine
before the war. The parents of the men and women in the third group were neither
Holocaust survivors nor had they lost any close relatives.

Open-ended interviews yielded ratings on 26 symptoms clustered into five
categories. neurotic traits, depressive syndrome, maladjustment, personality
disturbances, and delinquent traits. Soldiers in the second group were found to be
significantly more neurotic with a higher incidence of psychosis than the other
two groups. The first group had significantly more personality disturbances and
delinquent traits. These results are not consistent with the hypothesis that extent
of parental trauma is associated with degree and extent of psychopathology.
However, as Solkoff (1981) noted, the study was replete with methodological flaws
that seem to represent most of the literature in the area. First, there was no
evidence of standardization in the interview procedure and apparently parents were

present for only some of the interviews. Second, the author failed to recognize the sampling bias that was produced from selection of the sample from a clinical population. Third, the assumption that amount of time spent in the camps or the extent of traumatic experiences is not a relevant factor in evaluating overall trauma, has never been justified, and may, in fact, be totally invalid.

Another controlled study carried out in Canada by Sigal, Silver, Rakoff, and Ellin (1973) found that survivor children were significantly more disturbed on measures of psychological functioning such as Nettler's Alienation Scale (1957), modified versions of the Cornell Medical Index and the Anomia Scale (Srole, 1956), and the Behavior Problem Checklist. However, the sampling bias described above as well as the inappropriateness of the measures for the population and poor controls limit the meaningfulness of the results.

In a more recent study, Leon, Butcher, Kleinman, Goldberg, and Almagor (1981) compared the psychological adjustment of Holocaust survivors and their children with a control group of similar European and religious backgrounds. Despite the severe psychological and physical trauma suffered during the war, there was no significant psychopathology in either parent or child survivor groups. This study was significant in that it utilized a nonclinical sample solicited through the refugee files of Jewish agencies, rather than from families seeking treatment.

There were few Minnesota Multiphasic Personality Inventory (MMPI) or Mental Health Ratings differences between survivor and control parents, with the exception of increased endorsement of items involving somatic problems such as dizziness and fainting spells. The MMPI profiles of the survivor and control children were both within normal range and were not significantly different from one another. In addition, both groups of children reported general closeness and a sense of openness with their feelings. These results do not seem to support previous findings of prevalent psychopathology among survivor families (e.g., Bettelheim, 1960; Eitinger, 1961). In contrast to the survivors in these studies, the survivors evaluated by Leon et al. (1981) had been able to cope with the terrible experiences that they endured, and were able to lead productive lives and raise psychologically healthy children.

Despite the fact that this study stands out by its use of nonclinical subjects and multiple measures of psychological functioning, the results must be viewed in light of the obvious nonrepresentativeness of the sample. Almost 50 percent of those contacted refused to participate in the study; the possibility clearly exists that those who did agree were generally more psychologically well adjusted than those who refused. Thus, the authors' conclusion that their findings "clearly indicate that concentration camp and other survivors of World War II and their children as a group do not manifest serious psychological impairment" (p. 514) must be tempered in light of the above noted sampling problem. The findings do show, however, that severe psychopathology is not an inevitable consequence of Holocaust-related trauma, either for victims or their children.

Solkoff (1981), in his review of the literature on children of the Holocaust, admonishes researchers in the area to attend to the fundamental canons of a proper experimental design, which have indeed been neglected in most of the studies conducted thus far. He lists four factors that must be incorporated in future research: (*a*) carefully selected samples that are more representative of the population about which generalizations are being made; (*b*) carefully selected control groups that are properly matched with experimental groups on those variables that could produce differences in pathology; (c) descriptions of intrafamilial interactions, including both healthy and psychological impaired children; and (d) samples that are more fully described to facilitate replication. Data on variables such as age of parents when incarcerated, pretrauma cultural and psychological backgrounds of parents, types of camps in which parents were incarcerated, and immediate postrauma experiences of each parent should be collected and evaluated as possible moderators of obtained relationships.

SYMPTOMATOLOGY COMMON IN CHILDREN OF SURVIVORS

Although there seem to be commonalities in the psychopathology found in children of survivors, the lack of consistency and universality of the symptomatology precludes its classification as a syndrome per se. However, several symtoms have been found to be prevalent among children of survivors.

Guilt

Perhaps the most profound and universal symptoms among children of survivors is guilt. Wanderman (1975) identified the etiology of this guilt as arising from the expectation on the part of the survivors that the world, including their families, should make up for their enormous losses. Survivors tend to feel at some level that they have suffered enough and that they have a right to expect that the rest of their lives should be comfortable and free of problems. Implicit in this expectation is an attitude that expects and often demands perfection from those around them, especially their children.

Children of survivors often acutely feel this pressure to live up to their parents' unrealistic expectations of them. They may respond to this pressure in one of several ways (Barocas & Barocas, 1980). They may internalize the need to always be perfect—to never make mistakes or be "human"—and consequently be highly anxious, perfectionistic, and achievement oriented. Resentful of the pressure to compensate for the losses that their parents sustained, they may adopt a passive-aggressive style in interacting with their parents. They may also openly express their resentment and rebel against these expectation, as well as their parents. Regardless of how they respond, they still carry a huge burden of guilt; either because of their internal resentment ("How can I be mad at my parents after they've been through so much?") or because of their open defiance ("How can I rebel against my parents and cause them so much pain?").

Inability to Individuate

A significant problem that often occurs in survivor children is an inability to individuate and establish themselves apart from their families (Russell, 1980). Sigal et al. (1973) cite parental expectations of their children to give meaning to their otherwise empty and destroyed lives as the underlying mechanism of this problem. Since all of their own personal hopes and dreams are unattainable because of their shattered and irretrievable losses, survivors tend to funnel these wishes and needs for achievement into their children. Thus, a child of survivors may not be treated as an individual, but rather as a symbol of what the parents lack in their own lives, and what they hopeto attain through that child.

Barocas and Barocas (1973) explain the phenomenon as the parents' attempt to obtain their own identification through their children. By using their offspring as their extensions, the parents satisfy their own needs, which were never met by their parents. By doing so, however, they fail to allow their children to seek and explore their own needs, wishes, and dreams. As a consequence to parents' reliance on their children for dream fulfillment, children become overvalued and treated as precious objects. Parental fear of loss and separation anxiety only serve to accentuate this problem, and maintains the overprotective and restrictive rearing of their children, which is so common in survivor families. Consequently, survivor children tend to feel "swallowed up" by their parents' overnurturance and control of their lives. In the study by Sigal et al. (1973), children often presented with school problems, severe depression, and loss of control. The buildup of hostility that was present as a result of being overcontrolled seemed to manifest itself, according to the authors, in periodic impulses of aggression often directed at parents or parental figures.

Interpersonal Difficulties

Another problem that is common in survivor families is sibling quarreling and hostility. Sigal et al. (1973) interpreted this problem as being a result of the children being unable to express the anger that they feel toward their parents. Instead, they displace their anger and direct it toward the nearest person(s) around them, which are often their siblings. Steinitz and Szronyi (1975), however, maintain that the impoverished psychological resources of survivor parents tend to result in children whose needs are not met. Their personality structures, therefore, are predisposed to being unable to get along with others, especially those closest to them.

In social situations, children of survivors may be extremely introverted and completely withdrawn. Those who identify with their parents' distrust of the world and their fears and anxieties are equally suspicious of others and tend to be interpersonally ineffective. Many suffer from poor self-images and ambivalent feelings about being Jewish (Russell, 1980). Children of survivors, especially in the U. S., inevitably feel different because their parents are worlds apart from those of their peers. As opposed to their American friends, they usually have very small families, no grandparents, and parents who tend to only associate with other Europeans. Hence, these children grow up feeling isolated and different, especially in communities without large populations of survivor families.

INTERVENTION WITH SURVIVOR CHILDREN

The literature on psychotherapy with children of survivors is not as extensive as that dealing with their parents, primarily because the shift of attention has only recently begun to focus on the problems that they face. However, those authors that address this issue generally recommend some form of family therapy for survivor families. Since the primary goal of the family therapy approach is to initiate or improve lines of communication among family members (Haley, 1971), a therapeutic strategy that encourages healthy dialogue between parents and children may, indeed, be the treatment of choice. This is because many authors stress the importance of parents communicating their experiences to their children in an appropriate and nonfrightening manner (Russell, 1980; Krell, 1979, 1982).

Krell (1982) maintained that the high failure rates with children of survivors may be due to the lack of involvement of parents in therapy. Acknowledging the often intense resistance of survivor parents to involvement in their child's treatment, Krell suggests that in order to establish trust and rapport, parents be involved as collaborators in treatment, rather than patients. Children's reluctance to initiate psychotherapy was discussed, as well and attributed either to their failure to relate their problems with their parents' experiences during the Holocaust or their view of psychotherapy as being authoritarian, with expectations of being labeled or punished. Furthermore, Krell suggested that modifications of traditional psychotherapeutic approaches need to be developed for children of survivors in view of these therapeutic obstacles.

Such a modification has been suggested by this author. He has found a therapeutic strategy similar to the guided imagery described by Rimm and Masters (1979) to be helpful in alleviating problems such as isolation and difficulties with individuation. Through the use of relaxation and guided imagery, the therapist sends clients back to their families of origin, real or symbolic, in their European towns. They are encouraged to visualize and describe how their relatives may appear and to communicate with them verbally or nonverbally. The aim is to help the individual to go beyond the diminished immediate family in order to reduce their sense of isolation and dependence on their parents in establishing an identity. Research, however, remains to be done to evaluate this strategy's effectiveness and utility.

Many others have stressed the importance of the children of survivors' learning to differentiate between fantasies of what may have happened to their parents and what, in fact, did happen, especially in homes where parents were reluctant to communicate their experiences (e.g., Simitis, 1981; Axelrod et al., 1980; Newman, 1979). Thus, opening the lines of communication through family therapy may help the children to accurately understand their parents' experiences and to put them in their proper perspective. Davidson (1980) felt that a family approach is best because it reduces resistance generated by the parents' fear that their children will be taken away from them through therapy.

Therapy or self-help children of survivor groups have been started in major Jewish communities through the U. S., either as autonomous entities or through the auspices of a Jewish social agency. These groups attempt to utilize the therapeutic benefits of a group to facilitate cohesion, reduced isolation, and support among members. The effects of such groups on the functioning of participants has been evaluated in several studies. Fogelman and Savran (1979) organized nine groups of "well-functioning" Jewish children of survivors that were recruited through public advertisements. After an initial screening, groups were formed with individuals of different social and religious backgrounds, but whose parents had similar war experiences. The groups were time limited, and focused on content rather than process. According to the authors, this was due somewhat to their own anxiety and loss of objectivity as children of survivors in previous groups that they had led. They discussed common concerns of group members, the most common of which was a feeling of being scarred and different. Many had identity problems about being Jewish and were frequently conflicted about whether or not they wanted to hear about their parents' experiences. Another frequently stated feeling was guilt over the anger they felt towards their parents.

Danieli (1981) described several types of groups that were offered as part of the Group Project for Holocaust survivors and their children, initiated in 1975. She observed that participation in these groups, which included "awareness groups" and self-help, long-term therapy, and multifamily group approaches, seemed to reduce the isolation experienced by the members. For both parents and children, the groups provided new extended that are so often yearned for by those whose families were destroyed as a result of the Holocaust.

Trachtenberg and Davis (1978) used a support group of 4 men and 4 women between 24 and 31 years old, who met for 2 hours a week for 10 months to illustrate the concerns of children of survivors. Prominent themes included: vindication of parents' suffering, intrapunitiveness, blocked autonomy, depression, high need achievement, and communication problems with parents.

The authors noted that adolescence seemed to be a particularly difficult time for children of survivors, and suggested that this was so because it was the time of life that corresponded to their parents' traumatization. However, no mention was made of the fact that adolescence also happens to be the developmental stage in which issues of independence, autonomy, and control are significant, all of which are problematic in survivor families.

Kinsler (1981) described group psychotherapy that allowed children of survivors to share experiences and help each other to cope with the problems that they face. The format was semieducational, borrowing heavily from Family Life Education concepts, and later developing in an actual therapy group. Leary (1984) presented various themes that permeated her therapy groups with children of survivors. Group members tended to desire symbiosis and nurturance from other members. This was interpreted as their efforts to create the extended family that they never had. An important goal of these groups was to transform the shame and guilt that the members experienced into pride about their unique status as the second generation, and of being able to give their parents hope and a sense of meaning about their survival.

Finally, there have been recent objections over the literature's continuing emphasis on psychopathological characteristics of children of survivors, without any allusion to those who seem to have made satisfactory adjustment. It is no wonder that so many of these individuals have vociferously rejected the overgeneralized assertions and the overused and misapplied diagnostic labels of mental health professionals. It is true that most studies describe clinical samples, but still, their authors continue to commit a serious injustice to those children of survivors who have become productive, creative, and healthy individuals, by failing to include them as examples of prominent exceptions to the patient samples presented.

As a response to what many of them perceive as a gross overemphasis on pathology, children of survivors have joined together and organized national sociopolitical groups, an example of which is the International Network of Children of Jewish Holocaust Survivors which serves as their voice on political and social issues such as civil rights, Holocaust education in the schools, and the location and conviction of Nazi war criminals. These attempts at organizing themselves are efforts at going beyond the traditional focus on psychopathology and towards more productive endeavors.

CONCLUSION

It is generally accepted that because of their parents' past sufferings and mal-adaptive behaviors, children of survivors constitute a high-risk group for behavior disorders and are often in need of psychotherapeutic intervention. However, the literature on therapeutic strategies involving these individuals remains sparse, replete with speculation, and with little hard data presented. The importance of developing novel therapeutic strategies that take into consideration the unique characteristics of survivor families has not been sufficiently considered. Addition-ally, the recent emphasis on group interventions, despite their obvious salutory effects, may divert attention away from the study of equally important therapy process issues and individual differences between cases. Indeed, if the present dearth of case examples is indicative of the attempts at understanding survivors and their children as individuals instead of members of homogeneous groups, then the rapid shift towards groups may be at the expense of a deeper understand-ing of the individual survivor, child, or family unit.

In conclusion, those who are interested in furthering the study of the effects of the Holocaust can be involved in several areas of research that need to be developed. First, the scientific community still does not have a sufficiently clear understanding of the complex family dynamics and its diverse effects on children of survivors. Although attempts at classifying survivor families (e.g., Danieli, 1981) have been useful and informative, little has been done to explore therapeutic implications of a difference between families, as well as between individuals. Second, carefully delineated guidelines to assist clinicians in preparing for therapy with survivors and their families are needed to facilitate the therapeutic process. To this end, differences in cross-generation sequelae among children of survivors must be considered and treatment plans must be modified accordingly. Third, new therapeutic strategies with survivors and their families are desperately needed to circumvent the aforementioned difficulties that often arise. Finally, as children of survivors begin to raise families of their own, research on effects of their parents' experiences on their own children will have to be explored. It is with this topic that this chapter is concluded.

POSTSCRIPT: THE THIRD GENERATION

Since most children of survivors have reached adulthood and have begun to have children of their own, some authors are beginning to realize the importance of looking at the third generation. For example, Rosenthal and Rosenthal (1980) offered a case study of a seven-year-old male patient who developed symptoms similar to those of his grandmother, who had survived the Holocaust in hiding.

However, a more positive emphasis is beginning to emerge that focuses on helping grandchildren of survivors to understand their grandparents' experiences. Although Posner (1984) acknowledges the importance of educating all children, especially these youngsters, about the Holocaust and their unique family history, she stresses that the information shared should be appropriate to the child's level of development. For instance, younger children tend to ask broader questions such as "Did children die in the Holocaust?" Parents naturally tend to protect their children from the horrible truths of the survivors' experiences. However, it is crucial to encourage these questions and to answer them simply and honestly. Parents should also be aware of the vulnerability that such knowledge may create in small children, and be prepared to reassure them that what happened to their grandparents happened a long time ago and that they are safe now. As children grow older, their questions become more specific and personalized (i.e., "Was Grandpa in a concentration camp?"). Again, these questions should never be avoided, but instead answered straightforwardly and without anxiety or hesitation. Books such as *The Children We Remember* (Abells, 1983) and Klein's (1981) *Promise of a New Spring,* a symbolic presentation of the Holocaust, are recommended to initiate discussions with grandchildren of survivors in a nonthreatening manner that does not elicit the anxiety and tension that may normally accompany such an emotionally powered discussion.

REFERENCES

Abells, C. (1983). The children we remember. Rockville, MD: Kar-Ben Copies, Inc.

Axelrod, S., Schnipper, P., & Rau, J. (1980). Hospitalized offspring of Holocaust survivors. *Bulletin of the Menninger Clinic, 44,* 1-14.

Barocas, C., & Barocas, H. (1973). Manifestations of concentration camp effects on the second generation. *American Journal of Psychiatry, 130,* 821.

Barocas, H., & Barocas, C. (1980). Separation-individuation conflicts in children of Holocaust survivors. *Journal of Contemporary Psychotherapy, 11,* 6-14.

Bettelheim, B. (1960). *The informed threat.* Glencoe, IL: Free Press.

Chodoff, P. (1970). The German concentration camp as a psychological stressor. *Archives of General Psychiatry, 22,* 78-87.

Chodoff, P. (1980). Psychotherapy of the survivor. In J. Dimsdale (Ed.), *Survivors, victims, and perpetrators.* Washington, DC: Hemisphere.

Danieli, Y. (1981). Differing adaptational styles in families of survivors of the Nazi Holocaust. *Children Today, 10*(5), 6-10, 34-36.

Davidson, S. (1980). The clinical effects of massive psychic trauma in families of Holocaust survivors. *Journal of Marital and Family Therapy, 6,* 11-21.

DeGraaf, T. (1975). Pathological patterns of identification in families of survivors of the Holocaust. *Israel Annals of Psychiatry and Related Disciplines, 13,* 335-363.

Dimsdale, J. (1980). *Survivors, victims, and perpetrators.* Washington, DC: Hemisphere.

Eitinger, L. (1972). *Concentration camp survivors in Norway and Israel.* The Hague: Martinus Nijhoff.

Eitinger, L. (1961). Pathology of the concentration camp syndrome. *Archives of General Psychiatry, 5,* 374-377.

Fogelman, E., & Savran, B. (1979). Brief group therapy with offspring of Holocaust survivors: Leaders' reactions. *American Journal of Orthopsychiatry, 50,* 96-108.

Frankl, V. (1962). *Man's search for meaning.* Boston: Beacon Press.

Freyberg, J. T. (1980). Difficulties in separation-individuation as experienced by offspring of Nazi Holocaust survivors. *American Journal of Orthopsychiatry, 50*(1), 87-95.

Haley, J. (1971). (Ed.). *Changing families: A family therapy reader.* New York: Grune and Stratton.

Kinsler, F. (1981). Second-generation effects of the Holocaust: The effectiveness of group therapy in the resolution of the transmission of parental trauma. *Journal of Psychology and Judaism, 6,* 53-67.

Klein, G. (1981). *Promise of a new spring.* Chappaqua, NY: Rossel Books.

Klein, H. (1973). Children of the Holocaust. In E. J. Anthony & C. Koupernick (Eds.), *The child in his family: The international yearbook for child psychiatry and allied disciplines* (Vol. 1, pp. 393-409. Melbourne, FL: Krieger.

Klein, H., Zellermayer, J., & Sharan, J. (1963). Former concentration camp inmates on a psychiatric ward. *Archives of General Psychiatry, 8,* 334-342.

Krell, R. (1982). Family therapy with children of concentration camp survivors. *American Journal of Psychotherapy, 36,* 513-522.

Krell, R. (1979). Holocaust families: The survivors and their children. *Comprehensive Psychiatry, 20,* 560-568.

Leary, L. (1984). Presentation at First International Conference of Children of Holocaust Survivors, New York.

Leon, G. R., Butcher, J. N., Kleinman, M., Goldberg, A., & Almagor, M. (1981). Survivors of the Holocaust and their children: Current status and adjustment. *Journal of Personality and Social Psychology, 41,* 503–516.

Luchterhand, E. (1970). Early and late effects of imprisonment in Nazi concentration camps: Conflicting interpretations in survivors research. *Social Psychiatry, 5,* 102–110.

Nathan, T. S., Eitinger, L., & Winnik, H. Z. (1964). A psychiatric study of survivors of the Nazi Holocaust: A study of hospitalized patients. *Israel Annals of Psychiatry and Related Disciplines, 2,* 47–80.

Newman, L. (1979). Emotional disturbances in children of Holocaust survivors. *Social Casework: The Journal of Contemporary Social Work, 60,* 43–50.

Niederland, W. (1961). The psychiatric evaluation of emotional disorders in survivors of Nazi persecution. *Journal of the Hillside Hospital, 10,* 232–247.

Nettler, G. (1957). A measure of alienation. *American Sociological Review, 22,* 670–677.

Posner, S. (1984). Presentation at First International Conference of Children of Holocaust Survivors, New York.

Powers, P. (1983). Body image and weight loss. Unpublished doctoral dissertation, Virginia Commonwealth University, Richmond, VA.

Rimm, D. C., & Masters, J. C. (1979). *Behavior therapy: Techniques and empirical findings.* New York: Academic Press.

Rosenthal, P., & Rosenthal, S. (1980). Holocaust effect in the third generation: Child of another time. *American Journal of Psychotherapy, 34.* 572–580.

Russell, A. (1980). Late effects: Influence in the children of the concentration camp survivor. In J. Dimsdale (Ed.), *Survivors, victims, and perpetrators.* Washington, DC: Hemisphere.

Sigal, J. J., Silver, D., Rakoff, V., & Ellin, B. (1973). Some secondgeneration effects of the Nazi persecution. *American Journal of Orthopsychiatry, 43,* 320–327.

Simitis, I. (1981). Extreme traumatization as cumulative trauma: Psychoanalytic investigation of the effect of concentration camp experiences on survivors and their children. *Psychoanalytical Study-Child, 36,* 415–450.

Solkoff, N. (1981). Children of survivors of the Nazi Holocaust: A critical review of the literature. *American Journal of Orthopsychiatry, 51*(1), 29–42.

Srole, L. (1956). Social integration and certain corollaries: An explanatory study. *American Sociological Review, 21.* 709–761.

Steinitz, L., & Szonyi, D. (1975). (Eds.). *Living after the Holocaust: Reflections by the postwar generations in America.* New York: Bloch.

Trachtenberg, M., & Davis, M. (1978). Breaking silence: Serving children of Holocaust survivors. *Journal of Jewish Communal Service, 54,* 294–302.

Trautman, E. C. (1971). Fear and panic in Nazi-concentration camps. *International Journal of Social Psychiatry, 10,* 134–141.

Trossman, B. (1968). Adolescent children of concentration camp survivors. *Canadian Psychiatric Association Journal, 13,* 121–123.

Wanderman, E. (1975). Children and Families of Holocaust survivors: A psychological overview. In L. Steinitz & D. Szonyi (Eds.) *Living after the Holocaust: Reflections by the postwar generations in America.* New York: Bloch, pp. 115–123.

Author Index

Subject Index